Interventions to Reduce Bullying and Cyberbullying

Interventions to Reduce Bullying and Cyberbullying

Special Issue Editors

Peter K. Smith
Sheri Bauman
Dennis Wong

MDPI • Basel • Beijing • Wuhan • Barcelona • Belgrade

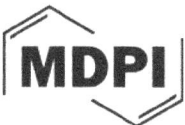

MDPI

Special Issue Editors

Peter K. Smith
University of London
UK

Sheri Bauman
University of Arizona
USA

Dennis Wong
City University of Hong Kong
Hong Kong

Editorial Office
MDPI
St. Alban-Anlage 66
4052 Basel, Switzerland

This is a reprint of articles from the Special Issue published online in the open access journal *International Journal of Environmental Research and Public Health* (ISSN 1660-4601) from 2018 to 2019 (available at: https://www.mdpi.com/journal/ijerph/special_issues/bullying_cyberbullying).

For citation purposes, cite each article independently as indicated on the article page online and as indicated below:

LastName, A.A.; LastName, B.B.; LastName, C.C. Article Title. *Journal Name* **Year**, *Article Number*, Page Range.

ISBN 978-3-03921-359-7 (Pbk)
ISBN 978-3-03921-360-3 (PDF)

Contents

About the Special Issue Editors

Peter K. Smith is Emeritus Professor of Psychology at the Unit for School and Family Studies, Goldsmiths, University of London, U.K. He is author of *Understanding School Bullying: Its Nature and Prevention Strategies* (Sage, 2014), and *The Psychology of School Bullying* (Routledge, 2019). He chaired COST Action IS0801 on Cyberbullying (2008–2012), the Indian-European Research Networking Programme on Bullying, Cyberbullying, and Pupil Safety and Well-Being (2012–2015).

Sheri Bauman is Professor of Counseling in the department of Disability and Psychoeducational Studies in the College of Education at the University of Arizona, Tucson, Arizona, USA. She is author of *Cyberbullying: What Counselors Need to Know* (American Counseling Association, 2008) and a new book, *Political Cyberbullying*, to be released in November 2019, and co-editor of the 2018 book, *Reducing Cyberbullying in Schools: International Evidence-Based Best Practice* (Elsevier). She is currently co-PI of a three-year funded project to student the effects of teaching practices on peer victimization and defending behaviors (National Science Foundation, 2019–2022, Dr. Jina Yoon, PI)).

Dennis Wong is Professor of Criminology and Social Work in the Department of Social and Behavioural Sciences, and Associate Dean of College of Liberal Arts and Social Sciences, City University of Hong Kong. He is honorary consultant on youth drugs abuse, school bullying, and offenders' rehabilitation for governmental organisations. He serves as board member for a number of non-governmental organisations and academic societies. He is well-known criminologist in the Greater China region and a life member of Asian Criminological Society. Apart from publishing articles in local and international journals, he has published books related to criminology, juvenile delinquency, school bullying, and restorative justice.

International Journal of
*Environmental Research
and Public Health*

MDPI

Editorial

Challenges and Opportunities of Anti-Bullying Intervention Programs

Peter K. Smith [1,*], Sheri Bauman [2] and Dennis Wong [3]

1   Department of Psychology, Goldsmiths, University of London, London SE14 6NW, UK
2   Department of Disability and Psychoeducational Studies, University of Arizona, Tucson, AZ 85721, USA;
     sherib@email.arizona.edu
3   Department of Social and Behavioural Sciences, City University of Hong Kong, Hong Kong, China;
     dennis.wong@cityu.edu.hk
*   Correspondence: p.smith@gold.ac.uk

Received: 13 May 2019; Accepted: 14 May 2019; Published: 22 May 2019

Over recent decades, bullying, and the more recent version of cyberbullying, have come to be recognized as important social and public health issues, generating an increasing volume of publications. It has been understood as a global, international issue, as evidenced in the UNESCO 2017 report on School Violence and Bullying: School Status Report. It has mainly been studied in schools, but it can occur in many contexts. Wherever it occurs, it can have harmful and pernicious effects, either short-term or long-term, for all involved including bystanders. For the victims especially, outcomes can include loss of self-esteem, depression, suicidal tendency, health problems, and reduced academic or work performance. Perpetrators, if unchallenged, can learn that this kind of abusive behavior can be carried out with impunity and continue on a pathway of antisocial behavior.

Most scholarship on bullying references the social-ecological model, which situates the individual at the center of concentric circles representing the various contexts in which the individual develops: Family and school, neighborhood, community and society, and historical time. As we move forward in this field, we need to examine how those larger, more distant layers impact the work done in schools.

From the origins of research on bullying, there have been attempts to intervene, noticeably in school settings. These are having some success, as evidenced by meta-analyses [1] and by collected contributions from across the globe [2,3]. An important phase in current research is to document successes and failures in anti-bullying interventions, and relate these to our rapidly growing knowledge base.

This Special Issue contains 14 contributions on the topic of interventions against bullying, including cyberbullying, and similar abusive behaviors, such as dating violence. There are also some papers in this Special Issue that assess positive or protective factors, such as well-being, self-efficacy, and school climate. Eight of the 14 contributions directly assess the effects of an intervention, with pre-/post-test designs and experimental and control groups. The other contributions examine a range of relevant topics, such as teacher attitudes, and pupils' confidence in intervening rather than being passive bystanders. Ten countries are represented among the authors, although both Spain and Italy make several contributions. Most of the articles are about secondary schools (pupils or teachers), but there are also contributions on early childhood, primary school, and university.

Many issues are highlighted in the contributions, but here we mention a few. One important aspect in interventions is whether bystanders (who often form a 'silent majority') feel empowered to act in a more prosocial way and defend a victim [4]. As shown in [5], this may depend in part on the pupil's own self-confidence, but also on wider aspects, such as class cohesion, or school climate. Victims too may or may not feel able to cope with bullying in effective ways; coping strategies can be enhanced as indicated in several studies [6–8].

Many interventions are broad-brush approaches given to a whole class or whole school. These can be valuable, but as shown in [9], they may be differentially effective for different pupils. Some pupils may need more targeted interventions, and it will be important to identify who they are as well as what kind of intervention is needed.

The actual interventions used at class or school level vary across particular programs [6–13]. However, they generally include some awareness-raising components, the role of bystanders, suggestions about coping strategies, and, in some cases, peer support elements in which other pupils can offer advice. However, for interventions against school bullying, teachers clearly have a vital and leading role; usually, they are delivering the anti-bullying programs. Several contributions focus on the teacher's role, including their attitude and confidence [14] and how their actions may be perceived by parents [15], or pupils [16]. One contribution [8] focusses on martial arts training, suggesting that traditional approaches focusing directly on bullying have had rather little success. In fact, direct approaches do have some success [1], but there is a balance to be struck between more general preventative approaches, and specific anti-bullying work—which is found already in some programs such as KiVa [7].

Unfortunately, the abuse of power is always going to be a temptation for some individuals who are in a powerful position—whether in schools or in the wider society. It is not going to be possible to 'eliminate' bullying. However, we can take actions to reduce its prevalence, to provide more effective help for victims, to assist bystanders to act positively, to encourage perpetrators to change their ways, and generally to improve safety and climate in schools and other settings [17,18]. This is likely to be especially important in schools, generally seen as the preparation for adult life.

On a more somber note, one of the corresponding authors, Anna Constanza Baldry, sadly died after her contribution [13] was accepted. Correspondence about this article should be addressed to one of her co-authors.

Author Contributions: All three authors shared equally in the editing of the articles in this Special Issue. The Editorial was drafted by Peter Smith and further edited and approved by Sheri Bauman and Dennis Wong.

Funding: This research received no external funding.

Conflicts of Interest: The authors declare no conflict of interest.

References

1. Gaffney, H.; Ttofi, M.M.; Farrington, D.P. Evaluating the effectiveness of school-bullying prevention programs: An updated meta-analytical review. *Aggress. Violent Behav.* **2019**, *45*, 111–133. [CrossRef]
2. Campbell, M.; Bauman, S. (Eds.) *Reducing Cyberbullying in Schools*; Elsevier: London, UK, 2018.
3. Smith, P.K. (Ed.) *Making an Impact on School Bullying: Interventions and Recommendations*; Routledge: London, UK, 2019.
4. Myers, C.-A.; Cowie, H. Cyberbullying across the lifespan of education: Issues and interventions from school to university. *Int. J. Environ. Res. Public Health* **2019**, *16*, 1217. [CrossRef] [PubMed]
5. Wachs, S.; Bilz, L.; Fischer, S.M.; Schubarth, W.; Wright, M.F. Students' willingness to intervene in bullying: Direct and indirect associations with classroom cohesion and self-efficacy. *Int. J. Environ. Res. Public Health* **2019**, *15*, 2577. [CrossRef] [PubMed]
6. Guarini, A.; Menin, D.; Menabo, L.; Brighi, A. RPC teacher-based program for improving coping strategies to deal with cyberbullying. *Int. J. Environ. Res. Public Health* **2019**, *16*, 948. [CrossRef] [PubMed]
7. Ortega-Barón, J.; Buelga, S.; Ayllón, E.; Martinez-Ferrer, B.; Cava, M.-J. Effects of intervention program Prev@cib on traditional bullying and cyberbullying. *Int. J. Environ. Res. Public Health* **2019**, *16*, 527. [CrossRef] [PubMed]
8. Moore, B.; Woodcock, S.; Dudley, D. Developing wellbeing through a randomised controlled trial of a martial arts based intervention: An alternative to the anti-bullying approach. *Int. J. Environ. Res. Public Health* **2019**, *16*, 81. [CrossRef] [PubMed]
9. Nocentini, A.; Palladino, B.E.; Menesini, E. For whom is anti-bullying intervention most effective? The role of temperament. *Int. J. Environ. Res. Public Health* **2019**, *16*, 388. [CrossRef] [PubMed]

10. Ferrer-Cascales, R.; Albaladejo-Blázquez, N.; Sánchez-SanSegundo, M.; Portilla-Tamarit, I.; Lordan, O.; Ruiz-Robledillo, N. Effectiveness of the TEI Program for bullying and cyberbullying reduction and school climate improvement. *Int. J. Environ. Res. Public Health* **2019**, *16*, 580. [CrossRef] [PubMed]

11. Del Rey, R.; Ortega-Ruiz, R.; Casas, J.A. Asegúrate: An intervention program against cyberbullying based on teachers' commitment and on design of its instructional materials. *Int. J. Environ. Res. Public Health* **2019**, *16*, 434. [CrossRef] [PubMed]

12. Muñoz-Fernández, N.; Ortega-Rivera, J.; Nocentini, A.; Menesini, E.; Sánchez-Jiménez, V. The efficacy of the "Date Adolescence" prevention program in the reduction of dating violence and bullying. *Int. J. Environ. Res. Public Health* **2019**, *16*, 408. [CrossRef] [PubMed]

13. Sorrentino, A.; Baldry, A.C.; Farrington, D.P. The efficacy of the Tabby improved prevention and intervention program in reducing cyberbullying and cybervictimization among students. *Int. J. Environ. Res. Public Health* **2019**, *15*, 2536. [CrossRef] [PubMed]

14. Begotto, T.; Tirassa, M.; Maran, D.A. Pre-service teachers' intervention in school bullying episodes with special education needs students: A research in Italian and Greek samples. *Int. J. Environ. Res. Public Health* **2019**, *15*, 1908. [CrossRef] [PubMed]

15. Lee, S.-H.; Ju, H.-J. Mothers' difficulties and expectations for intervention of bullying among young children in South Korea. *Int. J. Environ. Res. Public Health* **2019**, *16*, 924. [CrossRef] [PubMed]

16. Sjursø, I.R.; Fandrem, H.; O'Higgins Norman, J.; Roland, E. Teacher authority in long-lasting cases of bullying: A qualitative study from Norway and Ireland. *Int. J. Environ. Res. Public Health* **2019**, *16*, 1163. [CrossRef] [PubMed]

17. Villarejo-Carbillado, B.; Pulido, C.M.; de Botton, L.; Serradell, O. Dialogic model of prevention and resolution of conflicts: Evidence of the success of cyberbullying prevention in a primary school in Catalonia. *Int. J. Environ. Res. Public Health* **2019**, *16*, 918. [CrossRef] [PubMed]

18. Astor, R.A.; Benbenishty, R. *Bullying, School Violence, and Climate in Evolving Contexts*; Oxford University Press: New York, NY, USA, 2019.

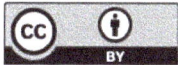

International Journal of
*Environmental Research
and Public Health*

MDPI

Article

Cyberbullying across the Lifespan of Education: Issues and Interventions from School to University

Carrie-Anne Myers [1],* and Helen Cowie [2]

1 Department of Sociology, City, University of London, London EC1V 0HB, UK
2 Department of Health and Medical Sciences, University of Surrey, Guildford GU2 7XH, UK;
   H.Cowie@surrey.ac.uk
* Correspondence: Carrie.Myers.1@city.ac.uk; Tel.: +44-207-040-4556

Received: 12 March 2019; Accepted: 2 April 2019; Published: 4 April 2019

Abstract: Research on cyberbullying amongst students has tended to be conducted separately within specific education institutional contexts, schools, further education (FE) and higher education (HE), neglecting a view that takes account of the entire educational lifespan. The present article addresses this gap in the literature, providing a novel take on examining its nature, social environments, legal consequences and potentially helpful interventions. To facilitate this, the article conceptualises cyberbullying in broad terms, recognising that it can take multiple forms of online and digital practice including: spreading rumours, ridiculing and/or demeaning another person, casting aspirations on the grounds of race, disability, gender, religion or sexual orientation; seeking revenge or deliberately embarrassing a person by posting intimate photos or videos about them without their consent; accessing another's social networking profiles with malicious intent and socially excluding a person from a social network or gaming site. This article demonstrates that harm from cyberbullying is a cause for concern for students at each developmental stage and that there are continuities in its appearance that need to be challenged at each point in the educational lifespan. And inaccurately, by university, the idea that 'nothing can be done' still is one of the main concerns for the victims. The article concludes with five key recommendations for future research and practice across the educational lifespan.

Keywords: cyberbullying; peer support; bystanders; moral disengagement; cyberbullying and the law; mental health; social environment; cyberbullying interventions; educational lifespan

1. The Nature of Cyberbullying

In the past decade, cyberbullying has emerged as a phenomenon at the school, college and university levels. Definitions of cyberbullying fall into two main categories. Some researchers view cyberbullying as a new form of traditional bullying, following the classical definition originally proposed by Olweus, which states that it is repeated over time, involves a power imbalance between perpetrator and target and has an intention to harm. In fact, Olweus, describes cyberbullying as "an overrated phenomenon", preferring to view it as simply an extension of traditional bullying into the virtual world. He argues that cyberbullying has low prevalence and that most of those who are being cyberbullied are also being bullied in traditional ways in the 'real' world [1].

By contrast, other researchers [2–4] consider that cyberbullying differs from traditional bullying in distinctive ways since it can invade all aspects of a target's privacy day and night, both at home and at the educational institution where the target studies. Furthermore, the perpetrators can choose to disguise their identity, so heightening the target students' insecurity about the quality of their relationships since they may not know which members of their peer group are involved in the cyberbullying. Additionally, if a harmful message "goes viral" through the actions of bystanders who forward the messages to others in their networks, the cybervictim's distress is compounded. Finally, if, in a 'one-off' attack, the action is severe, such as sharing a sexually explicit image of the victim, it transcends the boundaries of cyberbullying and in some countries becomes a criminal offence [3].

From this second perspective, like traditional face-to-face bullying, cyberbullying involves the deliberate intent to hurt a person or persons repeatedly over time. However, researchers such as Schulze-Krumbholz et al. found structural differences in cyberbullying when compared to traditional bullying with an absence of the "pure" cybervictim category in their sample of 6260 adolescents. In their study, they found that the perpetrators of cyberbullying reported that they had been bullied themselves in traditional ways. The researchers speculate that the anonymity of cyberbullying enabled these young people to fight back in ways that would be impossible face-to-face. This study confirms that there is some overlap between traditional and cyberbullying but that the latter has its own distinctive nature [6]. Boulton et al. conclude from their research into bullying at university that findings from traditional bullying should not be generalised to cyberbullying and vice versa. Furthermore, they argue, each broad category (whether bullying or cyberbullying) has sub-types of behaviour, each of which may be distinctive in its own right. They recommend a focus on attitudes towards the behaviour of both bullies and victims to predict whether a student will engage in bullying or cyberbullying in the future [2].

For the purpose of this article, we acknowledge the distinctive features of cyberbullying while at the same time accepting that to some extent there is an overlap between traditional and cyberbullying. In order to move the agenda along and look at continuities across the educational lifespan, and the ever-evolving nature of social media platforms, technology and the internet, we also argue that cyberbullying, as a stand-alone category, has to be considered in order to understand more deeply its potential for social and emotional harm to those directly involved as well as to the witnesses and bystanders. The objective of this paper is to address the following two research questions:

(1) To what extent has cyberbullying *across the lifespan of education*, that is from primary/elementary school, through college to university, been identified as an issue?
(2) What are the implications for educational establishments and educators to reduce and prevent cyberbullying across this learning lifespan?

2. Research Findings on Cyberbullying

Most of the research on cyberbullying has taken place in schools and we can gain a great deal of knowledge from this literature about the phenomenon [7]. More recently, there has been an upsurge of interest in cyberbullying among post-16 students, whether in further education (college) or higher education (university), for example, in Canada [8–10], in Finland [11,12], in the US [13] and in the UK [14]. The systematic review of cyberbullying among adults by Jenaro, Flores and Frias (2018) provides useful evidence on prevalence, contributing factors, short- and long-term impact and the role of bystanders. Although this review focuses on adults, in practice the authors found that most of the studies had been carried out in college student populations. They conclude that the impact of cyberbullying may be as severe amongst adult populations as amongst children but they note the buffering effect of personal and environmental factors, with emotional intelligence (in the individual) and social support (in the school and community environment) being the most influential variables [15].

Essentially, research into cyberbullying indicates negative immediate effects on the target with potentially harmful long-term impacts on psychosocial development, self-esteem, academic achievement and mental health [16–19]. For the students who are the targets of such bullying behaviours, the experience is unpleasant and distressing in the short term. However, for some there are longer term negative consequences for their mental health and their academic career. Bullying affects the target's self-esteem and often leads to social withdrawal from peer-group networks. Consequently, victims of cyberbullying run a heightened risk of mental health disorders, including depression and social anxiety [12,13]. For example, Schenk and Fremouw found that college student victims of cyberbullying were more likely than non-bullied peers to suffer from depression, anxiety and a range of psychosomatic complaints, as well as academic difficulties [20]. Research into the experiences of lesbian, gay, bi-sexual and transgendered (LGBT) students confirms the negative effect of bullying on the mental health of targets. One National Union of Students (NUS) survey [21] found that one in five lesbian, gay and bi-sexual (LGB) students and one in three transgendered (T) students reported at least one form of bullying on campus; many reported that they had to pass as 'straight' in order to protect themselves from homophobia and transphobia. Rivers and Valentine et al. report on the extremely negative effect that such treatment had on the mental health of staff and students [22,23]. In extremes, this could lead to suicide.

Cyberbullying involves many, if not all, of the children in a school class since not only the perpetrators and targets are affected but also the witnesses who view negative online messages and harmful video clips and who may in turn forward them to other people for their own amusement, regardless of the feelings of the victim. Cyberbullies are often rewarded for their online behaviour by the approval of the peer group. On the surface, they are the dominant ones with a côterie of admiring followers, but research indicates that the long-term outcomes for them are not good in terms of mental health, social competence and anti-social behaviour [24]. There is a high risk that they will continue to repeat their cyberbullying behaviour [25] since their popularity (which they value) is based on fear and intimidation rather than genuine friendship, making it highly likely that they will continue this method of relating to others as a means of acceptance in their peer group across the educational lifespan.

Cyberbullying among post-16 students continues to cause harmful effects on fellow students. It takes many forms, including such behaviours as: spreading nasty rumours on the grounds of race, disability, gender, religion and sexual orientation; ridiculing or demeaning a person; social exclusion; unwelcome sexual advances; stalking; threatening someone online; revealing personal information about a person that was shared in confidence [14]. West in two studies of cyberbullying among college students in the age-group 16–19 years, found that victims reported such disturbing behaviour as: being told to kill themselves; being sexually harassed; being taunted on account of their religion; being bullied on account of their sexual orientation; being attacked by a 'gang' of former friends on Twitter; having nasty comments posted online by a former romantic partner. The emotions experienced by the targets of bullying included anger, hurt, sadness, depression, embarrassment, anxiety, difficulty in concentrating, isolation, self-blame, fear, suicidal thoughts; victims also reported that the cyberbullying had an adverse effect on their capacity to study and on their ability to form social relationships online and in the real world. In the same study, the students who admitted to being cyberbullies reported reasons that included: fun; revenge; anger; jealousy; provocation; desire for power and status; freedom to behave in this way through the anonymity of the social media [26,27]. These findings are confirmed in a larger Canadian study ($N = 1925$) by Faucher et al. (2014) who also noted that women students were more vulnerable to attack through such forms of cyberbullying as "sexting", "morphing", "virtual rape" and "revenge porn" [9]. Phipps and Young made similar discoveries in their study of bullying and harassment among UK university students [28].

As indicated in many studies globally and across the educational lifespan, the effects of cyberbullying on mental health can be long-lasting [12,13,29,30]. The public nature of cyberbullying means that it can create a social context where cyberbullying is perceived as "normal" and "acceptable" ([5] p. 1172). Sexting (the exchange of online sexual images or videos) whether generated by others or self-generated, has contributed to recent increases in cyberbullying. This kind of material may begin within a close friendship group or couple but can quickly go viral and be circulated, without consent, to a much larger audience.

3. Cyberbullying across the Educational Lifespan

There is, a small, but growing, body of evidence to suggest that there is some continuity in being a bully or a victim from childhood through adolescence and into young adulthood [9,31,32]. Curwen et al. in a retrospective study of 186 university students who admitted to bullying their peers, found that, although there was an overall decrease in the incidence of verbal and physical bullying between high school and university, a substantial proportion of the student bullies in their study had also engaged in bullying behaviour at elementary and high school levels [33]. Chapell et al. found that over half of the adult bullies in their sample had also bullied others during childhood and adolescence. They conclude that this history of bullying indicates long-term benefits so that the behaviour becomes entrenched and continues to be a successful strategy for improving the bully's social status [34]. Not only that, there is evidence that bullies are popular amongst their peers and that bystanders are often indifferent to the suffering of the victims [25] and that this insensitivity to others' distress increases over time [35]. The impact on the victims is well documented within the school setting and is emerging as a core focus for looking at cyberbullying within the university sector [31]. The evidence indicates that, while cyberbullying behaviours follow the traditional bullying notions of an imbalance of power, with the added dimension of the internet, the anonymity of the behaviours gives 'more power' to the perpetrators and a greater feeling of helplessness to the victims. Additionally, the anonymity of the internet gives perceived power to former victims who can then take revenge on those who tormented them without the repercussions which would happen in a face-to-face context.

Furthermore, we also need to take account of the social contexts where the cyberbullying takes place. As Cassidy et al., argue: "Power imbalances are prevalent in the hierarchical context of universities: administrator to faculty member, senior to junior faculty, tenured to untenured, faculty to staff, supervisor to graduate student, instructor to student, not to mention imbalances based on gender, age, ethnicity, race, social status, and sexual orientation, which can permeate all of those relationships."([36], p. 2) Indeed, in their research into cyberbullying among students, faculty staff and administrators at four Canadian universities, they link their analysis of cyberbullying to the power and control model, adapted from the field of intimate partner violence, which considers behaviours such as "intimidation, threats, harmful language, social standing, exclusion and harassment in the exercise of power and control over another in a relationship." ([36], p. 2) Furthermore, they demonstrate that the internet and relevant communication technologies can be used to carry out any, or all, of these forms of behaviour. They conclude that "currently too many students and faculty are suffering the impacts of cyberbullying in isolation, frustrated with the attempts for solving their situations, without any clear guidelines to follow, and within the context of a university culture which benignly seems to tolerate such actions." ([36], p. 16).

Because of the global reach of the internet, social media platforms and any aggressive online behaviour such as cyberbullying, it follows that research within the university sector is global in its production. Increasingly, researchers in universities reach the same conclusion, namely that cyberbullying is a vast problem and that something has to be done about it [37,38].

4. The Role of the Bystander/Witness

Bullying is rarely something that happens only between two individuals, the bully and the victim. Rather, it happens in a social context where bystanders are fully aware of what is happening and take on distinctive participant roles, such as bully, victim, assistant, reinforcer, outsider and defender [39]. In fact, Salmivalli argues that bystanders/outsiders are trapped in a moral dilemma. Although they understand that bullying is wrong, they are acutely aware of their own need for security within the peer group [39]. Many bullies enjoy tormenting a vulnerable peer "for fun" and this can involve entertainment value for the onlookers [40]. The ways in which bystanders respond has a powerful impact on whether the cyberbullying continues or, even worse, goes viral. Through the actions of bystanders, a message that was intended for one other person or for a small group of close friends can quickly be sent to strangers without the permission of the target person. Too often, it is easier for the bystanders to enjoy the spectacle of another's distress than to challenge the bullies. Bystanders may even blame the victims for not being capable of defending themselves [41]. This indifference, or moral disengagement, is often justified on the grounds that the victim in some way deserved the treatment being meted out to them. In fact, by forwarding distressing images or videos, bystanders collude with the bullies and demonstrate that a process of moral disengagement has taken place [42].

The bystanders' lack of action to support the victim of cyberbullying can be explained in several ways. They may be afraid of becoming a target in turn if they challenge the bullies or defend the victim and they may justify their actions by rationalising them in terms of blaming the victim [35]. They may even admire the bullies and feel pride in the bullies' actions [43]. In turn, the actions of bystanders influence the behaviour of the wider peer group, for example, in whether to condone the cyberbullying or to defend the victim publicly.

However, many bystanders report feelings of discomfort and concern when they witness the occurrence of cyberbullying. Condeza et al. ([44], p. 44) report the following comments from witnesses of cyberbullying at a university in Chile:

"I felt powerless about the offenders' anonymity, and I felt ignorant because I did not know what to do." (female, second year)

"It angered me, but since it was not my friend, I cannot intervene." (male, second year)

Additionally, these researchers found that 44.5% of their sample of witnesses reported that they were afraid of becoming cybervictims if they intervened [44].

The problem has become so serious in the UK that Universities UK (UUK) has issued a report, *Changing the Culture*, on sexual violence, harassment and hate crime on campus with a list of recommendations, emphasising prevention, that all universities should take on board, which we will discuss below in the section on the complexities of cyberbullying and the law [45].

Victims' reactions to cyberbullying are crucial in understanding its incidence and impact. Some researchers argue that there are distinctive roles that can be assigned. For example, Cunningham et al surveyed 1004 university students and found that more than 60% of respondents reported involvement in cyberbullying in the following ways: 45.7% had been witnesses, 5.7% had been victims, 4.9% were perpetrator victims and 4.5% were perpetrators [46]. These are similar roles to the ones suggested by Salmivalli in her research on school bullying [39].

5. Victim Coping Strategies in Cyberbullying

Recent research considers cyberbullying in the university setting and its possible relationship with other personal and family variables. For example, Martinez-Monteagudo et al. consider the predictive capacity of the family environment and emotional intelligence in relation to cyberbullying among university students [47]. They sampled 1282 students and found that a deteriorated family environment increased the probability of being both a victim and a perpetrator of cyberbullying. Furthermore, they also found that the emotional intelligence of the students had a correlation with predicting the levels of participation in cyberbullying. They argue that: " . . . part of the problem of cyberbullying in the university setting may depend on the quality of the student's family relationships and EI level. These are variables that have yet to receive much attention from the scientific field. Thus, the family is seen to play a relevant role as a protective factor from cyberbullying, even in a university setting, controlling the behaviour of its members and the use of new technologies. Similarly, EI acts as a protective factor to prevent students from being victims as well as aggressors, highlighting the fundamental role exercised by emotional regulation in students. Thus, it is corroborated that both variables are relevant factors to be taken into consideration when developing social and educational policies, and when developing intervention programs to alleviate this problem." ([47] p. 224).

Such research demonstrates the continuities and patterns across the educational lifespan, but crucially also suggests that even though the students are at university, there is still an element of family involvement and engagement that will help the student if they become involved in a cyberbullying scenario. This is also pertinent since an increasing number of students choose to live at home whilst they study to keep down the costs and expenditure of being at university. Assumptions that students are over 18 and able to defend for themselves need to be challenged as positive relationships with the family emerge as a coping mechanism for involvement in cyberbullying, as they do for school students.

Attachments to members of the peer group are also significant, as McCloughlin et al. found in their survey of Australian adolescents [48]. Young people in this age-group have a strong need for social connectedness. Those who were more socially connected had better mental health than those who were not and had more effective defences against cyberbullying when it happened. The less young people feel socially connected to their peer group, the lower their self-esteem and the greater their sense of loneliness, both offline and online [49].

Gender also plays a very significant role in cyberbullying across the educational lifespan, notably at the university level. Cunningham et al., found that male students were more likely than their female counterparts to report as perpetrators or bully-victims [46], while Boulton et al., argued that the male undergraduates in their study viewed cyberbullying and those who perpetrate it, less negatively than the female students did [2].

Younger victims may try to fight back (often unsuccessfully) against the bullies or express their distress through tears and emotional displays, so risking further physical and psychological attacks from the bullies, and contempt from bystanders [50]. As victims progress through the educational lifespan, they are less likely to retaliate actively but are more likely to employ passive tactics, such as blocking or ignoring. As Kernaghan and Elwood argue in their qualitative study of cyberbullying during early adolescence, the cyberbullying event becomes a performance where the bystanders take the role of audience to a drama. The more the victims become distressed, the greater the entertainment and the less likely that bystanders will intervene to help [51]. Similarly, in focus groups, the adolescents in the study by Purdy and York reported that during an episode of cyberbullying, it is often easier to go along with the crowd since they were afraid that the bullies would turn on them [35]. Understandably, victims learn to disguise their true feelings. As children become adolescents, they are less likely to engage in fighting fire with fire, perhaps because of such negative experiences from peers and perceived inaction from adults. By the time cybervictims are at university, while they may have learned that aggressive retaliation achieves little, many have failed to find alternative coping strategies to reduce or prevent the cyberbullying [52].

A small number of studies indicate that the university sector could be better equipped to deal with cyberbullying, with lecturers and other staff becoming more proactive in helping. When considering victims of cyberbullying and how they deal with the situation whilst at university research is scant, in comparison to the school setting. Nonetheless there are some illuminating studies. For example, Orel et al., in a sample of 282 students, investigated the coping strategies the students would potentially use in response to future cyberbullying incidents. Blocking of the perpetrator was found to be the most common tactic considered [53], but does this passive tactic solve the problem?

Research from the school setting provides strong evidence that telling someone about being bullied is a crucial first step to resolving the problem, however, studies of college and university cyberbullying find that victims feel, at university, that telling someone about their situation will not result in a satisfactory outcome. For instance, Alqahtani et al., in their study of 165 university students found that 49% of students felt that their university could not or would not do anything about cyberbullying, even if it was reported; 47% felt that university staff would not believe or understand them even if they did complain or report what had happened [54]. Thus interventions that actively encourage children to tell someone that they are being cyberbullied, for example a member of staff from the pastoral care team, a school nurse or a peer supporter, are not being carried over to FE and HE levels so therefore are not being practiced across the educational lifespan.

6. The Victim-Offender Cycle

In Finland, Pörhölä [25,55] found that nearly half of those who reported being bullied at university had previously been subjected to school bullying. Retrospective studies, for example, Bauman and Newman in the US, also indicate that there is a high likelihood that university students who report being bullied were also bullied at junior and high school levels, but that being a stable victim from junior high to high school and then to university was more characteristic of male than female students [56].

However, the distinctive participant roles that are often researched and reported in more traditional forms of bullying [39] are not always as clear cut in cyberbullying incidents. Some researchers [2] have argued that it is almost impossible to make the distinction between the 'bully' and the 'victim' in the online world where cybervictims hide behind anonymity to become cyberbullies in revenge. Similarly, at secondary school level, Schultze-Krumbholz, et al., found that adolescents who bully others online are very likely to have been victims themselves [6]. Cyberbullying research confirms some degree of continuity across the educational lifespan but there are also discontinuities that need to be further investigated.

The discipline of criminology potentially offers useful insights since the 'victim/offender' cycle is played out in different criminal scenarios and the distinction between roles is not that clear cut. Decades of research have shown that there exists a connection between the perpetrator and the target, which has a number of complicated dynamics that need further investigation [57], with some arguing that the overlap is developmental in its nature and predictable from childhood [58] and others arguing that the relationship is so "intimately connected" that trying to understand victims and offenders as separate entities is not possible [59]. Clearly, the relationship between cyberbully and victim is key to understanding the wider cultural context and significance of the act [60] and is an area of further study that is needed when considering cyberbullying across the educational lifespan.

The victim/offender relationship is a difficult area to unpack when it comes to cyberbullying and research is beginning to show that it becomes even more difficult within the university sector because of the age and potential previous experience of all those who are involved. One way to begin to understand the complex interactions is to look at reactions to cyberbullying when it occurs. For example, Eristi and Akbulut surveyed 567 undergraduate students and 211 high school students. Among this sample they found that 170 (29.98%) of the undergraduates and 120 (56.87%) of the school aged students had been cyberbullied within the last six months prior to the study. They then considered and investigated the behavioural cyberbullying reactions of victimised students under four key factors, which were revenge, countermeasure, negotiation and avoidance. They also considered victimized students' emotional reactions as either internalizing (for example, 'fear', 'panic', 'anxiety' 'embarrassment' or 'guilt') or externalizing (for example, 'seeking revenge', 'getting aggressive' or 'angry'). Their research demonstrated that behavioural and emotional reactions varied according to gender and whether they were in school or at university [61]. Furthermore, computer self-efficacy and internet use were associated with different reaction types. They conclude that: "...new model and intervention proposals directed at reducing the unpleasant/damaging victimization consequences may better serve the goal of mitigating these consequences than descriptive investigations."([61], p. 9) Although this is a relatively large scale survey in an emerging field of investigation, it highlights, and adds to the debate, that victim reactions and retaliation processes must be included when considering how to understand cyberbullying across the educational lifespan.

7. Current Policy and the Role of the Law—The UK Context

The issues around law, the boundaries of responsibility and criminalization of behaviours are to be considered country by country, due to the nature of individual criminal justice systems. Here, we look at the UK as an example to highlight the minefield of problems that are emerging around cyberbullying and its intersection with crime. Although the authors acknowledge that there are many different laws and practices within other jurisdictions, focusing on one system will highlight the complexities of not tackling cyberbullying across the educational lifespan.

Within the UK, Advance HE, who were appointed as independent evaluators for the Office for Students (OfS) Catalyst-funded projects, were tasked with looking at 'what works' in student engagement in safeguarding projects following the UUK Changing the Culture Report [45] follow up report *Changing the Culture: One Year On* [62] and subsequent Catalyst funding to evaluate good practice across the sector. So far, they have identified the following as being the most effective ways to achieve this: firstly, "co-creation with students of training content and campaigns", secondly,

"Peer-to-peer learning or mentoring" and thirdly, "Collaboration with Student Unions." ([63], p. 2). They strongly recommend that students themselves should be encouraged to re-engage with practices, such as peer support and peer mentoring, that are commonplace in most primary and secondary schools in some form or another [64]. Perhaps rather than re-invent the wheel, the further and higher education systems need to reintroduce practices and policies to their students that the majority would have had some knowledge about whilst in their earlier years of their education.

Furthermore, UUK has now uncovered many issues that should be taken into consideration when focussing on sexual misconduct, hate crime and harassment, the original remit of *Changing the Culture* [45]. In October 2018 they held a round table event to explore the nature and scope of online harassment and cyberbullying within the university sector and to see what more can be done to prevent and respond to this form of hate crime. A report will follow in April 2019. Therefore, cyberbullying within universities is under consideration but it is still key to remember that any recommendations that are made are not mandatory as there is not a regulatory body that enforces universities to develop centralised policies. This is in contrast to schools and FE colleges that are required by law to have safeguarding practices in place and anti-bullying policies.

The problem here is the age of the students and, as has been argued in previous research, once students are at university, they are over the age of 18 and are legally adults, which brings with it challenges of responsibility and boundaries of policing [5]. It is worth noting here that although cyberbullying is not a criminal offence, there are a number of laws and relevant legislation that are used by the Crown Prosecution Service (CPS) to prosecute cases that involve online communication in England and Wales. These include: Offences Against the Person Act (1861), Protection from Harassment Act (1997), Malicious Communications Act (1988), The Crime and Disorder Act (1998) and the Serious Crime Act (2015) Students over the age of 18 can potentially be prosecuted for cyberbullying related offences. Since many students are unaware of this legislation, we recommend that education on the legal consequences of actions must be bought into the curriculum at a much earlier level. If behaviour is learned and repeated across the educational lifespan, the legal aspects need to be dealt with from the beginning, as soon as children and young people are able to understand the implications of what they are doing [49]. It would appear to be the case that certain communities within the wider society have a very high tolerance level for what is considered 'normal' or 'acceptable' in terms of violent behaviours. For example, within the UK amongst teenagers, sexting, upskirting and revenge porn have become particular causes for concern [5,65,66] and this is especially pertinent in the online world. The boundary between 'flirty' behaviour and crime is becoming even more blurred. Therefore, this needs to be factored in along with challenging a lack of knowledge about the law. It needs to be embedded in education, across the educational lifespan, with legal awareness training.

8. Intervening to Prevent and Reduce Cyberbullying

International evaluation studies [67,68] have systematically reviewed the successes and failures of interventions to combat bullying/cyberbullying at school level. For example, Ttofi and Farrington, in their meta-analysis of 44 school-based interventions carried out over a period of 25 years in Europe, Australia, America and South Africa, found that certain intervention programmes reduced rates of bullying others by 20–23% and victimisation by 17–20% [68]. The key components of such programmes included parent meetings and training, consistent disciplinary methods, classroom rules, school conferences and skilled classroom management by teachers. Smith et al. (2016) examined the effect of disciplinary methods and concluded that these needed to be non-punitive, negotiated by adults and children, and restorative in nature, with an emphasis on school safety for all, on the promotion of a positive school ethos, and positive relationships throughout the school. [67]. The evidence pointed to the effectiveness of sanctions that were perceived by the students as fair and reasonable, arising from a process of consultation in which members of the school community had taken part. Purdy and York, focussing on cyberbullying, argue that new ground rules are emerging concerning responsibility for action to counteract cyberbullying since the bullying frequently occurs at home during evenings and weekends when it is parents who have responsibility for their child's behaviour [35].

Within the school setting, bullying and cyberbullying interventions typically engage in a 'whole school' approach considering other factors such as the family and wider community in addressing the problem. Many schools across the world now adopt Social and Emotional Learning (SEL) programmes to enhance children's and young people's empathy for the distress of others and to create a more pro-social climate in the classroom and the school at large (for a comprehensive international overview, see [69]). An international review of successful and unsuccessful interventions [70] identified key components in the reduction of bullying, to include the creation of a whole-school policy against bullying and meetings/workshops with parents. Smith et al. (2016) identified the effectiveness of restorative methods within the school and the community in order to create a co-operative school climate with an emphasis on positive relationships and active participation on the part of students and staff in the creation and implementation of anti-bullying action [67]. Going one step further, Finne et al. argue that the dynamics of bullying are likely to persist in a school context if only superficial anti-bullying action is taken [71]. They argue that some form of rehabilitation needs to take place to change the quality of "peer ecology" ([71] p. 356) in the classroom. They argue that the moral disengagement that occurs when bullying persists creates a group norm that may well continue even when the active forms of bullying have ceased as a result of a successful intervention. Their model of relational rehabilitation takes three steps:

(1) *Ensuring teacher authority*: teachers play a crucial role through an authoritative teaching style that emphasises warmth, acceptance and tolerance. This can counteract the destructive power of the bullies;

(2) *Redistribution of social power and promoting a supportive classroom community*: In an abusive class community, power will have been wielded by the bullies. The teacher plays a crucial role in breaking up the previous hierarchies and creating a fairer social system that promotes friendship and prosocial behaviour. Such a class culture will be tolerant of difference and open to discussions about social inclusion and caring. The teacher plays an active part in helping the pupils to repair the damage that has been done.

(3) *Providing social and emotional learning (SEL) to the whole class*: Whole-class SEL programmes take a variety of forms but their essential principles concern the inclusion of all, the valuing of prosocial behaviour and the creation of a warm, supportive classroom community.

Similarly, in the college and university sector, the idea of rehabilitation is beginning to be discussed, with a growing emphasis on changing the culture to one of tolerance and community [62,72]. However, there is not to date the same level of coherence nor shared practice as appears at school level.

Whilst a number of studies focus on reporting the levels of cyberbullying across the educational lifespan, there are huge variations in how the problem should actually be tackled. Following the recommendations from cyberbullying within the school setting, research within the university sector is beginning to acknowledge that a very important and often neglected way to understand and deal with the problem is to engage with the students themselves. Cunningham et al (2015) stipulated that there were five key areas that need to be considered when tackling cyberbullying within the university sector:

(1) Emphasise the impact of cyberbullying on victims;
(2) Change cyberbullying prevention attitudes;
(3) Teach anti-cyberbullying strategies;
(4) Enable anonymous online reporting;
(5) Combine prevention with consequences ([46], p. 380).

These recommendations were made by the students themselves and the authors conclude that they would help when designing and implementing university anti-cyberbullying programmes.

Such research and subsequent recommendations indicate the need for a rather more complex whole university sector approach to tackling the problem than is currently available. Furthermore, the involvement of the students themselves is crucial, especially given the age of undergraduate students. They are adults and they need to be consulted in what works to reduce cyberbullying and thus make their learning environment more positive, especially in the light of the move to a heavy reliance on the online world for everything within the university sector, from online registration and timetables, to attendance monitoring, assignment submission and virtual learning environments. Universities continue to advance in adapting online systems and practices. Thus, it follows that mechanisms could also be introduced and improved to support students who have to use and engage with the online world.

9. Conclusions

To what extent has cyberbullying across the lifespan of education, that is from primary/elementary school, through college to university, been identified as an issue?

The evidence from the literature that we reviewed indicates that cyberbullying across the educational lifespan continues to be a critical issue for a proportion of students. Despite the wealth of high-quality research over three decades, the problem still needs to be addressed as a matter of urgency. Cyberbullying, to some extent, is a continuity and attitudes towards it need to change. While there are some overlaps with traditional bullying, there are clearly aspects unique to the online existence that have to be considered. Traditional anti-bullying interventions may not always be sufficient to capture the complexities of cyberbullying. The following gaps in knowledge need to be considered:

(1) One important gap concerns the widespread lack of knowledge amongst educators and their students about the legal consequences of cyberbullying behaviour across the educational lifespan.
(2) A second concerns the finding that cyberbullying is distressing at all stages of the educational lifespan but there is a lot of evidence now to support the view that cybervictims become less likely to report it as they reach FE and HE levels. The gap in understanding appears to be at university level and the assumption that students as young adults no longer need support in dealing with cyberbullying.
(3) Furthermore, the bystanders express less empathy and more moral disengagement the older they get, with university students showing the least sensitivity to peers' distress.
(4) Finally, by the time they reach adolescence and young adulthood cybervictims have run out of options for the help and support which they are more likely to get at primary school but which are less likely to feature as they progress through the educational lifespan They can resort to acceptance of their fate with all the attendant mental health difficulties that this entails *or* they can take revenge on their tormentors by becoming cyberbullies themselves. Neither is a good coping strategy. The gap here is we need more information on successful and unsuccessful strategies adopted by cybervictims across the educational lifespan.

What are the implications for educational establishments and educators to reduce and prevent cyberbullying across the educational lifespan?

Looking at cyberbullying in educational silos is not helpful. Students do not arrive at university and their problems begin. Rather, looking at education as a longitudinal journey is more helpful. Good practice could and should be shared amongst schools, colleges and universities in order to safeguard and educate students at all levels of their education. The following action points emerged from the literature search:

(1) At primary school level and to an extent at secondary level, schools are increasingly developing Social Emotional Learning (SEL) [69], restorative practices [73] or emotional rehabilitation [71] interventions to address the issue of cyberbullying, with an emphasis on the destructive nature of moral disengagement. Peer support systems are widespread [64]. Participant role theory is also

successfully used in Finland [39]. However, at FE and HE levels this is not happening. We have already mentioned the work that UUK [62] advocated around bystander training but to date this is only used in a few institutions and is yet to roll out across the sector. For those students that do identify as victims, there need to be improved systems, such as student welfare and counselling, to help them. Perhaps what need to be introduced at the FE and HE level are more comprehensive pastoral systems with appropriate training for the staff involved.

(2)   While there is a strong emphasis at school level on social skills, the development of empathy and the need for restorative practice to mediate in disputes, the legal aspects of cyberbullying are scarcely mentioned. By contrast, legal aspects of cyberbullying are increasingly on the agenda at FE and HE levels since the students are by now young adults. When cyberbullying incidents become criminal acts, the police are involved and legal proceedings may ensue. This indicates an imbalance at different levels of the educational lifespan. What is needed is legal awareness training across the educational lifespan.

(3)   There is strong evidence of both continuities and discontinuities in cyberbullying across the educational lifespan but, to date, there is little information on the nature of successful and unsuccessful coping strategies used by the targets of cyberbullying. Consequently, researchers and practitioners need to continue to collaborate to design methods for equipping future generations with the tools to navigate the internet safely and, in a socially positive way.

(4)   Primary and secondary schools have invested a great deal in counteracting the harmful effects of xenophobia, misogyny and homophobia; this is less evident at FE and HE levels. There should be considerably more sharing of expertise between schools, colleges and universities about interventions that are effective in this domain.

(5)   Finally, the literature indicates an urgent need to consider cyberbullying in its cultural context–its social and environmental ecology. The issue of moral disengagement is scarcely mentioned in the curriculum or in the pastoral care systems at HE and FE levels despite the evidence of cultural issues such as "laddism" [28], xenophobia [74], sexism [10,49] and homophobia [22] in FE and HE settings. Cyberbullying needs to be addressed and understood in all of its cultureal contexts across the educational lifespan.

One thing that is for certain is that the internet is not going to disappear. Technology will evolve, and more social media platforms will emerge. What this article shows is the urgent need to address certain gaps in the literature and implement successful interventions right across the educational lifespan to tackle cyberbullying.

Author Contributions: All authors contributed equally.

Conflicts of Interest: The authors declare no conflict of interest.

References

1.   Olweus, D. Cyberbullying: An overrated phenomenon? *Eur. J. Dev. Psychol.* **2012**, *9*, 520–538. [CrossRef]
2.   Boulton, M.; Lloyd, J.; Down, J.; Marx, H. Predicting Undergraduates' Self-Reported Engagement in Traditional and Cyberbullying from Attitudes. *Cyberpsychol. Behav. Soc. Netw.* **2012**, *15*, 141–147. [CrossRef]
3.   Kyriacou, C.; Zuin, A. Cyberbullying and moral disengagement: An analysis based on a social pedagogy of pastoral care in schools. *Pastor. Care Educ.* **2016**, *34*, 34–42. [CrossRef]
4.   Larranaga, E.; Yubero, S.; Navarro, R.; Ovejero, A. From traditional bullying to cyberbullying: Cybervictimization among higher education students. In *Cyberbullying at University in International Contexts*; Routledge: New York, NY, USA, 2019; pp. 99–111.
5.   Myers, C.-A.; Cowie, H. Bullying at University: The Social and Legal Contexts of Cyberbullying Among University Students. *J. Cross-Cult. Psychol.* **2017**, *48*, 1172–1182. [CrossRef]
6.   Schultze-Krumbholz, A.; Gobel, K.; Scheithauer, H.; Brighi, A.; Guarini, A.; Tsorbatzoudis, H.; Barkoukis, V.; Pyzalski, J.; Plichta, P.; Del Rey, R.; et al. A Comparison of Classification Approaches for Cyberbullying and Traditional Bullying Using Data from Six European Countries. *J. Sch. Violence* **2015**, *14*, 47–65. [CrossRef]

7. Smith, P.K.; Steffgen, G. (Eds.) *Cyberbullying through the New Media: Findings from an International Network, 1st Edition (Paperback)—Routledge*; Psychology Press: London, UK, 2013.

8. Cassidy, W.; Faucher, C.; Jackson, M. *Cyberbullying at University in International Contexts*; Routledge: London, UK, 2018; ISBN 978-1-351-74599-4.

9. Faucher, C.; Jackson, M.; Cassidy, W. Cyberbullying among University Students: Gendered Experiences, Impacts, and Perspectives. Available online: https://www.hindawi.com/journals/edri/2014/698545/ (accessed on 27 February 2019).

10. Shariff, S.; DeMartini, A. Cyberbullying and rape culture in universities: Defining the legal lines between fun and intentional harm. In *Bullying among University Studnets*; Routledge: London, UK, 2016; pp. 172–190.

11. Lappalainen, C.; Meriläinen, M.; Puhakka, H.; Sinkkonen, H.-M. Bullying among university students—Does it exist? *Finn. J. Youth Res.* **2011**, *29*, 64–80.

12. Sourander, A.; Klomek, A.B.; Ikonen, M.; Lindroos, J.; Luntamo, T.; Koskelainen, M.; Ristkari, T.; Helenius, H. Psychosocial Risk Factors Associated with Cyberbullying Among Adolescents: A Population-Based Study. *Arch. Gen. Psychiatry* **2010**, *67*, 720–728. [CrossRef]

13. Simmons, J.; Bauman, S.; Ives, J. Cyber-aggression among members of college fraternities and sororities in the United States. I. In *Bullying among University Students: Cross-National Perspectives*; Routledge: London, UK, 2016; pp. 93–109.

14. Cowie, H.; Myers, C.-A. *Bullying among University Students: Cross-National Perspectives*; Routledge: London, UK, 2016; ISBN 978-1-138-80926-0.

15. Jenaro, C.; Flores, N.; Frías, C.P. Systematic review of empirical studies on cyberbullying in adults: What we know and what we should investigate. *Aggress. Violent Behav.* **2018**, *38*, 113–122. [CrossRef]

16. Bates, S. Revenge Porn and Mental Health: A Qualitative Analysis of the Mental Health Effects of Revenge Porn on Female Survivors. *Fem. Criminol.* **2017**, *12*, 22–42. [CrossRef]

17. Cowie, H.; Myers, C.-A. *School Bullying and Mental Health: Risks, Intervention and Prevention*; Routledge: London, UK, 2018; ISBN 978-1-134-97743-7.

18. Lindsay, M.; Booth, J.M.; Messing, J.T.; Thaller, J. Experiences of Online Harassment Among Emerging Adults: Emotional Reactions and the Mediating Role of Fear. *J. Interpers. Violence* **2016**, *31*, 3174–3195. [CrossRef]

19. Walker, K.; Sleath, E. A systematic review of the current knowledge regarding revenge pornography and non-consensual sharing of sexually explicit media. *Aggress. Violent Behav.* **2017**, *36*, 9–24. [CrossRef]

20. Schenk, A.M.; Fremouw, W.J. Prevalence, psychological impact, and coping of cyberbully victims among college students. *J. Sch. Violence* **2012**, *11*, 21–37. [CrossRef]

21. National Union of Students Education beyond the Straight and Narrow. *LGBT Students' Experience in Higher Education*; NUS: London, UK, 2014.

22. Rivers, I. Homophobic and transphobic bullying in universities. In *Bullying Among University Students: Cross-national Perspectives*; Routledge: London, UK, 2016; pp. 48–60.

23. Valentine, G.; Wood, N.; Plummer, P. *The Experience of Lesbian, Gay, Bisexual and Trans Staff and Students in Higher Education*; Equality Challenge Unit: London, UK, 2009.

24. Colliety, P.; Royal, C.; Cowie, H. The unique role of the school nurse in the holistic care of the bully. *Br. J. Sch. Nurs.* **2016**, *11*, 443–449. [CrossRef]

25. Pörhölä, M. *Do the Roles of Bully and Victim Remain Stable from School to University? Theoretical Considerations*; Routledge: London, UK, 2016; ISBN 978-1-138-80925-3.

26. West, D. Prevalence of Cyberbullying amongst Students Aged 16–19 in Further Education. In Proceedings of the University of Birmingham School of Education Research Conference, Birmingham, UK, 1 December 2012.

27. West, D. An investigation into the prevalence of cyberbullying among students aged 16–19 in post-compulsory education. *Res. Post-Compuls. Educ.* **2015**, *20*, 96–112. [CrossRef]

28. Phipps, A.; Young, I. *That's What She Said: Women Students' Experiences of 'Lad Culture' in Higher Education*; NUS: London, UK, 2013.

29. Cassidy, W.; Faucher, C.; Jackson, M. Cyberbullying among youth: A comprehensive review of current international research and its implications and application to policy and practice. *Sch. Psychol. Int.* **2013**, *34*, 575–612. [CrossRef]

30. Giovazolias, T.; Malikiosi-Loizos, M. Bullying at Greek universities: An empirical study. In *Bullying among University Students: Cross-National Perspectives*; Routledge: London, UK, 2016; pp. 110–126.

31. Bauman, S.; Bellmore, A. New Directions in Cyberbullying Research. *J. Sch. Violence* **2015**, *14*, 1–10. [CrossRef]
32. Zalaquett, C.P.; Chatters, S.J. Cyberbullying in College: Frequency, Characteristics, and Practical Implications. *SAGE Open* **2014**, *4*, 2158244014526721. [CrossRef]
33. Curwen, T.; McNichol, J.S.; Sharpe, G.W. The Progression of Bullying from Elementary School to University. *Int. J. Humanit. Soc. Sci.* **2011**, *1*, 47–54.
34. Chapell, M.S.; Hasselman, S.L.; Kitchin, T.; Lomon, S.N.; MacIver, K.W.; Sarullo, P.L. Bullying in Elementary School, High School, and College. *Adolesc. San Diego Int. Q. Devoted Physiol. Psychol. Psychiatr. Sociol. Educ. Asp. Second Decade Hum. Life* **2006**, *41*, 633.
35. Purdy, N.; York, L. A critical investigation of the nature and extent of cyberbullying in two post-primary schools in Northern Ireland. *Pastor. Care Educ.* **2016**, *34*, 13–23. [CrossRef]
36. Cassidy, W.; Faucher, C.; Jackson, M. Adversity in University: Cyberbullying and Its Impacts on Students, Faculty and Administrators. *Int. J. Environ. Res. Public. Health* **2017**, *14*, 888. [CrossRef]
37. Souza, S.B.; Simão, A.M.V.; Ferreira, A.I.; Ferreira, P.C. University students' perceptions of campus climate, cyberbullying and cultural issues: Implications for theory and practice. *Stud. High. Educ.* **2018**, *43*, 2072–2087. [CrossRef]
38. Sam, D.L.; Bruce, D.; Agyemang, C.B.; Amponsah, B.; Arkorful, H. Cyberbullying Victimization among High School and University Students in Ghana. *Deviant Behav.* **2018**, 1–17. [CrossRef]
39. Salmivalli, C. Participant Roles in Bullying: How Can Peer Bystanders Be Utilized in Interventions? *Theory Pract.* **2014**, *53*, 286–292. [CrossRef]
40. Fluck, J. Why Do Students Bully? An Analysis of Motives Behind Violence in Schools. *Youth Soc.* **2017**, *49*, 567–587. [CrossRef]
41. Weber, M.; Ziegele, M.; Schnauber, A. Blaming the Victim: The Effects of Extraversion and Information Disclosure on Guilt Attributions in Cyberbullying. *Cyberpsychol. Behav. Soc. Netw.* **2013**, *16*, 254–259. [CrossRef]
42. Kyriacou, C.; Zuin, A. Cyberbullying bystanders and moral engagement: A psychosocial analysis for pastoral care. *Pastor. Care Educ.* **2018**, *36*, 99–111. [CrossRef]
43. Jones, S.E.; Manstead, A.S.R.; Livingstone, A.G. Ganging up or sticking together? Group processes and children's responses to text-message bullying. *Br. J. Psychol.* **2011**, *20*, 71–96.
44. Condeza, R.; Gallardo, G.; Pérez, P.R.; Gallardo, G.; Pérez, P.R. Experiences of Cyberbullying at a Chilean University: The Voices of Students. Available online: https://www.taylorfrancis.com/ (accessed on 27 February 2019).
45. Universities UK (UUK). *Changing the Culture: Report of the Universities UK Taskforce Examining Violence against Women, Harassment and Hate Crime Affecting University Students*; UUK: London, UK, 2016.
46. Cunningham, C.E.; Chen, Y.; Vaillancourt, T.; Rimas, H.; Deal, K.; Cunningham, L.J.; Ratcliffe, J. Modeling the anti-cyberbullying preferences of university students: Adaptive choice-based conjoint analysis. *Aggress. Behav.* **2015**, *41*, 369–385. [CrossRef]
47. Martinez-Monteagudo, M.C.; Delgado, M.C.; Ingles, C.J.; Garcia-Fernandez, J.M. Cyberbullying in the university setting. Relationship with family environment and emotional intelligence. *Comput. Hum. Behav.* **2019**, *91*, 220–225. [CrossRef]
48. McLouglin, L.; Spears, B.; Taddeo, C. The Importance of Social Connection for Cybervictims: How Connectedness and Technology Could Promote Mental Health and Wellbeing in Young People. *Int. J. Emot. Educ.* **2018**, *10*, 5–24.
49. Powell-Jones, Holly Bullying and social media. In *School Bullying and Mental Health: Risks, Intervention and Prevention*; Routledge: London, UK, 2018; pp. 115–129.
50. Mahady Wilton, M.M.; Craig, W.M.; Pepler, D.J. Emotional Regulation and Display in Classroom Victims of Bullying: Characteristic Expressions of Affect, Coping Styles and Relevant Contextual Factors. *Soc. Dev.* **2000**, *9*, 227–245. [CrossRef]
51. Kernaghan, D.; Elwood, J. All the (cyber) world's a stage: Framing cyberbullying as a performance. *Cyberpsychol. J. Psychosoc. Res. Cyberspace* **2013**, *7*. [CrossRef]
52. Perren, S.; Corcoran, L.; Cowie, H.; Dehue, F.; Garcia, D.; Guckin, C.M.; Sevcikova, A.; Tsatsou, P.; Völlink, T. Tackling Cyberbullying: Review of Empirical Evidence Regarding Successful Responses by Students, Parents, and Schools. *Int. J. Confl. Violence* **2012**, *6*, 283–292.

53. Alexandria, O.; Marilyn, C.; Kelly, W.; Eliza, L.; Melanie, K. Exploring University Students' Coping Strategy Intentions for Cyberbullying. *J. Interpers. Violence* **2017**, *32*, 446–462. [CrossRef]
54. Alqahtani, S.; Elbedour, S.; Freeman, K.; Ricks, E.; Reed, G.; Reed, K.W.; Merrick, J. Cyberbullying in Colleges and Universities: A Survey of Student Experiences and Attitudes about Cyberbullying. *Int. J. Child Adolesc. Health* **2018**, *11*, 73.
55. Pörhölä, M. Consequences of previous school-bullying experiences in young adulthood. In *Opiskelutenveys*; Duodecim: Helsinki, Finland, 2011; pp. 46–48.
56. Bauman, S.; Newman, M.L. Testing assumptions about cyberbullying: Perceived distress associated with acts of conventional and cyber bullying. *Psychol. Violence* **2013**, *3*, 27–38. [CrossRef]
57. Cuevas, C.A.; Finkelhor, D.; Turner, H.A.; Ormrod, R.K. Juvenile Delinquency and Victimization: A Theoretical Typology. *J. Interpers. Violence* **2007**, *22*, 1581–1602. [CrossRef]
58. Beckley, A.L.; Caspi, A.; Arseneault, L.; Barnes, J.C.; Fisher, H.L.; Harrington, H.; Houts, R.; Morgan, N.; Odgers, C.L.; Wertz, J.; et al. The Developmental Nature of the Victim-Offender Overlap. *J. Dev. Life-Course Criminol.* **2018**, *4*, 24–49. [CrossRef]
59. Jennings, W.G.; Piquero, A.R.; Reingle, J.M. On the overlap between victimization and offending: A review of the literature. *Aggress. Violent Behav.* **2012**, *17*, 16–26. [CrossRef]
60. Lauritsen, J.L.; Sampson, R.J.; Laub, J.H. The Link Between Offending and Victimization Among Adolescents. *Criminology* **1991**, *29*, 265–292. [CrossRef]
61. Erişti, B.; Akbulut, Y. Reactions to cyberbullying among high school and university students. *Soc. Sci. J.* **2018**. [CrossRef]
62. Universities UK (UUK). *Changing the Culture: One Year on—An Assessment of Strategies to Tackle Sexual Misconduct, Hate Crime and Harassment Affecting University Students*; UUK: London, UK, 2017.
63. Advance H.E. What do we know so far: What works in student safeguarding projects. In *Catalyst Student Safeguarding Evaluation: Briefing Note 2*; Advance HE: London, UK, 2018.
64. Cowie, H. Peer Support as an Intervention to Counteract School Bullying: Listen to the Children. *Child. Soc.* **2011**, *25*, 287–292. [CrossRef]
65. McGlynn, C.; Rackley, E.; Houghton, R. Beyond 'Revenge Porn': The Continuum of Image-Based Sexual Abuse. *Fem. Leg. Stud.* **2017**, *25*, 25–46. [CrossRef]
66. Ringrose, J.; Harvey, L.; Gill, R.; Livingstone, S. Teen girls, sexual double standards and 'sexting': Gendered value in digital image exchange. *Fem. Theory* **2013**, *14*, 305–323. [CrossRef]
67. Smith, P.K.; Thompson, F.; Craig, W.; Hong, I.; Slee, P.; Sullivan, K.; Green, V.A. Actions to Prevent Bullying in Western Countries. Available online: /core/books/school-bullying-in-different-cultures/actions-to-prevent-bullying-in-western-countries/87D264089B0737772D78292C5FCC8270 (accessed on 28 February 2019).
68. Ttofi, M.M.; Farrington, D.P. Effectiveness of school-based programs to reduce bullying: A systematic and meta-analytic review. *J. Exp. Criminol.* **2011**, *7*, 27–56. [CrossRef]
69. Cefai, C.; Bartolo, P.A.; Cavioni, V.; Downes, P. *Strengthening Social and Emotional Education as a Core Curricular Area Across the EU: A Review of the International Evidence*; European Union: Brussels, Belgium, 2018.
70. Ttofi, M.M.; Farrington, D. *School-Based Programs to Reduce Bullying and Victimization*; The Campbell Collaboration: Oslo, Norway, 2009.
71. Finne, J.; Roland, E.; Svartdal, F. Relational rehabilitation: Reducing the harmful effects of bullying. *Nord. Stud. Educ.* **2018**, *38*, 352–367. [CrossRef]
72. Keashley, L. In the e-presence of others: Understanding and developing constructive cyber-bystander action. In *Cyberbullying at University in International Contexts*; Routledge: New York, NY, USA, 2019; pp. 141–156.
73. Sellman, E. *Restorative Approaches to Conflict in Schools*, 1st ed.; Routledge: London, UK, 2014; ISBN 978-0-415-65611-5.
74. Aziz, R. The Research Students Experience. In *Bullying among University Students: Cross-National Perspectives*; Routledge: London, UK, 2016; pp. 21–32.

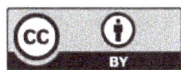

International Journal of
Environmental Research and Public Health

MDPI

Article

RPC Teacher-Based Program for Improving Coping Strategies to Deal with Cyberbullying

Annalisa Guarini [1,*], **Damiano Menin** [2], **Laura Menabò** [1] **and Antonella Brighi** [3]

[1] Department of Psychology, University of Bologna, 40127 Bologna, Italy; laura.menabo@studio.unibo.it
[2] Department of Education Studies "Giovanni Maria Bertin", University of Bologna, 40126 Bologna, Italy; damiano.menin2@unibo.it
[3] Faculty of Education, Free University of Bolzano, 39042 Brixen-Bressanone, Italy; antonella.brighi@unibz.it
* Correspondence: annalisa.guarini@unibo.it; Tel.: +39-051-2091869

Received: 31 January 2019; Accepted: 13 March 2019; Published: 16 March 2019

Abstract: Background: Cyberbullying is a serious threat to public health and teachers can play a key role in its detection, prevention and intervention. The present study evaluated the effectiveness of the RPC ("Relazioni per crescere"—Relationships to Grow) program, a short intervention, implemented at classroom level by trained teachers, aimed at improving awareness on cyberbullying and increasing proactive coping strategies to deal with cyberbullying behaviors. Method: The effectiveness of the RPC project was analyzed through an observational study (pre/post-intervention comparison), involving 898 Italian students of Lower Secondary schools (6th–8th grades). Results: Hierarchical logistic regression showed that after the intervention students were more likely to consider the different roles in cyberbullying (cyberbully, cybervictim, reinforce/assistant, defender and bystander/observer). In addition, hierarchical linear regressions highlighted an improvement of social coping and cognitive coping strategies after the intervention. Conclusions: RPC is a short, teacher-based program that can increase the awareness of cyberbullying among students and improves their effective coping strategies to address cyberbullying. Further research on the efficacy of short teacher-based programs would be worthwhile, given the limited financial and time resources of the schools, emphasizing the active and crucial role of teachers in tackling cyberbullying.

Keywords: cyberbullying; coping strategies; teacher based-intervention; adolescents

1. Introduction

Even if cyberbullying is a recent phenomenon described the first time 15 years ago, it is a widespread problem among students around the world [1] and it constitutes a serious public health issue, since it has been associated with a decrease in wellbeing and an increase in symptoms of depression, anxiety and low self-esteem [2–4]. Moreover, several episodes in the last 10 years have pointed out the extreme effects of victimization, such as suicide [5]. In addition, cyberbullying has an impact on the learning environment at school, negatively affecting the school climate [6].

At the international level, bullying and cyberbullying are considered forms of psychological and physical violence and they represent a violation of Article 9 of the UN Convention on the Rights of the Child (UNCRC). At the European level, there are no specific legal instruments targeting cyberbullying, but the EU has the role of coordinating and supporting the national initiatives of Country members and to promote Directives on victims' rights [7]. In Italy, both a law to contrast cyberbullying [8] and guidelines for schools [9] have been recently approved, since previous studies have shown that cyberbullying is a severe phenomenon in Italian schools. Indeed, a higher rate of cyberbullying among Italian students in comparison to Spanish and UK students was described [10,11]. A high incidence of cyberbullying among Italian students was confirmed by another European project, suggesting higher implication in cyberbullying in Poland, Italy and Greece compared to Spain, UK and Germany [12]. In addition, cyberbullying was described as a widespread phenomenon in Italy since similar incidences were found among different regions [13]. Finally, the phenomenon was already diffused (around 10%) among pre-adolescents as described by a large sample representative of the Italian Lower Secondary school population [14]. Starting from these results, the Italian law [8] aimed at preventing and identifying cyberbullying in all its forms. In particular, the Italian law stressed the relevance of, in each school, designating a teacher who can coordinate actions to prevent and contrast cyberbullying. This indication was integrated in the Italian Guidelines of Ministry of Education, Universities and Research [9], that suggest the need to implement a nationwide teacher training campaign in order to empower teachers' capacity to detect risky online behaviors and cyberbullying phenomena, adopting an interdisciplinary approach.

As acknowledged by the Italian enactments, the role of teacher is very crucial in identifying, preventing and intervening against cyberbullying. However, there is converging evidence that teachers do not perceive themselves to be adequately prepared for this task, suggesting that more research needs to be conducted in order to understand how schools and communities can intervene with cyberbullying [3,8–10]. In an Australian study, teachers reported to be less likely to recognize instances of cyberbullying, and were more uncertain about how to address bullying involving technology, compared to other forms of bullying [15]. Fewer than 10% of Australian secondary school staff reported feeling very skilled to deal with cyberbullying, while 50% felt poorly or not at all skilled to do so [16]. Other evidences showed that although teachers were aware they should do more to prevent cyberbullying [17] and they recognized cyberbullying as a problem, their perspectives and ideas on effective strategies to prevent cyberbullying were largely inconsistent and they highlighted the need for training on cyberbullying [15,18,19].

Concerning teacher training, very few interventions entirely delivered by teachers have been described in the literature. An example of a manual-based intervention entitled "Media Heroes" was implemented in Germany [20]. Teachers, after training, proposed several activities in their classes. The long version of the intervention (10 weeks) revealed a reduction of cyberbullying and an increase of affective empathy, while the short version (1 day) of the intervention showed a positive effect of cognitive empathy [20]. The Spanish "Asegúrate Program" was another example of targeted interventions against cyberbullying to be implemented by teachers, taking into account the theory of normative social behavior, self-regulation skills and the ideas/belief held by adolescents. Results showed a decrease in aggression and cyberaggression thanks to the intervention [21].

Alongside these specific intervention projects, modules for teachers' training have been included into "whole school" approaches to tackle bullying and cyberbullying. As an example, the Cyber-Friendly Schools (CFS) project was a comprehensive whole-school intervention against bullying and cyberbullying. In this program teachers implemented one third of the contents [22]. Additionally, the Tabby Improved Prevention and Intervention Program (TIPIP) was a whole school approach combining the Ecological System Theory and the Threat Assessment Approach. A teacher training module was one out of the four components of the project (teachers, parents, in class activities and online materials) and it aimed at describing the cyberbullying phenomenon, risk factors for students' involvement, how to prevent and manage cyberbullying, and legal issues [23]. The KiVa Antibullying Program consisted of both universal and focused actions with a particular attention to bystanders. A teacher training and a teacher's guide that provided step-by-step instructions for the curriculum lessons (20 h) were included in the program [24]. The KiVa program, developed to contrast bullying behaviors, has shown a good efficacy in reduction of cybervictimization and cyberbullying [24]. In the NoTrap! Program, a short training module for teachers was implemented too, even if the intervention was carried on through the peer educators' interventions [25].

Besides the specific components included in each intervention package, it should be taken into consideration what the prevention program is aimed at. A meta-analysis by Van Cleemput et al. [26] pointed out that many studies described a qualitative or quantitative evaluation of a prevention program aimed at reducing cyberbullying and cybervictimization among 10 to 18 year olds or at changing its proximal determinants (knowledge, attitudes, social skills, coping strategies). The outcomes of a program, indeed, can differ significantly across the different approaches, with some programs specifically aimed at obtaining a reduction of cyberbullying or cybervictimization rates, while other programs appear to be more focused on reducing the exposure to risk factors for cyberbullying and/or on improving protective factors, such as proactive and functional coping strategies. In this line, the strategy to invest in health promoting behaviors can be more beneficial [26], in light of the consideration that risk-reduction behavior is harder to change than health-promoting behavior, such as increasing appropriate coping skills [27].

For this purpose, it might be useful to consider what literature identifies as "effective" and "ineffective" coping strategies. Slee and Murray-Harvey [28] examined experts' views on the effectiveness of coping strategies utilized by Australian secondary school students and they found that items rated by the experts as "effective" and "ineffective" strongly aligned with the theoretical description of coping proposed by Lazarus [29]. Lazarus differentiated among problem-focused coping strategies (directed toward managing or altering the problem causing distress) and emotion-focused coping strategies (directed at regulating the emotional response). In the study by Slee and Murray-Harvey [28], behaviors like "talk to a school counselor" and "get support from others", which fall into the category of problem focused coping strategies, were rated by the experts as effective, while statements/actions like "see myself at fault" and "wish for a miracle", which were expressions of an emotion-focused coping style were generally rated as ineffective by the experts. The strategies adopted to cope with cyberbullying may influence the persistency of victimization [30–32], as well as its effect on mental health of the victim. Interventions should be designed to empower students by targeting their attitudes, problem solving skills, and their sense of control and to assist them to respond more effectively to being victimized [33,34].

To our knowledge, very few intervention programs aimed specifically at promoting and evaluating changes in students' coping strategies to cyberbullying, and none of them was fully delivered by teachers. Pieschl and Urbasik [35] found a significant increase in the use of technical coping styles, but they found no differences in the use of other coping styles (i.e., retaliation, proactive, withdrawal). Lam and Frydenberg [36] did not find significant changes in the use of productive coping styles, non-productive coping styles or seeking social support after the intervention.

The RPC program ("Relazioni per Crescere", "Relationships to Grow") was a universal, modularized and theoretically based intervention developed to help teachers in preventing and contrasting cyberbullying in their classes, through the promotion of health-related behaviors and by fostering positive relationships among students. It built on previous knowledge about potential risk and protective factors such as empathy and coping skills. This shift towards the consideration of protective factors besides the risk factors acknowledges the suggestions elaborated in the framework of Developmental Psychopathology [37,38].

The RPC is a short intervention program entirely delivered by teachers (6 h of teacher training; four activities proposed by teachers in their class during school hours; 1.5–2 h for each activity; 1 h of teacher supervision with expert psychologists). The program content is focused on the main following areas that, as suggested by a recent review [4], have been identified as the key components included in effective programs against cyberbullying.

1. Digital literacy. Risky information and communications technology (ICT) use was one of the main predictors of cyberbullying perpetration and cyberbullying victimization, as revealed by a recent meta-analysis [39]. High-risk actions such as sharing passwords, talking to strangers, and uploading intimate information on social networks made victims more vulnerable [40]. In addition, cyberbullying was also in comorbidity with other Internet risks, such as sextortion and online grooming [41].

2. Awareness raising and education on cyberbullying. Students needed to increase their awareness on cyberbullying, particularly for females [42]. Awareness-raising concerning the moral implications and the harm that can be caused to others by content manipulation, offensive

language, social exclusion, threats, etc., has proven to be effectively pursued by some programs as ConRed [43]. Awareness raising can also target the social dynamics of bullying and cyberbullying, since many students behave in ways that maintain, even fuel, the bullying behavior. This aspect has been particularly emphasized in the KiVa program [44].

3. Communication and social skills. Card and Hodges [45] found a lack of social skills/competence among the victims of violent bullying, and this may also be mirrored in cyberbullying [40]. Moreover, since cyberbullying arises frequently from face to face interactions at school, improving the social and communicative skills of the class-group could result in better relationships among students, thus also in a long term reduction of cyberbullying [46].

4. Empathy training. The need of empathy training in reducing cyberbullying behavior was highlighted by previous studies [47]. In particular both the cognitive empathy (recognizing and understanding another's emotional state) and the affective empathy (subjective state from emotional contagion) were inversely associated with cyberbullying [20].

5. Coping skills. Several types of coping strategies were described in relation to cyberbullying: confronting, technical solutions, supportive strategies and avoidant strategies [48]. Coping skills to deal with cyberbullying may exacerbate or may help to reduce the intensity of the aggression and can have significant associations with mental health. In the case of cyberbullying, it appeared that the negative consequences were influenced by the use of ineffective coping strategies, and the use of ineffective coping appeared to keep bullying and cyberbullying going [49]. Therefore, the intervention program aimed at improving proactive problem-focused coping strategies (cognitive or social) and to reduce passive/avoidant strategies.

Based on previous research results, the present paper examined the effects of RPC intervention based at the classroom level and implemented by trained teachers, aimed at improving awareness, and increasing proactive coping strategies. We hypothesized that this short intervention may increase students' knowledge of the phenomenon and improve students' coping skills in dealing with cyberbullying. In addition, a possible reduction of cyberbullying and cybervictimization was expected, even if this was not the aim of the intervention since this trend was not found by previous studies which proposed short interventions [20].

2. Methods

2.1. Participants

In the present study, 898 students filled in a questionnaire before and at the end of intervention. Students were recruited from 35 Public Lower Secondary schools from all the nine provinces of Emilia-Romagna region (North-Centre of Italy). Data of the Emilia-Romagna region revealed that 18% of students did not have an Italian citizenship (for more details see http://istruzioneer.gov.it/dati/fact-sheet/). According to the data of the HBSC Study [50], in the Emilia-Romagna region 64% of the students in the age range from 11 to 15 years lived with two parents. For what concerns the level of education of the parents, in the Emilia-Romagna region the results from the HBSC study [50] revealed that, in the range from 11 to 13 years of age, 31% of mothers had a University degree, 37% an Upper Secondary school degree, 12% a Vocational training qualification, 18% a Lower Secondary school degree, and 2% a Primary school certification. Fathers had lower levels of education compared to mothers: 26% of fathers had a University degree, 35% an Upper Secondary school degree, 13% a Vocational training qualification, 24% a Lower Secondary school degree, and 2% a Primary school certification. Concerning socioeconomic status (SES), the Family Affluence Scale revealed that the population of the Emilia-Romagna region was comprised of 17% in the low level, 53% in the medium level, and 30% in the high level. Data about the general SES of the families in Emilia-Romagna showed that this region reports families with higher levels of SES compared to the medium score of other Italian regions. As established by the Italian Ministry of Education [51], the subjects to be taught in Italian Lower Secondary schools are Italian, two other languages—English plus Spanish,

French or German—History, Geography, Math, Science, Music, Arts, Physical Education, Technologies. Preliminary skills of cyber literacy are included in Technologies.

Concerning the year level of our sample, 198 students attended the 6th grade (22%), 473 the 7th grade (53%), and 227 the 8th grade (25%). The age of participants ranged from 10 to 15 years (M = 12.15, SD = 0.83). The participants are a convenience sample, because the schools decided autonomously to take part to the intervention study and indicated to the research team which classes would have implemented the RPC program. The gender composition of the sample was balanced: 49% were females (*n* = 438) and 51% were males (*n* = 460). The data were collected from 2017 and 2018. No other anti-bullying programs have been carried out in the involved schools.

2.2. Questionnaire

The questionnaire consists of two different sections concerning cyberbullying and coping strategies.

Cyberbullying was assessed using two 11-item scales from the European Cyberbullying Intervention Project Questionnaire (ECIPQ; [2,12,20]). The questionnaire covered different behaviors including direct and indirect aggression and social exclusion online (e.g., "Someone spread rumors about me online"/"I spread rumors about someone online", "Someone created a fake account pretending to be me online"/"I created a fake account pretending to be someone else online"). Students were asked to answer to each item on a 5-points Likert scale (0 = never; 1 = one or two times; 2 = monthly; 3 = weekly; 4 = several times in the last week). Cronbach's alphas were respectively 0.82 and 0.83 for cyberbullying and cybervictimization scales. In addition, an open-ended question was asked in order to investigate the awareness of different roles involved in cyberbullying ("Who do you think is involved in an episode of cyberbullying?").

Strategies to cope with cyberbullying were assessed using an adapted and translated version of the "Coping with Bullying Questionnaire" [52]. The scale included four subscales, measuring respectively cognitive (10 items, e.g., "Think of different ways I could solve the problem"), social (eight items, e.g., "Ask a teacher for help with the cyberbullying"), passive (five items, e.g., "Wish a miracle would happen to stop the cyberbullying") and confrontational coping (four items, e.g., "Fight back"). Participants were asked to indicate their responses to real or hypothetical situations on each item on a 5-point Likert scale (from 0 = never to 4 = always). Cronbach's alphas were respectively 0.76 for cognitive and confrontational coping, 0.87 for social coping and 0.55 for passive coping. The last one was therefore excluded from further analysis since it was not a robust variable.

2.3. RPC Program

Teachers attended a training course (6 h) with expert psychologists concerning theoretical definitions of bullying and cyberbullying phenomena and the explanation of activities to carry out with their students. Teachers received also a manual with step-by-step descriptions of the activities and some materials that they could use in their classes. The following in-class activities were proposed by teachers (four activities; 1.5–2 h for each activity):

(1) Digital literacy. Using brainstorming, teachers debated with students' risks and opportunities of ICTs in order to improve safe use of technologies.
(2) Awareness raising and education on cyberbullying. Starting from different scenarios, students in small groups identified roles involved in cyberbullying and they co-constructed the definition of cyberbullying.
(3) Empathy training. Students experienced different roles in cyberbullying through a short role-playing in order to improve both cognitive empathy (recognizing another's emotional state) and affective empathy ("How I felt in this role").
(4) Coping skills. Students in small groups produced slogans to contrast cyberbullying taking into account the different roles involved in the phenomenon ("What can be useful for a victim? What

can a bystander do?"). The different types of coping strategies were analyzed, identifying which can be more effective in contrasting cyberbullying.

Communication and social skills were improved in all activities since dialog, discussion and negotiation among students were encouraged. At the end of each activity, students produced materials (posters, slogans, pictures) that allowed to both synthesize the contents and to keep the main messages for the class in the future. The activities were proposed by teachers in their classes within a two-month period. During these months 1 h of supervision of teacher activities was provided by expert psychologists in order to support teachers in the program implementation.

2.4. Coding

Participants were categorized into four groups based on cybervictimization and cyberbullying scores for descriptive purposes. Students who admitted to have perpetrated at least one type of online aggression on a monthly basis, or admitted to at least two different types of online aggression were considered as bullies [12]. Students who reported having suffered at least one type of online aggression on a monthly basis, or reported having suffered at least two different types of online aggression were considered as victims [12]. Based on this classification, participants were assigned to one of the four mutually exclusive groups: "Not Involved", "Pure Victims", "Pure Bullies" and "Bullies/Victims".

Average scores were calculated for each scale (cyberbullying, cybervictimization, social, cognitive and confrontational coping).

The coding of the open-ended question "Who do you think is involved in an episode of cyberbullying?" was performed using CAQDAS software NVivo (version 11, QSR International, Melbourne, Australia). Based on a priori definition of different roles involved in bullying [53], five categories were identified: bully, victim, reinforce/assistant, defender and bystander/outsider. For each category, two expert psychologists selected a set of semantically keywords.

Answers provided by participants to the open question in pre- and post-intervention were analyzed to quantify the occurrence of each category. Repetitions within the same answer were not considered. In addition, the number of empty answers and "I do not know" answers were counted.

2.5. Procedure and Study Design

A repeated measures design was adopted to investigate the effectiveness of the intervention. Students filled in online questionnaires during school hours. The first questionnaire was filled in during the week before the intervention (pre-intervention) and the second questionnaire within two weeks after the end of in-class activities (post-intervention). Teachers remained in the classrooms during the survey in order to clarify any questions or problems. All questionnaires were anonymous, and a nickname was chosen by the student and used for data collections (pre-intervention and post-intervention) in order to match the responses.

2.6. Ethics

The study protocol met the ethical guidelines for the protection of human participants, including adherence to the legal requirements of Italy, and received a formal approval by the Bioethics Committee, University of Bologna. Both parents gave their informed written consent for the participation to the study.

2.7. Statistical Analysis

Regression analyses were run using the lmerTest package under R version 3.5.2 (R Foundation for Statistical Computing, Vienna, Austria) and the significance level was set at 0.05. Multilevel linear regressions were fitted to inquire the potential changes in average scores for cyberbullying and coping-related variables after the intervention (cyberbullying, cybervictimization, social, cognitive and confrontational coping). The hierarchical structure of the data set was modeled by including a random intercept, with students nested in classes, nested in schools. Gender and age were included as predictors in the regressions in order to control for their potential effects.

Binary variables resulting from the coding of the question "Who do you think is involved in cyberbullying?" were analyzed via hierarchical logistic regressions, in order to assess whether the understanding of cyberbullying social dynamics varied following the intervention.

3. Results

3.1. Cyberbullying/Cybervictimization

Table 1 displays the distribution of participants across role-based groups. About 30% of participants, both in pre-intervention and post-intervention, were involved in cyberbullying as bully, victim, or bully-victim.

No significant changes in average scores for cyberbullying or cybervictimization were highlighted by multilevel regressions (Table 1). No gender- or age-related differences were found.

Table 1. Cyberbullying and cybervictimization before and after the intervention.

Cyberbullying	Pre-Intervention	Post-Intervention	t	β	p
Not Involved	601 (71.1%)	589 (70.1%)			
Pure Victims	124(14.7%)	128 (15.2%)			
Pure Bullies	43 (5.1%)	38 (4.5%)			
Bullies-Victims	77 (9.1%)	85 (10.1%)			
Cyberbullying	1.07 (0.17)	1.07 (0.20)	0.40	0.01	0.689
Cybervictimization	1.13 (0.29)	1.14 (0.30)	0.97	0.02	0.331

Note: No. (percentage) for role-based groups (percentage was calculated excluding missing values; 53 cases in the pre-intervention assessment and 58 cases in the post-intervention assessment); mean (SD) for cyberbullying and cybervictimization scores.

3.2. Awareness of Cyberbullying Social Dynamics

As displayed in Table 2, after the intervention the number of students mentioning keywords pertaining to the category victim was doubled (pre-intervention, 28.6%; post-intervention, 63.7%). Similarly, 66% of respondents ($n = 593$) recognized the role of the bully after the intervention, with a relevant increase compared with pre-intervention assessment (39.8%). The roles of reinforce/assistant and bystander/outsider were almost non-existent before the intervention (below 1%), while after the program the role of reinforce/assistant was acknowledged by 5.2% of participants and that of bystander/outsider by 12.9% of respondents. The number of those recognizing the role of defender increased from below 1% before the intervention to 2.2% after the intervention, but its occurrence was deemed too low for regression analyses. The number of those not answering the question decreased from 10.1% before the intervention to 3% after the intervention.

Table 2. Awareness of cyberbullying social dynamics before and after the intervention.

Roles	Pre-Intervention		Post-Intervention		Wald	b	p
	Yes	No	Yes	No			
Victim	257 (28.6%)	641 (71.4%)	572 (63.7%)	326 (36.3%)	13.01	2.08	<0.001
Bully	357 (39.8%)	541 (60.2%)	593 (66.0%)	305 (34.0%)	10.86	1.42	<0.001
Reinforce/Assistant	5 (0.6%)	893 (99.4%)	47 (5.2%)	851 (94.8%)	10.18	8.82	<0.001
Bystander/Outsider	7 (0.8%)	891 (99.2%)	116 (12.9%)	782 (87.1%)	13.81	10.83	<0.001
Defender	4 (0.4%)	894 (99.6%)	20 (2.2%)	878 (97.8%)			
Missing/No answer	91 (10.1%)	807 (89.9%)	27 (3.0%)	871 (97.0%)	−8.81	−4.85	<0.001

Note: Yes: No. (percentage) of the participants who mentioned at least once one of the words included in the respective category.

Hierarchical logistic regressions confirmed differences between the pre- and post-intervention surveys regarding the different roles in cyberbullying. After the intervention, participants were more likely to mention at least one word associated to the category victim, bully, reinforce/assistant, and bystander/outsider compared with the pre-intervention (Table 2). In addition, after the intervention, participants were found to be less likely to either not answer the question or answer "I don't know", compared to before the intervention (Table 2).

3.3. Coping Strategies

Hierarchical linear regressions highlighted some differences between the pre- and post-intervention surveys regarding coping strategies (see Table 3 for descriptive statistics).

Table 3. Coping strategies before and after the intervention.

Coping Strategies	Pre-Intervention	Post-Intervention	*t*	*β*	*p*
Social Coping	1.70 (1.08)	1.89 (1.06)	5.11	0.10	<0.001
Cognitive Coping	1.47 (0.77)	1.58 (0.74)	3.55	0.07	<0.001
Confrontational Coping	1.89 (1.18)	1.98 (1.12)	1.45	0.03	0.147

Note: Mean (SD) for each category.

As highlighted in Table 3, the score for social coping was higher in the post-intervention assessment, compared with the pre-intervention assessment. Social coping also displayed higher scores for girls compared to boys, t (1642) = 7.51, $β = 0.12$, $p < 0.001$. A post-intervention increase was also found for cognitive coping (Table 3). Cognitive coping also highlighted a gender difference, with girls having higher scores than boys, t (4997) = 4.15, $β = 0.11$, $p < 0.001$.

Confrontational coping did not change significantly after the intervention, highlighting only a positive association with age, t (1673) = 2.21, $β = 0.07$, $p = 0.028$.

4. Discussion

The present study evaluated the effectiveness of the RPC program, a short intervention, implemented at the classroom level by trained teachers, aimed at improving awareness of cyberbullying and increasing proactive coping strategies in dealing with cyberbullying. We also analyzed a possible reduction of cyberbullying and cybervictimization behaviors.

Concerning the awareness of cyberbullying, the RPC program increased students' knowledge of the social dynamic of cyberbullying, making them more aware of the interplay among the different roles involved in this phenomenon. Indeed, at the open question "Who do you think is involved in an episode of cyberbullying?" students showed to identify, after in-class activities, the different roles involved in cyberbullying and they were more aware that cyberbullying was a group phenomenon characterized by the following roles: cyberbully, cybervictim, reinforce and assistant, defenders and bystanders/outsiders [53]. The awareness that cyberbullying was a group process and a social phenomenon [53], pointed out the important role of bystanders: this was the first step to promote responsibility in the class and to change the normative rules that may also support and foster aggressive behaviors online [44].

The RPC program also showed a significant improvement of students' coping skills in dealing with cyberbullying. Coping refers to "conscious efforts individuals use to regulate emotion, cognition, behavior, internal states, or situation to reduce threat" [54]. The coping process starts with threat appraisal, i.e., the perceptions of how stressful the event is for the individual. According to Transactional Model of Stress and Coping [55], appraisal happens at two levels: one is the primary appraisal, which assesses the situation in order to determine whether it is a threat; the secondary appraisal assesses the changeability of the situation (or the possibility to change it) along with the individual's resources to manage the associated stress. These cognitive appraisals determine the coping style selected. In light of our results, where an increase of the problem-focused strategies emerged after the intervention, we may hypothesize that a better knowledge of the cyberbullying phenomenon may have influenced the coping strategies chosen to deal with it. Indeed, a clearer picture of the social dynamics implied in this phenomenon, as shown by the qualitative analysis of the different roles involved in cyberbullying, may have facilitated the two levels of the appraisal process: (a) by providing the students with information helpful to detect the malicious intention behind certain messages; (b) by providing them with a set of resources to deal with it, including those available in the school environment (i.e., peers, teachers, the school policy). This may have led students to indicate more effective coping strategies as the ones we have reported: asking for help to friends, teachers and parents (knowing that there are teachers prepared to support), thinking about how to solve the situation. These strategies showed to be more available for girls than for males before the intervention (as reported in the literature [56]), but increased for both the genders after the intervention. The adoption of assertive coping, such as the confrontational one, was not influenced significantly by the intervention. This latter emphasizes the victim's attempt to assume an active position with respect to the bully. Specifically, this strategy involves seeking a direct but not aggressive confrontation with the bully in order to stop his/her behavior [57], and it is widely used in cases where the source of the bullying is known [58,59], and in less serious cases of online harassment [60]. It would be relevant to explore the use of this coping strategy in relation to the intensity of the cyberbullying suffered by the victims.

Concerning the effect of the RPC program on the reduction of cyberbullying and cybervictimization, we found that the prevalence of the phenomenon was stable between pre- and post-intervention. Our results revealed that a short intervention (8 h in class), as the RPC program, can improve the awareness of the phenomenon and increase the use of effective coping strategies, but it did not have an effect on the reduction of rates of cyberbullying. Our findings were in line with the results of the short Media Heroes intervention [20]. Indeed, while the long-term (10 weeks) "Media Heroes" program was effective in reducing cyberbullying and promoting affective empathy, the short Media Heroes (1 day, four sessions of 90 min) program was not effective in reducing cyberbullying, reporting a significant effect only on cognitive empathy. Other programs targeted for teachers that described an effect on the reduction of cyberbullying were more extensive (eight sessions for the "Asegúrate Program" [21]). In addition, the RPC program cannot be compared to other programs using a "whole school approach" ([22–24]). These programs, in fact, even if they were effective in reducing cyberbullying [61], were expensive and required high support from the schools as well as a great time investment. Unfortunately, as suggested by educators, even if some programs were promising, time constraints, lack of colleagues' support and uncooperative parents could limit their effect [62]. For this reason, a short program, as RPC, could be a valid tool to increase the awareness of the cyberbullying phenomenon and to promote effective coping strategies. The promising results, however, suggest the efficacy of the RPC programme should be analyzed in a long-term follow-up; if the results obtained in such a short intervention would remain stable in a longer period, this would improve its cost/benefit ratio.

Limitations

The first limitation was the study design. An observational study was carried out with an analysis of change between pre- and post-intervention phases. The absence of a control group did not allow the investigation of both the effect of maturation and the role of increased awareness. Several studies revealed that cyberbullying increased in control groups, suggesting that without an intervention the phenomenon could grow [20]. Other studies suggested that the intervention modified the awareness, attitude and self-perceptions in dealing with bullying and cyberbullying [63]. Further studies with the RPC program should be carried out using a quasi-experimental design with a control group, since, as suggested by a recent review [4] research at a school does allow true randomization. The collection of a control group could help to understand the effect of the RPC program on cybervictimization and perpetration, taking into account the effect of maturation and the role of awareness.

A second limitation of the present study was that only the global effect of the intervention was analyzed, without disentangling the effects of specific components of the interventions. As suggested by a recent review and meta-analysis [61] this is a very important challenge, since even if we know that prevention and intervention programs for cyberbullying are effective, we need to explain which specific components of the intervention are more relevant.

The third limitation concerned the implementation of the intervention: dosage and fidelity. Even if all students involved in the present research took part into the four in-class activities, we did not know if the teachers used all the materials proposed and followed the suggestions from the manual. A more complex index of implementation should be added in further research, since individual and interpersonal factors are important for successful implementation of the program [44].

Measures of SES background were not collected directly in the present study. More detailed information would be useful in further studies to improve the generalization of our findings and for understanding the role of these variables in moderating the effect of intervention.

The last limitation of the present study was the selective focus on cyberbullying behaviors. We decided this selective focus following the indication of Italian law [8]. We also needed to implement a short program that could have been suitable for teachers during their curricular hours (Reading/Spelling, Maths, etc.), since no extra hours were available for intervention projects. However, since the cyberbullying phenomenon has comorbidities with other behaviors such as bullying and sextortion [64], we can hypothesize that programs also including activities to contrast these phenomena, could be more effective in reducing cyberbullying [24]. In addition, the lack of specific questions about sextortion and online sexual victimization could have contributed to underestimating the cybervictimization, mainly among females [65].

5. Conclusions

RPC is a short and friendly program targeted at teachers that increases the awareness on cyberbullying among students and improves their effective coping strategies to address cyberbullying. Programs like RPC should be part of the schools' daily activities proposed by teachers. Teacher-based and short interventions can sometimes be the only possibility to trigger schools' initiatives to prevent cyberbullying, since this kind of intervention may fit with the limited financial and time resources of the schools. In addition, it may respond, at least in Italy, to the recommendations enacted by the Ministry of Education concerning the active involvement of teachers in actions against cyberbullying.

Author Contributions: Conceptualization, A.G. and A.B.; Data curation, D.M.; Formal analysis, D.M. and L.M.; Funding acquisition, A.G.; Methodology, D.M. and L.M.; Project administration, A.G.; Supervision, A.G. and A.B.; Writing—original draft, A.G.; Writing—review & editing, D.M., L.M. and A.B.

Funding: This research was granted by "IC Ozzano dell'Emilia (Bologna)" with the Grant entitled "Formare per prevenire. L'educazione ai new media per la prevenzione dei fenomeni del bullismo e cyberbullismo" (Coordinator of the Department of Psychology, Annalisa Guarini).

Acknowledgments: The authors are grateful to the teachers, the students and they families that took part to the research. Thanks to the psychologists (Sandra Maria Elena Nicoletti, Felicia Roga and Luana Fusaro) of the SERES Service (Department of Psychology, Coordinator Annalisa Guarini) who carried on the training with teachers. Thanks also to the Regional School Office of Emilia-Romagna Region for supporting the research.

Conflicts of Interest: The authors declare no conflict of interest.

References

1. Zych, I.; Ortega-Ruiz, R.; Del Rey, R. Systematic review of theoretical studies on bullying and cyberbullying: Facts, knowledge, prevention, and intervention. *Aggress. Viol. Behav.* **2015**, *23*, 1–21. [CrossRef]
2. Brighi, A.; Melotti, G.; Guarini, A.; Genta, M.L.; Ortega, R.; Mora-Merchán, J.; Smith, P.K.; Thompson, F. Self-Esteem and Loneliness in Relation to Cyberbullying in Three European Countries. In *Cyberbullying in the Global Playground*; Li, Q., Cross, D., Smith, P.K., Eds.; Wiley-Blackwell: Oxford, UK, 2012; pp. 32–56, ISBN 978-1-119-95448-4.

3. Espelage, D.L.; Hong, J.S. Cyberbullying Prevention and Intervention Efforts: Current Knowledge and Future Directions. *Can. J. Psychiatry* **2017**, *62*, 374–380. [CrossRef] [PubMed]

4. Hutson, E.; Kelly, S.; Militello, L.K. Systematic Review of Cyberbullying Interventions for Youth and Parents With Implications for Evidence-Based Practice: Cyberbullying Interventions for Individual Youth and Parents. *Worldviews Evid.-Based Nurs.* **2018**, *15*, 72–79. [CrossRef] [PubMed]

5. Hinduja, S.; Patchin, J.W. Bullying, Cyberbullying, and Suicide. *Arch. Suicide Res.* **2010**, *14*, 206–221. [CrossRef]

6. Hinduja, S.; Patchin, J.W. Cyberbullying: A Review of the Legal Issues Facing Educators. *Prev. School Fail. Altern. Educ. Child. Youth* **2011**, *55*, 71–78. [CrossRef]

7. European Union. Policy Department C: Citizens' Rights and Constitutional Affairs. Cyberbullying among Young People. Available online: http://www.europarl.europa.eu/RegData/etudes/STUD/2016/571367/IPOL_STU(2016)571367_EN.pdf (accessed on 15 December 2018).

8. Italian Cyberbullying Law N. 71/2017. *Disposizioni a tutela dei minori per la prevenzione ed il contrasto del fenomeno del cyberbullismo*; Gazzetta Ufficiale della Repubblica Italiana: Roma, Italy, 2017.

9. MIUR (Italian Ministry of Education, University and Research). *Aggiornamento Linee di Orientamento per la prevenzione e il contrasto del cyberbullismo*. Available online: http://www.miur.gov.it/documents/20182/0/Linee+Guida+Bullismo+-+2017.pdf/4df7c320-e98f-4417-9c31-9100fd63e2be?version=1.0 (accessed on 10 December 2018).

10. Genta, M.L.; Smith, P.K.; Ortega-Ruiz, R.; Brighi, A.; Guarini, A.; Thompson, F.; Tippett, N.; Mora-Merchàn, J.; Calmaestra, J. Comparative Aspect of Cyberbullying in Italy, England and Spain: Findings From a DAPHNE Project. In *Cyberbullying in the Global Playground. Research from International Perspectives*; Li, Q., Smith, C.D., Eds.; Blackwell Publishing Ltd.: New York, NY, USA, 2012; pp. 15–31.

11. Ortega, R.; Elipe, P.; Mora-Merchán, J.A.; Genta, M.L.; Brighi, A.; Guarini, A.; Smith, P.K.; Thompson, F.; Tippett, N. The Emotional Impact of Bullying and Cyberbullying on Victims: A European Cross-National Study: Emotional Impact of Bullying and Cyberbullying. *Aggress. Behav.* **2012**, *38*, 342–356. [CrossRef] [PubMed]

12. Del Rey, R.; Casas, J.A.; Ortega-Ruiz, R.; Schultze-Krumbholz, A.; Scheithauer, H.; Smith, P.; Thompson, F.; Barkoukis, V.; Tsorbatzoudis, H.; Brighi, A.; et al. Structural validation and cross-cultural robustness of the European Cyberbullying Intervention Project Questionnaire. *Comput. Hum. Behav.* **2015**, *50*, 141–147. [CrossRef]

13. Brighi, A.; Guarini, A.; Palermiti, A.L.; Bartolo, M.G.; Genta, M.L. Victimization in traditional bullying and cyberbullying among Italian preadolescents. An investigation in Emilia Romagna, Tuscany and Calabria. *Età Evolutiva* **2011**, *33*, 38–48.

14. Vieno, A.; Gini, G.; Lenzi, M.; Pozzoli, T.; Canale, N.; Santinello, M. Cybervictimization and somatic and psychological symptoms among Italian middle school students. *Eur. J. Public Health* **2015**, *25*, 433–437. [CrossRef]

15. Cross, D.; Shaw, T.; Hearn, L.; Epstein, M.; Monks, H.; Lester, L.; Thomas, L. *Australian Covert. Bullying Prevalence Study (ACBPS)*; Child Health Promotion Research Centre, Edith Cowan University: Perth, Australia, 2009.

16. Barnes, A.; Cross, D.; Lester, L.; Hearn, L.; Epstein, M.; Monks, H. The Invisibility of Covert Bullying Among Students: Challenges for School Intervention. *Aust. J. Guid. Couns.* **2012**, *22*, 206–226. [CrossRef]

17. Green, V.A.; Johnston, M.; Mattioni, L.; Prior, T.; Harcourt, S.; Lynch, T. Who is responsible for addressing cyberbullying? Perspectives from teachers and senior managers. *Int. J. School & Educ. Psychol.* **2017**, *5*, 100–114. [CrossRef]

18. DeSmet, A.; Aelterman, N.; Bastiaensens, S.; Van Cleemput, K.; Poels, K.; Vandebosch, H.; Cardon, G.; De Bourdeaudhuij, I. Secondary school educators' perceptions and practices in handling cyberbullying among adolescents: A cluster analysis. *Comput. Educ.* **2015**, *88*, 192–201. [CrossRef]

19. Macaulay, P.J.R.; Betts, L.R.; Stiller, J.; Kellezi, B. Perceptions and responses towards cyberbullying: A systematic review of teachers in the education system. *Aggress. Viol. Behav.* **2018**, *43*, 1–12. [CrossRef]

20. Schultze-Krumbholz, A.; Schultze, M.; Zagorscak, P.; Wölfer, R.; Scheithauer, H. Feeling cybervictims' pain: The Effect of Empathy Training on Cyberbullying. *Aggress. Behav.* **2016**, *42*, 147–156. [CrossRef]

21. Del-Rey-Alamillo, R.; Mora-Merchán, J.A.; Casas, J.-A.; Ortega-Ruiz, R.; Elipe, P. "Asegúrate" Program: Effects on cyber-aggression and its risk factors. *Comunicar* **2018**, *26*, 39–48. [CrossRef]

22. Cross, D.; Shaw, T.; Hadwen, K.; Cardoso, P.; Slee, P.; Roberts, C.; Thomas, L.; Barnes, A. Longitudinal impact of the Cyber Friendly Schools program on adolescents' cyberbullying behavior: Impact of the Cyber Friendly Schools Program. *Aggress. Behav.* **2016**, *42*, 166–180. [CrossRef] [PubMed]

23. Sorrentino, A.; Baldry, A.; Farrington, D. The Efficacy of the Tabby Improved Prevention and Intervention Program in Reducing Cyberbullying and Cybervictimization among Students. *Int. J. Environ. Res. Public Health* **2018**, *15*, 2536. [CrossRef]

24. Williford, A.; Elledge, L.C.; Boulton, A.J.; DePaolis, K.J.; Little, T.D.; Salmivalli, C. Effects of the KiVa Antibullying Program on Cyberbullying and Cybervictimization Frequency Among Finnish Youth. *J. Clin. Child Adolesc. Psychol.* **2013**, *42*, 820–833. [CrossRef]

25. Palladino, B.E.; Nocentini, A.; Menesini, E. Evidence-based intervention against bullying and cyberbullying: Evaluation of the NoTrap! program in two independent trials: Evaluation of the NoTrap! Program. *Aggress. Behav.* **2016**, *42*, 194–206. [CrossRef]

26. Van Cleemput, K.; DeSmet, A.; Vandebosch, H.; Bastiaensens, S. A systematic review and meta-analysis of the efficacy of cyberbullying prevention programs. Presented at the Etmaal van de Communicatiewetenschap, Wageningen, NL, USA, 3–4 February 2014.

27. Adriaanse, M.A.; Vinkers, C.D.W.; De Ridder, D.T.D.; Hox, J.J.; De Wit, J.B.F. Do implementation intentions help to eat a healthy diet? A systematic review and meta-analysis of the empirical evidence. *Appetite* **2011**, *56*, 183–193. [CrossRef]

28. Slee, P. Murray-Harvey R Experts' views on students' strategies for copying with bullying. Presented at the ISRA XV111 World Meeting, Budapest, Hungary, 8–13 July 2008; pp. 8–13.

29. Lazarus, R.S. Hope: An Emotion and a Vital Coping Resource Against Despair. *Soc. Res.* **1999**, *66*, 653–678.

30. Kochenderfer, B.J.; Ladd, G.W. Victimized children's responses to peers' aggression: Behaviors associated with reduced versus continued victimization. *Dev. Psychopathol.* **1997**, *9*. [CrossRef]

31. Smith, P.K.; Talamelli, L.; Cowie, H.; Naylor, P.; Chauhan, P. Profiles of non-victims, escaped victims, continuing victims and new victims of school bullying. *Br. J. Educ. Psychol.* **2004**, *74*, 565–581. [CrossRef] [PubMed]

32. Kanetsuna, T.; Smith, P.K.; Morita, Y. Coping with bullying at school: Children's recommended strategies and attitudes to school-based interventions in England and Japan. *Aggress. Behav.* **2006**, *32*, 570–580. [CrossRef]

33. Terranova, A.M. Factors that Influence Children's Responses to Peer Victimization. *Child Youth Care Forum* **2009**, *38*, 253–271. [CrossRef]

34. Skrzypiec, G.; Slee, P.; Murray-Harvey, R.; Pereira, B. School bullying by one or more ways: Does it matter and how do students cope? *School Psychol. Int.* **2011**, *32*, 288–311. [CrossRef]

35. Pieschl, S.; Urbasik, S. Does the cyber bullying prevention program surf-fair work? An evaluation study. In *From Cyberbullying to Cyber Safety: Issue and Approach in Educational Context*; Internet Policies and Issues: Privacy and Identity Protection; Ria Hanewald; Nova Science Publishers Inc.: Hauppauge, NY, USA, 2013; pp. 205–224.

36. Lam, C.W.C.; Frydenberg, E. Coping in the Cyberworld: Program Implementation and Evaluation—A Pilot Project. *Aust. J. Guid. Couns.* **2009**, *19*, 196–215. [CrossRef]

37. Mohaupt, S. Review Article: Resilience and Social Exclusion. *Soc. Policy Soc.* **2009**, *8*, 63. [CrossRef]

38. Rutter, M. Resilience as a dynamic concept. *Dev. Psychopathol.* **2012**, *24*, 335–344. [CrossRef]

39. Chen, L.; Ho, S.S.; Lwin, M.O. A meta-analysis of factors predicting cyberbullying perpetration and victimization: From the social cognitive and media effects approach. *New Media Soc.* **2017**, *19*, 1194–1213. [CrossRef]

40. Gradinger, P.; Strohmeier, D.; Schiller, E.M.; Stefanek, E.; Spiel, C. Cyber-victimization and popularity in early adolescence: Stability and predictive associations. *Eur. J. Dev. Psychol.* **2012**, *9*, 228–243. [CrossRef]

41. Machimbarrena, J.M.; Calvete, E.; Fernández-González, L.; Álvarez-Bardón, A.; Álvarez-Fernández, L.; González-Cabrera, J. Internet Risks: An Overview of Victimization in Cyberbullying, Cyber Dating Abuse, Sexting, Online Grooming and Problematic Internet Use. *Int. J. Environ. Res. Public Health* **2018**, *15*, 2471. [CrossRef]

42. Elçi, A.; Seçkin, Z. Cyberbullying Awareness for Mitigating Consequences in Higher Education. *J. Interpers. Viol.* **2019**, *34*, 946–960. [CrossRef] [PubMed]

43. Del-Rey-Alamillo, R.; Casas, J.-A.; Ortega-Ruiz, R. The ConRed Program, an Evidence-based Practice. *Comunicar* **2012**, *20*, 129–138. [CrossRef]

44. Haataja, A.; Ahtola, A.; Poskiparta, E.; Salmivalli, C. A process view on implementing an antibullying curriculum: How teachers differ and what explains the variation. *School Psychol. Q.* **2015**, *30*, 564–576. [CrossRef] [PubMed]

45. Card, N.A.; Isaacs, J.; Hodges, E.V.E. Multiple Contextual Levels of Risk for Peer Victimization: A Review with Implications for Prevention and Intervention Efforts. In *School Violence and Primary Prevention*; Miller, T.W., Ed.; Springer: New York, NY, USA, 2008; pp. 125–153, ISBN 978-0-387-75660-8.

46. Ortega-Ruiz, R. Knowing, Building and Living Together on Internet and Social Networks: The ConRed Cyberbullying Prevention Program. *Soc. Netw.* **2012**, *6*, 11. [CrossRef]

47. Ang, R.P.; Goh, D.H. Cyberbullying Among Adolescents: The Role of Affective and Cognitive Empathy, and Gender. *Child Psychiatry Hum. Dev.* **2010**, *41*, 387–397. [CrossRef] [PubMed]

48. Perren, S.; Corcoran, L.; Cowie, H.; Dehue, F.; Garcia, D.; Guckin, C.M.; Sevcikova, A.; Tsatsou, P.; Völlink, T. Tackling Cyberbullying: Review of Empirical Evidence Regarding Successful Responses by Students, Parents, and Schools. *Int. J. Confl. Viol.* **2012**, *6*, 10. [CrossRef]

49. Jacobs, N.C.L.; Dehue, F.; Völlink, T.; Lechner, L. Determinants of adolescents' ineffective and improved coping with cyberbullying: A Delphi study. *J. Adolesc.* **2014**, *37*, 373–385. [CrossRef]

50. HBSC, Health Behavior in School-Aged Children. Stili di vita e salute degli adolescenti. I risultati della sorveglianza HBSC Italia 2014. Regione Emilia-Romagna. 2016. Available online: https://salute.regione. emilia-romagna.it/documentazione/rapporti/rapporto-stili-di-vita-e-salute-degli-adolescenti-i-risultati-della-sorveglianza-hbsc-2014-in-emilia-romagna-2016/at_download/file/HBSC_RER_2016.pdf (accessed on 15 December 2018).

51. MIUR (Italian Ministry of Education, University and Research). Decreto 16 novembre 2012, 254. Available online: http://www.gazzettaufficiale.it/eli/id/2013/02/05/13G00034/sg (accessed on 15 December 2018).

52. Murray-Harvey, R.; Skrzypiec, G.; Slee, P.T. Effective and Ineffective Coping With Bullying Strategies as Assessed by Informed Professionals and Their Use by Victimised Students. *Aust. J. Guid. Couns.* **2012**, *22*, 122–138. [CrossRef]

53. Salmivalli, C.; Lagerspetz, K.; Björkqvist, K.; Österman, K.; Kaukiainen, A. Bullying as a group process: Participant roles and their relations to social status within the group. *Aggress. Behav.* **1996**, *22*, 1–15. [CrossRef]

54. Raskauskas, J.; Huynh, A. The process of coping with cyberbullying: A systematic review. *Aggress. Viol. Behav.* **2015**, *23*, 118–125. [CrossRef]

55. Lazarus, R.S.; Folkman, S. Coping and adaptation. In *Handbook of Behavioral Medicine*; Guilford Press: New York, NY, USA, 1985; pp. 282–325.

56. Frisén, A.; Berne, S.; Marin, L. Swedish pupils' suggested coping strategies if cyberbullied: Differences related to age and gender. *Scand. J. Psychol.* **2014**, *55*, 578–584. [CrossRef] [PubMed]

57. Aricak, T.; Siyahhan, S.; Uzunhasanoglu, A.; Saribeyoglu, S.; Ciplak, S.; Yilmaz, N.; Memmedov, C. Cyberbullying among Turkish Adolescents. *CyberPsychol. Behav.* **2008**, *11*, 253–261. [CrossRef] [PubMed]

58. Huang, Y.; Chou, C. An analysis of multiple factors of cyberbullying among junior high school students in Taiwan. *Comput. Hum. Behav.* **2010**, *26*, 1581–1590. [CrossRef]

59. Price, M.; Dalgleish, J. Cyberbullying Experiences, impacts and coping strategies as described by Australian young people. *Youth Stud. Aust.* **2010**, *29*, 51.

60. Machackova, H.; Dedkova, L.; Mezulanikova, K. Brief report: The bystander effect in cyberbullying incidents. *J. Adolesc.* **2015**, *43*, 96–99. [CrossRef] [PubMed]

61. Gaffney, H.; Farrington, D.P.; Espelage, D.L.; Ttofi, M.M. Are cyberbullying intervention and prevention programs effective? A systematic and meta-analytical review. *Aggress. Viol. Behav.* **2018**. [CrossRef]

62. Cunningham, C.E.; Rimas, H.; Mielko, S.; Mapp, C.; Cunningham, L.; Buchanan, D.; Vaillancourt, T.; Chen, Y.; Deal, K.; Marcus, M. What Limits the Effectiveness of Antibullying Programs? A Thematic Analysis of the Perspective of Teachers. *J. School Viol.* **2016**, *15*, 460–482. [CrossRef]

63. Merrell, K.W.; Gueldner, B.A.; Ross, W.S. How Effective Are School Bullying Intervention Programs? A Meta-Analysis of Intervention Research. *School Psychol. Q.* **2008**, *23*, 26–42. [CrossRef]

64. Wolak, J.; Finkelhor, D.; Walsh, W.; Treitman, L. Sextortion of Minors: Characteristics and Dynamics. *J. Adolesc. Health* **2018**, *62*, 72–79. [CrossRef] [PubMed]

65. Zetterström Dahlqvist, H.; Gillander Gådin, K. Online sexual victimization in youth: Predictors and cross-sectional associations with depressive symptoms. *Eur. J. Public Health* **2018**, *28*, 1018–1023. [CrossRef] [PubMed]

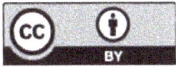

International Journal of
*Environmental Research
and Public Health*

MDPI

Article

Mothers' Difficulties and Expectations for Intervention of Bullying among Young Children in South Korea

Seung-ha Lee * and Hyun-jung Ju

Department of Early Childhood Education, Chung-Ang University, Seoul 06974, Korea; jhj834@gmail.com
* Correspondence: seungha94@cau.ac.kr

Received: 16 January 2019; Accepted: 11 March 2019; Published: 14 March 2019

Abstract: This study investigated the difficulties of mothers in coping with the bullying of their children and their expectations concerning bullying intervention for young children in South Korea. Twenty mothers with young children were interviewed. Interviews were transcribed in Korean. Nvivo 12 software was used to analyze the data. Four themes emerged: "mothers' coping strategies", "problems of interventions", "expectations of interventions", and "developmentally appropriate interventions for young children". Each theme was divided into categories and further into subcategories. Mothers used diverse strategies to intervene when their children were bullied and showed dissatisfaction with the current intervention system. Their expectations for interventions for young children were explained in terms of familial, school, and local/governmental levels. These results emphasized that intervention policies for bullying among young children should be urgently established, and intervention programs need to consider the developmental characteristics of young children.

Keywords: Bullying; intervention; young children; South Korea; hakkyo-pokryuk; prevention

1. Introduction

Bullying is defined as an aggressive behavior that is repeated on a targeted person who has difficulty defending themself [1]. Bullying research has heavily focused on mid-childhood and adolescence; however, studies have shown that bullying clearly exists among young children [2–4]. Characteristics of bullying in early childhood differ from those in middle childhood or adolescence; they are less likely to be repeated on a targeted person, and children are less-likely to perceive an imbalance of power. Additionally, the bullying behavior of young children tends to show low stability, especially in terms of the victim role [4–6]. Due to the different characteristics of bullying in early childhood, researchers have suggested diverse terms such as unjustified aggression [5] or precursory bullying [6]. Kirves and Sajanieme [7] reported that 12.6% of daycare children were directly involved in bullying and even 3-year-old children were able to identify bullying and distinguish bullying from quarrelling.

1.1. Coping Strategies of Young Children

Young children cope with bullying in varied ways. In Monks et al., 4–6-year-old children coped with bullying by most frequently telling an adult, followed by fighting back, getting a friend to help, walking away, crying, and giving something up to the aggressor [5]. Similarly, Reunamo and colleagues interviewed 761 young children about coping strategies in bullying situations [8]. Their results showed that among the children's responses, 70% engaged in participative strategies, that is, doing something to remedy the situation (e.g., telling the teacher, defending oneself, asking to play together, or settling the quarrel, etc.). Sixteen percent showed withdrawal strategies (e.g., going away, telling a teacher or mother, leaving, playing alone, or crying), 6.8% of uncertain strategies (e.g., not knowing what to do, or doing nothing), and 5.1% of dominant strategies (e.g., pushing bullies far away, hitting or teasing back) were shown. Only 1.6% of the children's responses did not care about the bullying (e.g., "I don't care", "I will be in peace"). Therefore, the majority of young children asked for support from adults and some children used ineffective strategies (e.g., fighting back or passive reaction). These results suggest that adults need to play a role in stopping bullying among young children. In other words, young children should be guided to employ appropriate and effective coping strategies by adults.

1.2. Intervention Program for Bullying in Early Childhood

Intervention programs have been developed to prevent bullying among young children [9–11]. These have generally focused on increasing the social emotional competence and assertive skills of children, and training teachers to cope with children's bullying. One of the most well-known programs is the Bernese Prevention Program against Victimization (Be-Prox) developed by Alsaker in Switzerland [9]. It focuses on enhancing teachers' competence in managing bullying among young children. This program increases teachers' sensitivity to bullying, enhances their skills, and helps establish principles for positive peer interactions. Additionally, parental involvement is encouraged during its implementation. Be-Prox has shown positive effects on decreasing bullying [12]. Additionally, the Early Childhood Friendships Project (ECFP) in the U.S.A. [11,13] was designed as a classroom-based program for young children and consists of a series of content for reducing physical and relational bullying and victimization, and increasing prosocial behaviors. Implementation of this program led to significant decreases in bullying and victimization [13].

These programs have generally focused on young children or their teachers. This is critical for intervention since children and teachers are directly involved in the bullying situation in preschool settings. However, many studies have shown that the family environment and parenting practices influence bullying, thus parents and families should be included in the intervention programs [14–19].

1.3. Parental Involvement in Stopping Bullying

Parents can play an important role in reducing bullying because parenting style is related to children's bullying experiences in school, and parents' attention to school bullying is involved with intervention effectiveness [19]. Lereya et al. conducted a meta-analysis of 70 studies about parenting in relation to peer victimization [17]. They showed that being in the role of the bully and the bully/victim were related to negative parenting, whereas positive parenting practices (e.g., communication with children, warmth, affectionate relationships, parental involvement and support, and supervision) were protective against being a bully or a bully/victim.

Additionally, studies have emphasized that parental involvement is an important factor to maximize the effects of intervention programs [20,21]. The parents' understanding of bullying may affect whether they respond effectively and appropriately to their child when they disclose victimization [22]. Parental attention and attitude toward bullying, and information or knowledge of intervention can help children cope with bullying effectively [21,23–25].

Involving parents in children's bullying is important, but parents need appropriate information and training because not all adult mediation and coping strategies are helpful for reducing bullying. Fekkes et al. showed that some children who reported their victimization to adults received help, but some children reported that the situations stayed the same or became worse after reporting these incidents to adults [26]. Additionally, some adults told children to seek revenge, inaction, or ignoring the behavior, however, these strategies are not recommended by research [27].

Parents may recognize children's bullying earlier than the school [21]. They may be aware of their children's different moods and negative emotions. Young children often did not properly report their victimization experiences to their parents because of their limited language abilities, or desire to continue to play with the aggressor. Parents were aware of their children's negative feelings, but often dismissed their children were being victimized [28].

Parents' experiences related to the bullying of their children may impact the strategies they use to intervene. Our previous study indicated that mothers of young children showed different attitudes toward the bullying of their children, depending on whether their children were the aggressor or the victim and whether relations among the mothers were close or not. The mothers of the aggressors or mothers close to the aggressors' mothers tended to be more generous with regard to the situation whereas the victims' mothers or mothers close to the victims' mothers did not [28].

Intervention programs sometimes include parental involvement, however, parents have only been involved to a limited extent [20,29]. Only a few studies on prevention/intervention programs for young children have evaluated their effectiveness, which has been typically measured by school staff or pupils [12,13]. Parents have been rarely involved in evaluating the effects of intervention programs. Thus, it is not known how parents view the effectiveness of bullying prevention/intervention program or policies. Furthermore, the effectiveness of intervention can be seen differently by perspectives. For example, pupils felt that the coping program was not enough to prevent bullying whereas school staff believed that it was adequate [30].

Elucidating parents' opinions may fill gaps concerning the perception of intervention effectiveness. Specifically, by involving parents in this research, differences between theory and practice could be explained, and we might better understand whether parents' views differ from those of the researchers or policymakers. This can allow us to understand if some interventions are seen as ineffective by parents. This study focused on the experiences and expectations of bullying interventions among mothers of young children. Furthermore, this study explored the mothers' perceptions rather than the fathers, since mothers tend to be more deeply engaged in the care of their children than fathers in South Korea [31].

1.4. Bullying Interventions in South Korea

The South Korean government has endeavored to reduce school bullying which can be explained by two mainstreams. The first was the establishment of the "*Hakkyo-pokryuk* (school violence) Prevention and Countermeasure Act" and the second was a national project, *Wee*, which is an integrated system for school safety.

In South Korea, all schools have to follow the *Hakkyo-pokryuk* Prevention and Countermeasure Act, which has many articles within it. Among them, two representative articles are described. First, as a proactive policy, schools must provide education about the prevention of school bullying more than once a semester. Second, as a reactive policy, every school must have a committee to prevent and intervene in cases of school bullying ("the *Hakkyo-pokryuk* intervention committee"). This committee may consist of teachers, psychologists, representative parents, medical doctors, or lawyers. Half of the committee members are to be parents of school children who are elected by other parents. If bullying occurs, a committee meeting is held. The children or parents of the children involved in the situation may also attend if required. The committee members discuss the situation and decide upon a solution for the victim and the aggressor. If the problem cannot be solved within the school, the school can seek mediation from local education authorities. Additionally, a child can report his/her victimization directly to the police over the phone (i.e., call 117, a specialized phone number for helping victims of school bullying) or via the Internet (http://www.safe182.go.kr/index.do). In these cases, the police are involved and they often collaborate with school officials to solve the problem. Therefore, *Hakkyo-pokryuk* can be solved by either the school officials or local police, but is more likely to be solved by school officials.

The *Wee* project can be both a proactive and reactive strategy against bullying. It was launched in 2008 by the government and includes a multi-support service network among schools, educational authorities, and local communities, who collaborate to promote student safety and healthy school lives. They support and counsel students on a variety of difficulties. Bullying is one of the main issues of the *Wee* project.

There are three levels of the *Wee* project: the *Wee* class at the school level, *Wee* center at the local educational authority level, and the *Wee* school at the city or province level. The *Wee* project can also be connected to the *Hakkyo-pokryuk* intervention committee or police, for example, bullies can be sent to the *Wee* class, *Wee* center, or *Wee* school after the decision of the committee or police. Currently in South Korea, 55% of schools have a *Wee* class [32], which is located within the school. This is a place for student counseling. The *Wee* class holds regular office hours, and students can visit to talk about their issues. The *Wee* center belongs to the local educational authorities. When schools cannot solve their students' problems such as bullying, dropping-out, and behavioral or psychological problems, local education authorities intervene. The *Wee* school is a boarding school for high-risk students, which includes psychological treatment, academic education, and special programs for helping adapt for school.

Positive effects of the *Wee* class have been reported. Schools with the *Wee* class had lower bullying and victimization rates compared to those that did not, and this effect was significant among schools that have had the *Wee* class for more than one year [33]. Additionally, schools with a *Wee* class more frequently implemented prevention programs for students when compared to those that did not [34]. However, there is no intervention policy, and no programs for bullying in kindergarten/daycare centers in South Korea. Only elementary-, middle-, and high-school students have been participants in the *Wee* project. Prosocial elements or moral values (i.e., sharing, kindness, cooperation, fairness, etc.) are included in the curriculum in early childhood settings followed by the "Character Education Promotion Act" in South Korea. This includes preventive practices for bullying from a broad perspective, but no specific intervention efforts have addressed bullying among young children.

Lower elementary school students are less likely to be the focus of intervention programs. Moreover, bullying among lower elementary school pupils has rarely been focused on. The South Korean government has investigated the experience of *Hakkyo-pokryuk* for all students from upper elementary school, middle school, and high school students every year, but not among lower elementary school pupils. Thus, it is not known how many children from lower elementary school grades are involved in bullying. Additionally, considering that most young children belong to an educational institution in South Korea [35], there is an urgent need to investigate bullying among young children to establish appropriate interventions.

This study aimed to investigate difficulties, experiences, and expectations of mothers about anti-bullying interventions in early childhood education settings. The aims of this study were to explore: (1) What interventions were used when young children were involved in bullying? (2) What difficulties were experienced while intervening? and (3) What were the mothers' expectations of these interventions?

2. Methods

2.1. Participants

Twenty mothers living in Seoul and Gyeonggi Province in South Korea participated in this study. Snowball sampling was used. Mothers who were familiar with the authors and who had experienced the bullying of their children were interviewed and then asked to make introductions to other mothers with similar experiences. Participants were aged 32–47 years, married, and all had 1–3 children aged 1–16 years (at least one child was aged 3–5 years). Most mothers were college or university graduates (one mother was a high-school graduate).

This study conceptualized early childhood from birth to eight years old [36]. In this age range, children in kindergarten, daycare centers, and lower elementary school level were included. These children were exposed to bullying, but their bullying experiences have hardly been investigated in research.

2.2. Procedure

Semi-structured interviews were conducted. There were 13 individual interviews (M1, M2, M3, M7, M8, M9, M10, M11, M12, M15, M16, M17, and M18) and three focus group interviews; each group consisted of 2–3 mothers (Focus group 1: M4, M5, M6; Focus group 2: M13, 14; Focus group 3: M19, M20). In many cases, individual interviews were conducted, but depending on the mothers' schedules, familiarity with the other mothers, and their wishes, a focus group method was also used. These methods provided fruitful information about the mothers' perceptions of the bullying interventions. The interviewee (second author) did not use specific terms when the interview began. This was intentional because there are several terms used in South Korea corresponding to the term bullying in Western cultures such as *gipdan-ttadolim* (group isolation), *gipdan-goerophim* (group bullying), *hakkyo-pokryuk* (school violence), and *wang-ta* (social exclusion). Each term indicates a slightly different meaning [37]. If the interviewer used a certain term, this may have resulted in biased comments. The terms related to bullying were only used when participants used the term first. Instead, cartoons describing several types of bullying behaviors were shown to the participants, which have been widely used to examine the concept of bullying across cultures [38]. In this study, six cartoons were used, and each cartoon described different types of aggression: physical individual aggression (hitting a smaller person), verbal aggression (saying nasty things), indirect physical aggression (breaking another's ruler), physical group aggression (several children hitting a child), direct/relational aggression (not allowing someone to play with others), and indirect/relational aggression (spreading a rumor). Next, the participants were asked about their thoughts using the following questions:

- Has your child ever experienced (or have you ever heard about) these behaviors? If so, how did you intervene to stop them?
- What difficulties did you have while intervening in the bullying?
- Have you received any informal or formal support to intervene in the bullying of your children? If so, what support was provided? Who or where did you get help? Were they helpful for you to solve the problem?
- Do you have any expectations or wishes for stopping young children's bullying?
- What are needed to stop young children's bullying?
- What types of intervention can be helpful? Who or which institution should provide the intervention?

Interviews took approximately 60–120 min and were held in the participants' homes or at cafés near their homes. After the interviews, each mother was given a gift card equivalent to 18 U.S Dollars as compensation for their participation.

Some patterns were repeated after ten to eleven mothers were interviewed. However, we conducted more interviews as there were still many patterns that newly appeared. The mothers' responses or comments were diverse, depending on the bullying experiences of their children. We finished the data collection at the twentieth mother (sixteenth interview) because we recognized that the data had already reached saturation; the interviews did not add any new patterns, and we judged that plentiful information had been obtained.

2.3. Ethical Issues

Using an exempt self-determination tool of Chung-Ang University, this study did not require IRB approval. The exemption criteria are that a study should not include children or adults who may not be legally, mentally, or cognitively competent to consent. Additionally, a study should not include the sensitive information of individuals (the Personal Information Protection Act 23 in South Korea). Sensitive information includes data that relates to an individual's ideology, political views, health, sexual life, or other information that could seriously damage one's private life. This study did not include any such information.

The purpose and methods of the study were explained to potential participants. The list of interview questions was distributed to the mothers before their participation; therefore, they could decide whether to participate after reading the list. Among the 23 mothers whom the author contacted, three mothers decided not to participate; two had not experienced bullying of their children, and one had scheduling conflicts. After this process, the mothers' written consent was obtained. Most mothers showed open attitudes and talked actively about their experiences. The participants' anonymity was respected by using random labels to identify the mothers. For example, M1 was used to indicate Mother 1. In addition, when the children's names were mentioned, they were only reported as a letter of the alphabet (e.g., A, B, C, and so on).

2.4. Qualitative Analysis

All interviews were recorded and transcribed. Nvivo 12 software (QSR International, Victoria, Australia) was used to analyze the data. The grounded theory of Strauss and Corbin [39] was used for the coding process. First, in open coding, the *concepts* of the sentences were extracted. Based on similarities or commonalities among the concepts, the concepts were combined into higher-order code, called *categories*. During the categorizing, the concepts and quotes coded to the concepts were revisited many times, and their suitability was consistently checked. Next, axial coding to compare and contrast among the categories was conducted. Linkages between the categories were made. Some categories were conceptually lower, and included in other categories; in this case, they were classified into subcategories. Finally, in finding overall concepts, a core category was identified. The categories were broken down, queried, and comprised into a higher construct [40]. The most representative and overall concept, *themes* were labelled. Memos and conceptual ideas arising during the course of analysis were written and used through all procedures of the analysis [41].

Through this process, four themes emerged. The authors independently processed the data coding and then held discussions. If discrepancies emerged among the authors, the data and analysis were revisited, and the authors endeavored to find the underlying meaning of the data. To increase the validity and reliability of the analysis process, an independent researcher participated in the process. This individual reviewed whether the mothers' quotes were coded reliably, and scrutinized the appropriateness of the classification among codes, categories (and subcategories), and themes. Finally, the independent researcher verified whether the analysis represented the phenomena. If disagreements arose, these were further discussed between the researcher and the authors until a consensus was reached.

3. Results

The four themes "mothers' coping strategies", "problems of interventions", "expectations of interventions" and "developmentally appropriate interventions for young children" emerged.

3.1. Theme 1. Mothers' Coping Strategies

Mothers used diverse intervention strategies to cope with their children's bullying/victimization. These were explained by four categories: "direct intervention strategies", "indirect intervention strategies", "no response or do not know", and "deciding to intervene".

3.1.1. Category 1-1. Direct Intervention Strategies

'Direct intervention strategies' means that mothers intervene in the bullying/victimization situation directly by telling a teacher, meeting with the bullies or bullies' mothers, or bringing their child to the counseling center for psychological treatment. Sometimes, these strategies were used together.

"I met the aggressor's mom, I phoned her and asked to meet. I told her that I can't sleep whenever I see my child's wound." (M14).

"It was really severe and frequent. I told a teacher and asked not to be in the same class with my girl and that child (aggressor)." (M20).

"One girl told *F*, 'You weren't in my class, you have come from the other kindergarten, you are not my friend!' So, *F* cried every day and didn't want to go to kindergarten, I went to kindergarten with *F* and stayed at *F*'s side every day." (M6).

"I brought *T* to the counseling center which was run by an NGO, *T* received counseling for three times." (M20).

3.1.2. Category 1-2. Indirect Intervention Strategies

Indirect intervention strategies refer to intervening in the situation through the children. This was the most frequent response reported by mothers. Mothers used active and passive indirect strategies. The subcategories "active-indirect strategies" and "passive-indirect strategies" explained the category.

Subcategory 1-2-1. Active-Indirect Strategies

Mothers explained that children have to do something to reduce the bullying, so they taught their children what to do, or they learned coping strategies to teach their children.

Generally, mothers used positive strategies such as teaching social and emotional skills to their children to react appropriately; these skills related to solving peer-conflict positively, maintaining relationships, increasing empathy, and communication skills.

"I said to *B*, 'Put yourself in the other child's shoes' . . . then *B* told me, 'He (she) would feel bad . . . ' then *B* seems to think that she should not do it next time." (M2).

"I told *P*, 'You approach slowly and say something to her, rather than just look at her without words'." (M16).

Additionally, some mothers wished their children would not exaggerate and tell just as it is.

"I didn't imagine at all that my child did do that, I believed 'My girl is really innocent, naive, and a real child' . . . But I found out that she made up stories when she was in a disadvantageous position... I saw it, so I told her to say as it is . . . If a teacher asks you, just tell only what you see." (M19).

Mothers noted that adults needed to support children to solve problems by themselves rather than directly intervening in their children's relationship problems.

"Adults' intervening should be wise, if we want to intervene, indirect coaching is better. If we do directly intervene in the relationships among children, children's conflict moves to conflicts among parents of the children." (M11).

In some cases, mothers instructed their children to react in the same way to the aggressors (i.e., revenge).

"When *E* was hit for the first time, I said, 'You should hit the child next time. You hit the child as much as you were pained' . . . *E* hit the other child, I asked 'How did you feel?' *E* said, 'It wasn't good'." (M5).

Additionally, mothers learned from other mothers or obtained information through the Internet concerning how to respond to their child's victimization.

"I searched books first, psychological books in the library. I lack parenting skills. I studied how to raise a boy, and watched TV programs related to parenting . . . I searched information through the Internet related to 'a bully' . . . " (M18).

Subcategory 1-2-2. Passive indirect strategies

Sometimes mothers told their children to ignore or avoid the aggressor and play with other children.

"Make other friends first, and get along with [that] child later." (M2).

3.1.3. Category 1-3. No Response or Do Not Know

Some mothers trusted the mother of the other child or did not know how to do. Sometimes they just put up with it.

"I just thought, 'It is children's matter' . . . I trusted her [the aggressor's mother]." (M8).

"I didn't know what to do. I didn't have wisdom, or experiences about this. I didn't know the situation enough. I just have my child's words . . . I didn't know what will happen, what to do... I felt helpless." (M16).

"I don't have any certain answer. I can't say to S, 'You hit as the child did to you' nor 'Just stay and do not hit back' . . . so I told S, 'Ask help from an adult' . . . but the teacher says, 'Do not tattle' . . . There is nothing S can do . . . so I don't have any words for S . . . I am helpless... Do I have to say to S, 'Run away?' it is so sad, very sad . . . I really do not know how to tell S." (M19).

"My boy was hit on his face really seriously in kindergarten. I really wanted to rush to the child and do something to him/her. I have never hit my child. I was sleepless for a week . . . but I thought something more serious like an accident might happen while he grows up so I did not express my negative feelings to him." (M14).

These reactions are important because the mothers' lack of responses did not mean that they did not care about the situation. Rather, it can be interpreted as an "inability" to react although they wanted to act against the victimization of their children. Mothers did not react because they thought that their child may be agitated or made more anxious by their emotional responses. The mothers' rational responses may be appropriate; however, they could have acted by teaching children or seeking help from others.

3.1.4. Category 1-4. Deciding to Intervene

This category describes how mothers used the diverse coping strategies explained above. The subcategories are "understanding the situation correctly" and "discrepancy between mother and father on intervention strategies".

Subcategory 1-4-1. Understanding the Situation Correctly

They emphasized that understanding the situation correctly was most critical and the type of strategy differed in each bullying situation.

Understanding the bullying situation correctly was frequently mentioned; this was important for the mothers before acting or using an intervention.

"I phoned the aggressor's mom, and told the story . . . later, I found that she heard a completely different story from her son. If I didn't know the truth, I would have asked the *Hakkyo-pokryuk* intervention committee." (M19).

Mothers used various strategies such as direct and indirect intervention strategies depending on the bullying situation, and its severity. Additionally, several interventions could be used together.

"At first, I listen to my child's words, and lead my child to understand the other child's mind. 'Why the child did it to you?' If it doesn't get resolved, adults need to help such as teachers, and the other child's mom. Adults need to interfere in the issue . . . If this doesn't work, I will leave the kindergarten or school." (M17).

Subcategory 1-4-2. Discrepancy between Mother and Father on Intervention Strategies

Discrepancies in the desired means of intervention arose between mothers and fathers. The discrepancies influenced mothers to decide on appropriate intervention strategies. Some mothers complained that their husbands did not respond thoughtfully on this matter.

"Fathers often do not think this as serious. They think 'Children are grown up like that.' Mothers are upset. I am really agonized when my child comes home with cry." (M3).

In contrast, some mothers explained the difficulty of dealing with the strong reactions of their husband, so sometimes they told only part of the stories to their husbands because they were afraid that the situation would become much more severe, or difficult to manage.

"I did not tell my husband about the details. Men do not stay silent as do women. They protest vigorously, they check whether the situation is administrative or lawful. That is why teachers are cautious to tell fathers. Men bear in mind and react strongly in a sudden. Mothers care of relationships, but fathers do not . . . I am anxious that he is gone too far." (M10).

M10 mentioned anxiety over the reaction of her husband, but she did not seem to be negative to the active reaction of her husband. The fathers' active reaction seemed to make the mothers relieved, even if it was sometimes an over-reaction. In contrast, the fathers' indifference was problematic for the mothers to manage the matter.

3.2. Theme 2. Problems of Interventions

The theme "problems of interventions" included problems and difficulties with the current intervention policies and programs. Problems were related to the counseling center and school/preschools such as kindergarten, daycare centers, or both. The two categories "counseling center/psychiatry-related" and "school-related" explained this theme.

3.2.1. Category 2-1. Counseling Center/Psychiatry-Related

The mothers used counseling centers, which can be run by the local authorities or government, or run by professionals in child development centers, and visited child-psychiatric clinics. Regarding the counseling centers and psychiatrists, the mothers complained about the difficulty of access. Furthermore, follow-up treatment was not conducted at those centers therefore the effectiveness was only temporary. The four subcategories of "lack of counseling centers", "physical and psychological distance", "high costs", and "temporary effect" explained this category.

Subcategory 2-1-1. Lack of Counseling Centers

"There are few places to get support. There is little information about counseling centers." (M2).

Subcategory 2-1-2. Physical and Psychological Distance

Physical distance to the center made it difficult for the mothers to visit.

"It is far from my home, I hesitated whether I need to bring my child to that far, I asked myself 'Is my child that serious to go that far?'" (M1).

Due to the psychological distance, mothers expected the problem to be solved within the school/kindergarten.

"The Center is a third party, they don't know our children as the kindergarten does, it feels disconnected from us." (M11).

Subcategory 2-1-3. High Costs

High costs were a problem that prevented some mothers from visiting psychiatric clinics. Some mothers hesitated in using these services because of the costs, but some mothers were willing to pay for it as long as the psychology or behavior of their children could be improved:

"I heard that it was 100,000 won [around 89 U.S dollars] per psychiatric counseling session. A friend of mine [aggressor's mom] said 'It is not a waste if my boy could grow up righteously. It is better than being a bad person later.'" (M9).

Subcategory 2-1-4. Temporary Effect

Mothers reported on the effectiveness of counseling or psychiatric treatment. However, the effectiveness was seen as temporary.

"If the treatment of a psychiatrist is effective, the expensive fee is fine, but the effects don't last long... During treatment, the child looks fine, but as time goes by, the effects are fizzled out." (M2)

3.2.2. Category 2-2. School-Related

This category explains the mothers' difficulty or dissatisfaction related to school or preschool intervention. The four subcategories of "lack of knowledge", "stigma", "superficiality", and "teachers' stress" explained the category.

Subcategory 2-2-1. Lack of Knowledge

The lack of knowledge about bullying was frequently explained in terms of class teachers and the organization of the committee members of *Hakkyo-pokryuk*. *Wee* class teachers (who were involved only in counseling pupils at the schools) were professional counsellors; however class teachers were not experts. Teachers in kindergarten or daycare centers were not aware of *Hakkyo-pokryuk* or bullying. Mothers pointed out the problems with members of the committee. Most schools have committee members who are parents and only sometimes have professionals such as lawyers or doctors. This resulted in lack of knowledge of the *Hakkyo-pokryuk* intervention committee.

"The *Hakkyo-pokryuk* intervention committee is not for solving children's problems in school, rather it looks like a place for expression of parents' own opinions." (M16).

"Often the committee members are parents. Thus, some committee members who are parents may be biased to judge the bullying situation." (M14).

Additionally, kindergarten teachers' unskillful intervening techniques for bullying made the situation worse.

"In the kindergarten there was a child who is developmentally advanced. He bullied other children, so teachers suggested sending the child to upper class where one-year older children belonged. The suggestion was formally shown without parental admission. Mothers did not agree of it. Teachers suggested the solution clumsily." (M9).

The untrained teachers and unprofessional members of the *Hakkyo-pokryuk* intervention committee led to many problems and caused parents' emotional distress rather than solving the conflict reasonably.

Subcategory 2-2-2. Stigma

Lack of knowledge about bullying among the school/preschool staff can generate stigma among children who are "trouble-makers". The lack of management of the intervention system may have contributed to the problem.

"L's cousin said that *Wee class* is a kind of threat which is used by teacher. 'If you keep doing like that, you may be sent to *Wee class*' ... The teacher of my child says, 'You can go *Wee class* if anyone needs to, you can talk whatever you want and play there' ... but teachers in other schools say, '*Wee class* children! Come here and follow me', they bring the children to *Wee class*." (M20).

"If *W* and *Y* fights, the committee is held, even if they were 1st graders, but the situation is spread even to fourth and fifth graders, their names, class, etc. .... Then, the aggressor would be fine because other children will not bother or tease him/her. Victim is seen as pitiful to the children. The aggressor is stigmatized as a bad child among mothers in the committee." (M14).

Subcategory 2-2-3. Superficiality

Mothers reported that the intervention system was superficial because it did not correct bad behavior nor did it address the children's motive for bullying.

"I don't think it is a good idea to make children apologize to each other in public, I have never seen them do it sincerely." (M17).

"A policeman comes up in the *Hakkyo-pokryuk* intervention committee and greets mothers, but I do not trust him/her at all. It is like a 'performance', to show someone. I don't want it. Rather, they should approach children friendly 'Hey, I am here, whenever you feel afraid, call me' ... " (M14).

"It does not grasp problems, each child (victim or aggressor) has his/her inside. It does not analyze nor lead children to reconciliation. It neither teach nor guide children. Rather it does 'this is your fault,' 'this is teacher's fault.' Children's victimization is problem, but also parents who do behave like that (in the committee) are problem." (M16).

Mothers distrusted the solutions such as forcing apologies between the children or just judging the children's fault without being aware of their minds. It is doubtful whether adults have a strong will to solve children's problems. Alternatively, adults in the committee might not know appropriate, efficient, and helpful ways to assist the children. Particularly, the procedure of the committee was problematic, and this may come from a lack of knowledge about bullying among the committee members.

Subcategory 2-2-4. Teachers' Stress

Although mothers complained of the teachers' lack of knowledge to cope with bullying, they also appreciated the level of stress that teachers experience may distract their attention from bullying and interrupt the development of coping skills for bullying. Teachers experienced a lack of support in the workplace as well as stress due to their interactions with parents.

"Teachers got hurt from parents. I have heard that teachers cry. Teachers in daycare centers do not have break time, they do not have annual leave, they cannot manage the work related to bank because banks close at 4 pm. If they confront mothers on the way to the bank, that can be gossip among mothers. So I have heard that they disguised when they need to go out." (M9).

"My friend is a school teacher. When the committee of *hakkyo-pokryuk* was held, the parents assaulted her, she was so stressful that she got herpes zoster. The day after, the parents apologized her. What is that! Humiliating a teacher in front of other parents and saying sorry next day." (M16).

3.3. Theme 3. Expectations of Intervention

The mothers' expectations of interventions comprised three levels: the categories "family level", "school level", and "local authorities/government level" explained the mothers' expectations. In addition, "pessimistic for prevention/intervention" was indicated.

3.3.1. Category 3-1. Family Level

Mothers emphasized an affectionate home environment and its role in children's character development. Four subcategories of "parental responsibility", "affection and attention", "character and moral education", and "self-reliance" explained the category.

Subcategory 3-1-1. Parental Responsibility

Mothers should be careful about the behavior of their children; and should not overreact about their children's victimization.

"Parents are better not to be sensitive. If they are, children would keep reflecting it. I expect my child is not a sensitive soul." (M17).

Early discovery of a child's problem is the responsibility of their parents.

"Mothers should find a child's problem such as anxiety or violent characteristics as early as possible, she may bring the child to a psychological therapist." (M4).

Subcategory 3-1-2. Affection and Attention

Parents' affection and attention concerning children's daily lives are fundamental.

"Parents must care for children. They have to pay attention to their children, always ... They have to ask themselves 'Is my child doing well in school?' ... Mothers' role is most important until a child grows up as a member of society. I am keen to my child and support him/her." (M12).

However, one mother reported that "ignorance is bliss". She was afraid of being neurotic if she knew all of the details about the story. M9 seemed to avoid the situation and was distressed about her child being bullied.

"Sometimes, if mothers do not know, children can have opportunity to make relationships with others, then they can solve the problem by themselves. If I hear the story from other mothers, I am inquisitive and ask my child to check, 'How was that child today?' ... If I know something, which can make me anxious. I hope I do not know and my child does well." (M9).

Subcategory 3-1-3. Character and Moral Education

Mothers emphasized character and moral education at home. This can be achieved by increasing the ability of children to empathize. Conflicts among young children occur over very trivial things, therefore adults need to teach children the means to obtain what they want without damaging relationships or others' emotions.

"Actually, in kindergartens, children want to have toys which others have. Then they can fight ... I says to *P*, 'A friend may want the toy you want ... you should not take out what others have. You should get along with others. You have to acknowledge what others want' ... The other day, *P* pushed another child ... I keep saying 'That is wrong and bad behavior' until *P* understands." (M16)

Additionally, character education should be specific rather than the rote learning of 'good things'.

"Preventive strategies are too wide to inform them one by one ... They should go with character education ... Just simply saying, 'You should not play with *X*' is not specific because my child can be both aggressor or victim. So, character education is fundamental to prevent these behaviors... I teach my child proper behaviors." (M12).

Subcategory 3-1-4. Self-Reliance

Mothers highlighted children's self-reliance; they must learn coping skills against bullying, because it could happen throughout their lives.

"I will teach *G* to have autonomy, and self-reliance. *G* should express himself/herself, like 'You must not do that to me' ... Mothers cannot solve everything though they can help ... A child should stand up to the aggressor." (M7).

3.3.2. Category 3-2. School Level

At the school level, teachers were the most important in terms of preventing bullying. In addition, a change of curriculum was suggested. The category was explained in terms of the five subcategories: "teachers' role", "increasing number of teachers, *Wee* class teachers, and counsellors", "collaboration among mothers, teachers, and psychiatrists/counsellors", "providing more opportunity for plays and physical activities", and "social education programs".

Subcategory 3-2-1. Teachers' Role

There were many comments about the importance of teachers. Mothers mostly emphasized that teachers were very influential, especially for young children.

"Teachers' intervening is most effective because parents' and teachers' words are influential for young children." (M17).

"The best solution among several strategies I tried was to ask the teacher. It was definite and the firmest solution because the teacher acknowledged the situation very accurately." (M16).

Subcategory 3-2-2. Increasing Number of Teachers, Wee Class Teachers, and Counsellors

Mothers understood the teachers' difficulty in caring for many children in one class and they felt children would have more opportunities for counseling if the teacher–child ratio decreased.

"More teachers are needed ... If the ratio of teacher-child is low, teachers would take care of children better." (M15).

"Teacher-Assistants are necessary. If a child wants to go to the nursing room, there needs to be someone who brings the child there. Also, the TA could check whether a child really goes to the nursing room, or goes to play around." (M19).

"One counselor in one school is really lacking, it doesn't make sense." (M10).

The number of professionals should be increased within educational institutions to make it easier to take care of children and supervise bullying.

Subcategory 3-2-3. Collaboration among Mothers, Teachers, and Psychologists/Counsellors

Mothers, teachers, psychiatrists/counsellors can support each other as they each have a unique role:

"If a teacher mediates well between mothers, the victim's mother could understand the situation, but if the teacher leaves mothers to meet and talk by themselves, the mothers couldn't solve it. They are just on their children's sides. They may be emotional . . . Teachers could be in between aggressor's and victim's mothers. Teachers balance the situation, but mothers believe their children's words." (M20).

"A school nurse is dispatched in every school, similarly, psychological counselors may join in the incident and do what kindergarten teachers cannot do. They can work together." (M8).

Subcategory 3-2-4. Providing More Opportunity for Plays and Physical Activities

Mothers expected a diminishing number of academic classes and an increase in more free play with peers, which can help with the children's social and emotional development.

"I want group play more, not individual play in kindergarten." (M9).

"I wish elementary school curriculum focused on morality or diversity rather than on study. *G* learns English three times per week in the daycare center, but I think playing is better than that . . . playing, running . . . " (M7).

Subcategory 3-2-5. Social Education Programs

A social education program needs to be accentuated from early childhood.

"I think making relationships is necessary for children. They have to develop their competence for it. School needs to teach this. People all have different characteristics, so children should learn about that and respect it." (M5).

"Children have to know the possible consequences which can be caused by certain behavior. The program related to *Hakkyo-pokryuk* show this. Why not kindergarten?" (M12).

Most mothers suggested various ways to resolve conflicts through social education rather than punishing strategies. There was one mother who mentioned her experience that the intervention strategies could differ among mothers.

"Some mothers insisted punishment whereas some mothers said that it was too harsh. Some react strongly, other mothers step back. I have heard that there were more mothers who wanted to leave the issue to the school." (M2).

3.3.3. Category 3-3. Local Authorities and Government Level

Mothers' expectations of local authorities or the government covered a wide range of interventions. This was explained by the three subcategories of "establishing counseling places", "improving the sense of community", and "systematic and sustainable public interventions".

Subcategory 3-3-1. Establishing Counseling Places

Mothers expected places where they could talk about their difficulties related to their children within the preschool or their local areas.

"If a child is victimized, centers which manage parents' stress and difficulty would be helpful. They can tell us other cases, then we may feel, 'Oh this is not only my issue, other people also have similar difficulty . . . Then sometimes we can find a solution by ourselves." (M10).

Subcategory 3-3-2. Improving the Sense of Community

Parents needed to consider other families' perspectives. Parents' selfishness made the situation worse.

"Parents generally think 'My child does well, why did the other child do that?' This may elicit an aggressive attitude toward others. My child can be wrong. It is better not to think only from my child's perspective." (M16).

Parents needed to communicate and understand each other during parent meetings.

"Mothers are looking for a breakthrough. It is not for just a simple chat, it should be more educational to see things positively and change their thinking . . . That kind of meeting is needed." (M18).

Peaceful and relaxing local places would be helpful for families' happiness or harmony; families can refresh and relieve their stress by visiting places such as parks, gardens, and playgrounds, which may provide opportunities to communicate between family members and increase a sense of belonging to the local community.

"A new playground in a forest near my block was built, and family gardening was open. We played there many times. Providing something to local people is better than receiving a superficial message like 'report to police' from the local office. I and husband shared our thoughts with our children." (M9).

Subcategory 3-3-3. Systematic and Sustainable Public Interventions

Mothers required that collaboration among home, school, and government levels of care should be systematized. A coping manual for bullying was necessary.

"I think there must be a manual in educational institution such as stage 1, stage 2, etc. So, teachers can follow the manual if an accident happens. For example, stage 1. Calling parents, stage 2. something, and stage 3 . . . " (M4).

All interventions should be consistent and sustainable.

"I guess there must be education related to this in public institutions. Daycare centers can search and use those educational programs, even once a semester or once a month. Fire alarm safety training is regularly done though it hardly happens actually. But, there are very few social education things like emotional education, and peer relationships, though these things happen in everyday life." (M11).

"I expect that teachers might tell children about this matter regularly." (M20).

"From early childhood including low grade in elementary school we should have our eyes on *goerophim* . . . Caring and educating children only at home is not enough, schools and home have to counter this issue together . . . I hope the local community helps much more . . . I wish there were many home related activities such as visiting a home regularly, family connected program, or encouraging fathers' participation on parenting . . . These things finally decrease *goerophim* because the family becomes happy." (M3).

3.3.4. Category 3-4. Pessimistic for Prevention/Intervention

Some mothers showed pessimistic attitudes toward the intervention or prevention efforts. They thought that bullying could happen anywhere, and that bullies always exist unless all families are affective and all parents provide warm parenting, which does not actually exist. They felt that institutions could not solve the fundamental causes of bullying.

"If my child is victimized, it cannot be solved by the support from kindergarten or school... I would invite the aggressor, be nice him/her, ask 'what do you like?' and then at later 'how do you think about my child?' An opportunity is needed to solve the problem at first stage but these cannot be done by teachers or school staff." (M8).

"Is prevention possible? I think it is not, because home atmosphere or parenting style may affect children's behavior in schools. So, to prevent bullying, changing family or parents is essential but this is almost impossible ... These children exist wherever, and whenever. However, interventions to stop bullying are necessary. Counseling centers or supporting places should be located within the institution." (M1).

The mothers were doubtful and pessimistic about preventing bullying. However, they had their own ideas about how to solve the problem such as inviting the aggressor or establishing support centers. M8 was opposed to support from institutions whereas M1 believed it was necessary to stop bullying.

3.4. Theme 4. Developmentally Appropriate Intervention for Young Children

Mothers strongly suggested the need for a program that included contents of young children's social-emotional, and psychological developmental status. These were described by the three categories "using various resources", "consideration of concepts and terms", and 'ways of expression and language ability".

3.4.1. Category 4-1. Using Various Resources: Real Objects, Materials, Videos, Puppets, Storytelling

Mothers explained that social skills were essential for children. To increase the children's social skills, various materials were suggested such as videos, puppets, and storytelling using hypothetical situations.

"I am not sure whether the videos exist ... those show peer relationships among young children ... Social relationships programs are necessary ... The materials could be used both at home or in kindergarten. Teachers or mothers are able to educate with the materials- fairy tales, or video, dramas ... " (M11).

"Use like a role play, or storytelling, puppets. Children could tell their experiences related to the story which the teacher tells." (M20).

Making and showing educational videos for young children was most commonly mentioned by mothers. The videos should show situations that children may experience in their daily lives, thus explaining what bullying is and how to cope with it.

"The program should specify children's peer conflict situation. Just saying 'hitting is bad' is not enough ... Using examples of the situation would be helpful." (M5).

3.4.2. Category 4-2. Consideration of Concepts and Terms

As the young children's concept of *Hakkyo-pokryuk* was unclear, it was unsuitable for them to be educated using the term.

"I have heard that one child reported 'He/she was hit' to the police. He/she could have told this to his/her teacher. He/she did not consider its severity and just directly phoned to police, the problem became very big." (M6).

"Young children do not know what *Hakkyo-pokryuk* is, but, they use the term even if a friend teases them a little. So, the term is regarded as not serious to them." (M19).

"The first grade in elementary school looks like an extension of kindergarten. The first graders are very similar to kindergarteners ... The term *Hakkyo-pokryuk* has strong nuance to young children." (M20).

Acknowledging the severity of aggressive behavior is an important issue because it affects judging whether it is bullying, and whether it needs to be reported to the police. Young children seem to have difficulty in distinguishing *Hakkyo-pokryuk* from other aggressive behavior such as fights.

This is why various materials should be used to help young children in their understanding of bullying.

3.4.3. Category 4-3. Ways of Expression and Language Ability

As young children are not fully able to express their experiences with language, other ways to express their emotions and experiences should be considered.

"Children in lower grades in elementary school have difficulty with counseling because they are clumsy when expressing themselves. Art therapy or psychological therapy would be better for them, once or twice a month. A program that lets us know children's inside may be helpful. There is nothing." (M2).

As both a proactive and reactive strategy, understanding children's psychology is important, especially among young children whose language is restricted. This is also why the *Hakkyo-pokryuk* intervention committee may be not appropriate for lower grades in elementary school pupils as the committee sometimes requires the children to explain the situation.

4. Discussion

This study investigated mothers' experiences and expectations concerning bullying interventions among young children. Mothers used their own coping strategies, which had not been learned in public or systematically. They intervened in their children's bullying either directly or indirectly. The coping strategies mothers used in order to intervene in their children's bullying were sometimes effective and sometimes ineffective. The most problematic issue was having 'no information' about bullying and intervention programs for young children. At the elementary school level, mothers were anxious regarding less specialized teachers on *Hakkyo-pokryuk*. This may lead to children being stigmatized and may mistrust intervention systems. In kindergarten/daycare centers, the lack of places for counseling and lack of knowledge about bullying amongst the teachers were the main problems. Mothers showed their expectations with regard to intervention for young children from multi-contexts (i.e., family, school, and local/governmental level). These results provide many academic and political implications for the intervention of bullying among children.

4.1. Mothers' Intervention Strategies

The mothers predominantly used indirect intervention strategies such as teaching children social skills, assertiveness, or appropriate behavior. They sometimes used direct strategies by asking teachers for help or contacting the aggressor's mother. These strategies could be used together depending on the severity or repetition of the situation.

Mothers felt responsible for solving their children's bullying/victimization problems, but they often felt helpless because they felt unprepared to solve these problems. Mothers who did not respond to their children's bullying did not mean to convey that they did not care; rather, these mothers did not know what to do. This implies that institutional interventions should actively support mothers. Moreover, the mothers' strategies were made at a personal level, and not at an institutional or public level. There are no public manuals to inform mothers, and few places for mothers to visit for support. As Axford et al. [10] explained, successful intervention at the individual level is difficult to achieve and is more likely to be reactive than proactive.

4.2. Disappointment with the Intervention

Mothers pointed out the lack of a system or facilities that could offer them help. At the preschool level, this was more problematic because the mothers of children in kindergarten/daycare centers relied on teachers or counseling centers/psychiatric clinics. There was no formal network or system to solve these problems at the preschool level. Counseling centers or psychiatric clinics were not easy to access due to high costs, psychological distance as well as physical distance. Additionally, mothers felt that the intervention effects were temporary. The temporary effects may have resulted because the intervention strategies used by the mothers were disconnected; discussing the problem with the teacher and visiting counseling centers operated independently, although there is a need for them to work together to boost effectiveness.

Lack of knowledge about bullying among teachers was consistently noted as a main problem with the interventions. Kindergarten/daycare centers tried to mediate bullying among children, but the teachers were typically unaware of the instructions and had not been educated on how to teach children appropriate coping strategies when bullying occurred. At the elementary school level, a lack of knowledge about bullying among teachers was part of the incompetent management of the *Hakkyo-pokryuk* intervention committee and *Wee* class. Moreover, many parents serving on the committee did not have specialized knowledge about bullying, therefore their decisions were not considered credible to other mothers. The incompetence of teachers or school staff may lead to the stigmatization of children involved in the incidents, which may negatively affect the children's willingness to participate in the intervention programs.

Developmental consideration for younger groups was shown. Lower grade students in elementary school were often excluded from the intervention program. Their bullying behavior was sometimes managed by teachers or parents and was sometimes dealt with by the *Hakkyo-pokryuk* intervention committee. However, the committee does not seem to be appropriate for young children since it was designed for older children.

4.3. Mothers' Expectations for Intervention

Mothers expressed their many expectations related to the intervention policy and programs for bullying. These were explained in terms of the family, school, and at the local authorities/governmental level, which is consistent with developmental ecological perspectives [16]. In bullying, individual and contextual factors are interrelated from a proximal system (children's parents, friends, etc.) to a broader context such as cultural norms and beliefs. Therefore, for a prevention program, multi-level contextual factors should be considered [16,42,43].

According to the mothers we interviewed, the most fundamental prevention method was within the family, particularly that of parental affection and character education, which has been stressed in previous studies [17]. Affectionate parenting styles allow children to talk freely to their parents about their difficulties, which provides them with chances to learn coping skills to prevent further victimization [42,44]. Additionally, regular communication between children, teachers, and parents is important to prevent and intervene in bullying as 25% of bullied children do not tell adults, which may exacerbate victimization [26].

For young children, self-reliance was emphasized as they may confront similar or more severe bullying situations as they grow older. This is similar to teaching assertiveness to young children as an important strategy [45,46]. Mothers expected that the problem would be solved within the preschool as the preschool staff know their children well. This reflects that training for teachers about bullying is necessary, which has been emphasized in many studies [47,48].

The most reliable intervention mentioned by the mothers was the teachers' competence. Mothers seemed to rely on the teachers' competence to solve the problem as a mediator. For mothers, teachers are physically and psychologically closer to their children than counselors or psychiatrists. Training teachers in preschool is effective in sustaining the effectiveness of the intervention because teachers consistently care for children at least for one year whereas counsellors are connected only for a short time.

Therefore, a systematic manual should be established, which means developing a protocol specifying the process or stages about how teachers or parents can respond when bullying takes place. For example, at Stage 1, teachers should pay attention to the situation and the children's words. In Stage 2, teachers should decide what kind of intervention is appropriate for the situation. For example, the model for conflict mediation suggested by Kostelnik et al. [49] might be useful (i.e., initiate the mediation process → clarify each child's perspective → sum up, generate alternatives → agree on solution → reinforce the problem-solving process → follow through). Teachers should also determine whether the children should be separated (if they are harming each other), and whether parents should be told. In Stage 3, if these efforts fail, teachers can be connected to specialized institutions or counseling centers. For this, a local network between schools/preschools and counseling centers/child psychiatrists needs to be created, and access must be easy and welcoming for mothers.

More professionals should be included in the *Hakkyo-pokryuk* committee, and the government should strictly control these criteria. Alternatively, a third party such as the local authorities should intervene when necessary. This may lead mothers to view interventions as more authoritative and effective. Smith also suggested considering the balance between school policy and action centrally [48] (p. 421).

The superficiality of the intervention program was pointed out. To prevent further bullying, it is fundamental to find out the reason for the bullying behavior and the course of the incident rather than judging fault. Furthermore, bullying and victimization are often related among young children [3,4,50]. Similarly, many mothers in this study viewed the young aggressor as a possible victim of negative parenting or a deprived home environment. One mother in this study reported her experience about some mothers insisting on punishing the aggressor. However, most mothers of young children in this study were less likely to blame children involved in the bullying. Rather, they considered that the parents of aggressive children should be changed and suggested that social support was needed for good parenting skills and a positive family atmosphere to the change home environment.

This corresponds to the theory of the restorative approach. The basic assumption of the restorative approach is to resolve conflict, compensate hurt, and rebuild good relationships rather than blaming bullies. Bullies acknowledge the consequences of their behavior, empathize with the victim's emotions, and compensate for the victim's pain [51]. Intervention programs using a restorative approach have been shown to be effective [52].

One mother said, "Children are still young. Deciding who are bullies and victims is adults' judgment. Asking them to reenact the situation is not appropriate. It is caused by adults' emotion (who are upset for the situation). Children are not that mature yet." (M14). This implies that intervention policies should be based on the children's perspectives. Adults develop intervention systems. They wish to clarify and solve the incident through many formal processes and system; how distinguish aggressor from victim, and how make them take responsibility of their behavior, which is retribution justice [51,53]. It is important to prevent bullying by viewing bullying from the children's perspective, which is very important, especially for younger children.

Few studies have suggested a restorative approach for young children's bullying, however, it is not clear how it could be applied in young children's bullying intervention. For example, circle time could be considered where a teacher can discuss the issue to elicit a solution with a whole class.

Social and moral education were emphasized. This is not new as it has been consistently and widely included in bullying prevention programs [54]. In particular, the home is a vital place for shaping one's character, personality, and school is an optimal place for practicing social skills with diverse individuals. This implies that the cooperation of families and schools are necessary, therefore, intervention program for families should be developed.

In South Korea, social and character education have predominantly been achieved through informal curriculum (i.e., latent curriculum) in schools/preschools rather than through special courses or academic subjects. However, social and moral education need to be arranged in formal education so that they can be emphasized consistently on a regular basis. Through social education at school, children may practice and develop their social skills with many peers. Since young children's language abilities, emotional competence, and social skills are still developing, schools or preschools need to teach them to develop and practice their skills and abilities, thus young children are able to solve their conflicts more peacefully and in socially acceptable ways. For example, SEL (Social and Emotional Learning) programs are widely used to develop emotional ability and decrease behavioral problems [55]. SEL has been developed as a school-based program from kindergarten to high school and it has been shown to be effective for students' social and emotional well-being [54].

The effectiveness of SEL has been shown for reducing aggression though the program is not directly related to bullying behavior [56,57].

Increasing the number of counseling centers for parents and children is required. There are no specific programs for bullying prevention/intervention. At the preschool level, an establishment corresponding to the *Wee* class is needed, which could be located within the preschool or within the larger community.

There has been much debate on the effectiveness of "bullying-focused" solutions, or more general solutions based on relationships and school climate and improving 'conviencia' (in Spanish, implies respect and co-existence) [51] (p. 327). Current intervention systems in South Korea (i.e., the *Hakkyo-pokryuk* intervention committee, *Wee* class) are closer to a "bullying-focused" solution. Moreover, these do not seem to function effectively unless the school staff are trained. Social and character education needs to be formalized to maintain its sustainability, whereas the procedure in the *Hakkyo-pokryuk* intervention committee is superficial and lacks substantive content, so the proactive system should be fortified. Young children's developmental characteristics do not fit into the bullying-focused system, and they have difficulties in controlling their desires and behaviors without appropriate social and moral knowledge and guidance. This study indicates that the focus of intervention for young children should be shifted from a reactive to proactive means.

4.4. Suggestions for Intervention for Young Children

(1) Family-based intervention program

Family-based intervention programs are crucial. Most mothers have difficulties in coping with bullying situations. The program should include general proactive to specific reactive solutions; knowledge about effective parenting styles, character/moral education, and coping manuals for bullying.

Generally in South Korea, schools/preschools regularly distribute a newsletter to parents, which covers a wide range of issues in schools/preschools; however, this is not sufficient for preventing bullying. More active programs or school policy are required (e.g., parent meetings and education about bullying). The FSFF (Friendly Schools Friendly Families) could be a good example [58] as it focuses on parents' attitudes, knowledge, and their self-efficacy to help children with bullying. Its effectiveness was maximized when high-intensity intervention was made at the whole-school level and family level [59]. Increasing parents' awareness of bullying was performed through diverse ways such as newsletters, booklets, songs, referral information, parent workshops, parent–child communication sheets, and class–home activities [59]. These activities may be useful for developing bullying interventions for parents.

Additionally, Butler and Platt developed a structured family therapy model to help by incorporating the families, teachers, and therapists. School counselors and teachers are part of the family therapy, and therapists are connected to the school directly during treatment. In this family based intervention program, the collaboration between professionals and parents is strongly emphasized [29]. Local authorities or government could help to establish the network between professionals, teachers, and parents, and they could also offer these programs to the local communities.

(2) Establishing intervention policy and program for young children

Increasing the teachers' specialization is an urgent issue as they require professional knowledge regarding bullying. Policies regarding the bullying of young children as well as for teachers are required. In South Korea, pre-service teachers in university or college must complete a course about school bullying prevention and intervention in university or college. Pre-service teachers in early childhood also take this course, but they learn about bullying at higher levels and do not learn about bullying in preschool. Thus, anti-bullying training in early childhood education should be separately established. Furthermore, for in-service teachers in preschools, education about bullying should be implemented on a regular basis.

Intervention programs should distinguish the lower grade students from those in the upper grades in elementary school. Although both of these grades attend elementary school, however, the developmental characteristics of the lower grade students are partly overlapped by those of the kindergarteners. Their behavior could include a wide spectrum from light conflict to severe violence. There also needs to be an academic consensus about the term for bullying among young children in South Korea.

Intervention policies and programs should reflect a non-punitive approach (i.e., a restorative approach) and include knowledge and skills to understand their motives for bullying, and their developmental and psychological status. Further studies are necessary to develop this.

(3) Governmental support for prevention

Many findings noted in this study require government support and public awareness; interventions may involve increasing counseling centers, teachers, and supervisors, awakening people's attention regarding the issue, and developing intervention program for teachers, parents, and children. Social support should help families and create a friendly and generous atmosphere among the parents. Prevention and intervention regarding bullying is an issue to be addressed by the whole community. Fortifying interventions does not necessarily lead to a reduction in bullying incidents. Proactive strategies may be the best solution for reducing bullying. The number of preventive services should be increased. Social emotional, or moral education are not optional, but necessary. Additionally, this should be arranged as part of the formal curriculum, meaning that preventive education will be provided on a regular basis. As Smith indicated, whatever the intervention policy, sanctions, and actions, the anti-bullying action should be effective, and for effectiveness, sustainability is truly essential [48].

5. Limitations

There are limitations in this study. First, the teachers' perspectives were not included, which may be helpful for understanding why some teachers were considered incompetent by the interviewed mothers. Comparisons of the perceptions between teachers and mothers could also be useful to develop training programs for parents and teachers. Further study is needed to clarify how teachers perceive situations of young children's bullying.

Second, the results should be carefully considered for generalization because this study was conducted with a limited sample and within a limited cultural context. This study did not investigate the fathers' perceptions. Future research is required to understand the father's perspectives and influences. Additionally, many participants in this study were relatively highly educated (college or higher). Although this was not intended by the authors, this may partly be caused by snowball sampling; the mothers introduced other mothers that they knew. This might have increased the similarity among the participants. Moreover, it is not clear whether the mothers' dissatisfaction and difficulties in this study can be found in other cultures. Therefore, a cross-cultural study would be useful for investigating whether the findings are similar in other cultures.

Third, cyberbullying among young children was not included in this study. Most children aged four to eight years old have the Internet access at home and the majority of them use computers for writing letters or chatting in The Netherlands [60]. In South Korea, 51% of children under nine years old have their own mobile phone and 85% of children under nine years of age used a smartphone or computer with access to the Internet [61].

Research on the parental awareness of young children's cyberbullying is particularly important as cyberbullying can occur over smartphones, so the parents' role in closely monitoring their children's use of technology is important [62]. Therefore, investigating the parental perception of use of technology or cyberbullying by young children is anticipated.

6. Conclusions

Acts and laws directly reflecting school bullying and prevention/intervention systems at a national level have been established in South Korea. However, the balance between the public intervention system and school ownership for dealing with bullying incidents should be considered. Systematic and public support is necessary, and long-term interventions are needed. Smith highlighted that continuing pressure on schools and policy makers is necessary to reduce bullying. Otherwise, other priorities than reducing bullying may be present, and some pressure could come from parents [48] (p. 422).

This study showed the importance of parental involvement through their voices, and emphasized the collaboration between homes, schools, and society. Additionally, it proposed a direction of intervention for young children's bullying. Finally, it may provide information for cultures with similar circumstances to that in South Korea where bullying interventions for young children have not been researched thoroughly.

Author Contributions: Conceptualization, H-j.J.; Data curation, S-h.L and H-j.J.; Formal analysis, S-h.L and H-j.J.; Investigation: H-j.J.; Methodology, S-h.L; Resources, S-h.L.; Writing original draft: S-h.L.; Writing—review & editing: S-h.L and H-j.J.

Funding: This research received no external funding.

Conflicts of Interest: The authors declare no conflict of interest.

References

1. Olweus, D. *Bullying at School: What We Know and What We Can Do*; Blackwell Publishing Ltd.: Oxford, UK, 1993; ISBN 978-0631192411.
2. Kochenderfer-Ladd, B. Identification of Aggressive and Asocial Victims and the Stability of Their Peer Victimization. *Merrill-Palmer Q.* **2003**, *49*, 410–425. [CrossRef]
3. Lee, S.H.; Smith, P.K.; Monks, C.P. Participant roles in peer-victimization among young children in South Korea: Peer-, self-, and teacher-nominations. *Aggress. Behav.* **2016**, *42*, 287–298. [CrossRef] [PubMed]
4. Monks, C.P.; Smith, P.K.; Swettenham, J. Aggressors, victims, and defenders in preschool: Peer, self-, and teacher reports. *Merrill-Palmer Q.* **2003**, *49*, 453–469. [CrossRef]
5. Monks, C.; Ortega Ruiz, R.; Torrado Val, E. Unjustified aggression in preschool. *Aggress. Behav. Off. J. Int. Soc. Res. Aggress.* **2002**, *28*, 458–476. [CrossRef]
6. Levine, E.; Tamburrino, M. Bullying among young children: Strategies for prevention. *Early Child. Educ. J.* **2014**, *42*, 271–278. [CrossRef]
7. Kirves, L.; Sajaniemi, N. Bullying in early educational settings. *Early Child Dev. Care* **2012**, *182*, 383–400. [CrossRef]
8. Reunamo, J.; Kalliomaa, M.; Repo, L.; Salminen, E.; Lee, H.; Wang, L. Children's strategies in addressing bullying situations in day care and preschool. *Early Child Dev. Care* **2015**, *185*, 952–967. [CrossRef]
9. Alsaker, F.D. Bernese programme against victimisation in kindergarten and elementary school. In *Bullying in Schools: How Successful Can Interventions Be?* Smith, P.K., Pepler, D., Rigby, K., Eds.; Cambridge University Press: Cambridge, UK, 2004; pp. 289–306. ISBN 978-0-521-53803-0.
10. Committee for Children. Second Step: Social-Emotional Skills for Early Learning. 2014. Available online: http://www.secondstep.org/Portals/0/EL/Research/EL_Review_Research.pdf (accessed on 10 January 2019).
11. Ostrov, J.M.; Massetti, G.M.; Stauffacher, K.; Godleski, S.A.; Hart, K.C.; Karch, K.M.; Mullins, A.D.; Ries, E.E. An intervention for relational and physical aggression in early childhood: A preliminary study. *Early Child. Res. Q.* **2009**, *24*, 15–28. [CrossRef]
12. Alsaker, F.D.; Valkanover, S. Early diagnosis and prevention of victimization in kindergarten. In *Peer Harassment in School: The Plight of the Vulnerable and Victimized*; Juvonen, J., Graham, S., Eds.; Guilford: London, UK, 2001; pp. 175–195. ISBN 1-57230-627-0.
13. Ostrov, J.M.; Godleski, S.A.; Kamper-DeMarco, K.E.; Blakely-McClure, S.J.; Celenza, L. Replication and extension of the early childhood friendship project: Effects on physical and relational bullying. *Sch. Psychol. Rev.* **2015**, *44*, 445–463. [CrossRef]

14. Gómez-Ortiz, O.; Romera, E.M.; Ortega-Ruiz, R. Parenting styles and bullying. The mediating role of parental psychological aggression and physical punishment. *Child Abus. Negl.* **2016**, *51*, 132–143. [CrossRef] [PubMed]

15. Holt, M.K.; Kaufman Kantor, G.; Finkelhor, D. Parent/child concordance about bullying involvement and family characteristics related to bullying and peer victimization. *J. Sch. Violence* **2008**, *8*, 42–63. [CrossRef]

16. Hong, J.; Espelage, D.L. A review of research on bullying and peer victimization in school: An ecological system analysis. *Aggress. Violent Behav.* **2012**, *17*, 311–322. [CrossRef]

17. Lereya, S.T.; Samara, M.; Wolke, D.D. Parenting behavior and the risk of becoming a victim and a bully/victim: A meta-analysis study. *Child Abus. Negl.* **2013**, *37*, 1091–1108. [CrossRef]

18. Nocentini, A.; Fiorentini, G.; Di Paola, L.; Menesini, E. Parents, family characteristics and bullying behavior: A systematic review. *Aggress. Violent Behav.* **2018**. [CrossRef]

19. Axford, N.; Farrington, D.P.; Clarkson, S.; Bjornstad, G.J.; Wrigley, Z.; Hutchings, J. Involving parents in school-based programmes to prevent and reduce bullying: What effect does it have? *J. Child. Serv.* **2015**, *10*, 242–251. [CrossRef]

20. Ahmed, E.; Braithwaite, V. Bullying and victimization: Cause for concern for both families and schools. *Soc. Psychol. Educ.* **2004**, *7*, 35–54. [CrossRef]

21. Eslea, M.; Smith, P.K. The long-term effectiveness of anti-bullying work in primary schools. *Educ. Res.* **1998**, *40*, 203–218. [CrossRef]

22. Mishna, F. A qualitative study of bullying from multiple perspectives. *Child. Sch.* **2004**, *26*, 234–247. [CrossRef]

23. Eslea, M.; Smith, P.K. Pupil and parent attitudes towards bullying in primary schools. *Eur. J. Psychol. Educ.* **2000**, *15*, 207–219. [CrossRef]

24. Pepler, D.; Smith, P.K.; Rigby, K. Looking back and looking forward: Implications for making interventions work effectively. In *Bullying in Schools: How Successful Can Interventions Be?* Smith, P.K., Pepler, D., Rigby, K., Eds.; Cambridge University Press: Cambridge, UK, 2004; pp. 307–324. ISBN 978-0-521-53803-0.

25. Farrington, D.P.; Ttofi, M.M. School-based programs to reduce bullying and victimization. *Campbell Collab.* **2009**, *6*, 1–149. [CrossRef]

26. Fekkes, M.; Pijpers, F.I.; Verloove-Vanhorick, S.P. Bullying: Who does what, when and where? Involvement of children, teachers and parents in bullying behavior. *Health Educ. Res.* **2004**, *20*, 81–91. [CrossRef]

27. Lovegrove, P.J.; Bellmore, A.D.; Green, J.G.; Jens, K.; Ostrov, J.M. "My voice is not going to be silent": What can parents do about children's bullying? *J. Sch. Violence* **2013**, *12*, 253–267. [CrossRef]

28. Ju, H.; Lee, S. Mothers' Perceptions of the Phenomenon of Bullying among Young Children in South Korea. *Soc. Sci.* **2019**, *8*. [CrossRef]

29. Butler, J.L.; Lynn Platt, R.A. Bullying: A family and school system treatment model. *Am. J. Fam. Ther.* **2007**, *36*, 18–29. [CrossRef]

30. Bradshaw, C.P.; Sawyer, A.L.; O'Brennan, L.M. Bullying and peer victimization at school: Perceptual differences between students and school staff. *Sch. Psychol. Rev.* **2007**, *36*, 361.

31. Hong, Y.-J.; Kangyi, L. The effect of parenting stress on social interactive parenting with a focus on Korean employed mothers' parenting support from ecological contexts. *Child. Youth Serv. Rev.* **2019**, *96*, 308–315. [CrossRef]

32. Lee, D. *A Study on the Policy Evaluation of the Wee Project-Focused on the Stage of Policy Process*; Korea National University of Education: Chung-Buk, Korea, 2017.

33. Kim, S.; Kim, J. An Analysis of Effectiveness of Wee project: Focused on High School. *Korean J. Policy Anal. Eval.* **2014**, *24*, 115–281.

34. Sim, J.; Lee, K. The effects of the "Wee Class" on the students involved in school Violence. *Korea Educ. Rev.* **2016**, *22*, 255–281.

35. Park, J.; Park, C.; Eom, J. *Mid-to-Long Term Forecasts of the Demand and Fiscal Spending for Early Childhood Education and Childcare*; Korean Institute of Child Care and Education: Seoul, Korea, 2015.

36. OECD. Early Learning and Development: Common Understanding. 2015. Available online: http://www.oecd.org/education/school/ECEC-Network-Common-Understandings-on-Early-Learning-and-Development.pdf (accessed on 15 January 2019).

37. Lee, S.; Smith, P.K.; Monks, C.P. Meaning and usage of a term for bullying-like phenomena in South Korea: A lifespan perspective. *J. Lang. Soc. Psychol.* **2012**, *31*, 342–349. [CrossRef]

38. Smith, P.K.; Cowie, H.; Olafsson, R.F.; Liefooghe, A.P. Definitions of bullying: A comparison of terms used, and age and gender differences, in a Fourteen–Country international comparison. *Child Dev.* **2002**, *73*, 1119–1133. [CrossRef]

39. Strauss, A.L.; Corbin, J.M. *Basics of Qualitative Research: Techniques and Procedures for Developing Grounded Theory*; SAGE: Thousand Oaks, CA, UAS, 1998; ISBN 9780803959392.

40. Coolican, H. *Research Methods and Statistics in Psychology*; Hodder & Stoughton; Hudder Arnold: London, UK, 2004; ISBN 0340812583.

41. Walker, D.; Florence, M. Grounded theory: An exploration of process and procedure. *Qual. Health Res.* **2006**, *16*, 547–559. [CrossRef] [PubMed]

42. Cassidy, W.; Faucher, C.; Jackson, M. What Parents Can Do to Prevent Cyberbullying: Students' and Educators' Perspectives. *Soc. Sci.* **2018**, *7*, 251. [CrossRef]

43. Gibson, J.E.; Polad, S.; Flaspohler, P.D.; Watts, V. Social Emotional Learning and Bullying Prevention: Why and How Integrated Implementation May Work. In *Contemporary Perspectives on Research on Bullying and Victimization in Early Childhood Education*; Saracho, O., Ed.; IAP: Charlotte, NC, USA, 2016; pp. 295–330.

44. Wright, M.; Wachs, S. Does Parental Mediation Moderate the Longitudinal Association among Bystanders and Perpetrators and Victims of Cyberbullying? *Soc. Sci.* **2018**, *7*, 231. [CrossRef]

45. Camodeca, M.; Goossens, F.A. Aggression, social cognitions, anger and sadness in bullies and victims. *J. Child Psychol. Psychiatry* **2005**, *46*, 186–197. [CrossRef] [PubMed]

46. Smith, P.K.; Sharp, S. *School Bullying: Insights and Perspectives*; Routledge: London, UK, 1994.

47. Hanish, L.D.; Kochenderfer-Ladd, B.; Fabes, R.A.; Martin, C.L.; Denning, D. Bullying among young children: The influence of peers and teachers. In *Bullying in American Schools: A Social-Ecological Perspective on Prevention and Intervention*; Espelage, D., Swearer, S.M., Eds.; Lawrence Erlbaum Associates: London, UK, 2004; pp. 141–160. ISBN 1-4106-0970-7.

48. Smith, P.K. Why interventions to reduce bullying and violence in schools may (or may not) succeed: Comments on this Special Section. *Int. J. Behav. Dev.* **2011**, *35*, 419–423. [CrossRef]

49. Kostelnik, M.; Soderman, A.; Whiren, A.; Rupiper, M.; Gregory, K. *Guiding Children's Social Development and Learning: Theory and Skills*; Cengage Learning: Boston, UK, 2014; ISBN 978-1285743707.

50. Monks, C.; Smith, P.K. Peer, self and teacher nominations of participant roles taken in victimisation by five-and eight-year-olds. *J. Aggress. Confl. Peace Res.* **2010**, *2*, 4–14. [CrossRef]

51. Smith, P.K.; Thompson, F.; Craig, W.; Hong, R.; Slee, P.; Sullivan, K.; Green, V.A. Actions to prevent bullying in western countries. In *School Bullying in Different Cultures. Eastern and Western Perspective*; Smith, P.K., Kwak, K., Toda, T., Eds.; Cambridge University Press: Cambridge, UK, 2016; pp. 301–333. ISBN 1107031893.

52. Thompson, F.; Smith, P.K. The use and effectiveness of anti-bullying strategies in schools. In *DFE-RR098*; DfE: London, UK, 2011.

53. Sellman, E. Building bridges: Preparing children for secondary school. *Pastor. Care Educ.* **2000**, *18*, 27–29. [CrossRef]

54. Saracho, O.N. Bullying prevention strategies in early childhood education. *Early Child. Educ. J.* **2017**, *45*, 453–460. [CrossRef]

55. Hoffman, D.M. Reflecting on social emotional learning: A critical perspective on trends in the United States. *Rev. Educ. Res.* **2009**, *79*, 533–556. [CrossRef]

56. Durlak, J.A.; Weissberg, R.P.; Dymnicki, A.B.; Taylor, R.D.; Schellinger, K.B. The impact of enhancing students' social and emotional learning: A meta-analysis of school-based universal interventions. *Child Dev.* **2011**, *82*, 405–432. [CrossRef]

57. Joseph, G.E.; Strain, P.S. Enhancing emotional vocabulary in young children. *Young Except. Child.* **2003**, *6*, 18–26. [CrossRef]

58. Cross, D.; Waters, S.; Pearce, N.; Shaw, T.; Hall, M.; Erceg, E.; Burns, S.; Roberts, C.; Hamilton, G. The Friendly Schools Friendly Families programme: Three-year bullying behaviour outcomes in primary school children. *Int. J. Educ. Res.* **2012**, *53*, 394–406. [CrossRef]

59. Cross, D.; Lester, L.; Pearce, N.; Barnes, A.; Beatty, S. A group randomized controlled trial evaluating parent involvement in whole school actions to reduce bullying. *J. Educ. Res.* **2018**, *111*, 255–267. [CrossRef]

60. McKenney, S.; Voogt, J. Technology and young children: How 4–7 years old perceive their own use of computers. *Comput. Hum. Behav.* **2010**, *26*, 656–664. [CrossRef]

61. Doh, N.; Bea, Y.; Lee, Y.; Lee, Y.; Kim, M.; Lim, J.; Kim, H. *A Longitudinal Study of Korean Children's Development*; Institute of Child Care and Education: Seoul, Korea, 2017; ISBN 979-11-87952-56-5 93330.
62. Kowalski, R.M.; Giumetti, G.W. Cyberbullying among children 0 to 8 years. In *Contemporary Perspectives on Research on Bullying and Victimization in Early Childhood Education*; Saracho, O., Ed.; IAP: Charlotte, NC, USA, 2016; pp. 157–175. ISBN 978-1-68123-596-7.

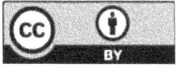

International Journal of
Environmental Research and Public Health

MDPI

Article

Dialogic Model of Prevention and Resolution of Conflicts: Evidence of the Success of Cyberbullying Prevention in a Primary School in Catalonia

Beatriz Villarejo-Carballido [1,*], Cristina M. Pulido [2], Lena de Botton [3] and Olga Serradell [4]

[1] Faculty of Psychology and Education, University of Deusto, 48007 Bilbao, Spain
[2] Department of Journalism and Communication Studies, Universitat Autònoma de Barcelona, 08193 Bellaterra, Spain; cristina.pulido@uab.cat
[3] Department of Sociology, Universitat de Barcelona, 08034 Barcelona, Spain; lenadebotton@ub.edu
[4] Department of Sociology, Universitat Autònoma de Barcelona, 08193 Bellaterra, Spain; olga.serradell@uab.cat
* Correspondence: beatriz.villarejo@deusto.es; Tel.: +34-944-139-003

Received: 30 December 2018; Accepted: 6 March 2019; Published: 14 March 2019

Abstract: This article analyses the evidence obtained from the application of the dialogic model of prevention and resolution of conflicts to eradicate cyberbullying behaviour in a primary school in Catalonia. The Dialogic Prevention Model is one of the successful educational actions identified by INCLUD-ED (FP6 research project). This case study, based on communicative methodology, includes the results obtained from documentary analysis, communicative observations and in-depth interviews. The evidence collected indicates that the implementation of this type of model can help to overcome cyberbullying; children are more confident to reject violence, students support the victims more and the whole community is involved in Zero Tolerance to violence.

Keywords: cyberbullying; intervention; school; minors; families; teachers; successful educational action

---

1. Introduction

Data on the prevalence of cyberbullying among minors indicate an urgent need for scientific evidence regarding how to prevent such bullying as early as possible [1–3], particularly in primary and secondary school. There is abundant scientific literature [4–6] that describes how cyberbullying affects young people in different countries. However, there is less scientific literature that describes successful prevention programmes. As indicated by Della Cioppa, O'Neil and Craig [7], there is a current need to develop educational interventions aimed at overcoming cyberbullying based on prevention programmes that have been scientifically proven to be successful. To this end, Della Cioppa et al. [7] evaluated 20 prevention programmes, few of which had been previously evaluated and even fewer of which use scientific evidence. Those programmes that achieved scientifically acceptable results coincided with involving the educational community as a whole or incorporating contexts beyond the school [7].

Recently, the systematic and meta-analytical review conducted by Gaffney et al. [8] provided evidence of the effectiveness of some cyberbullying prevention programmes. This study focused on the analysis of 24 publications; most of them used randomised controlled trials to evaluate cyberbullying prevention programmes and the other ones were quasi-experimental designs with before and after measures. Some of the contributions selected for advancing in this field are related to the fact that the evaluated programmes presented evidence of reducing cyberbullying. However, there is a research need to identify the components of intervention programmes which are most effective in reducing cyberbullying and victimisation and to explain the influence of overlapping offline and online victimisation [8].

The objective of this article is to respond to this urgent research need. Based on an analysis of the scientific literature, the elements that a prevention programme must include to guarantee favourable results were identified. Our in-depth study of the scientific literature focused on prevention programmes based on the behaviour of "bystanders", which in our context is translated as the role of "observers" or "spectators". In addition, we examined models of community intervention and presented the results of the application of the dialogic model of prevention and resolution of conflicts (DMPRC, hereinafter) [9] in a specific case. This model has been endorsed as a successful educational initiative by the integrated research project INCLUD-ED of the European Commission's sixth Framework Programme. INCLUD-ED is the only social sciences research project on the European Commission's list of the ten most successful research projects in Europe [10]. In addition to this, a qualitative case study was conducted using a communicative method [9].

1.1. Children's Media Use, A Balance Approach

Minors today live in a media-inundated society. As noted by Aguaded [11], the most intelligent and rewarding response to such a society requires the development of media competence. The concern of families has increased in recent years due to the use that minors make of media and the risks such use involves. As indicated by Livingstone et al. [12], it has become impossible for parents to prohibit the use of media. Thus, according to studies conducted by Livingstone and colleagues, families and schools should seek to maximise the opportunities to use media for learning and fun. It is necessary to minimise the risks and invest in the education of families with the aim of creating common strategies, face the risks and increase the positive use of media. We must also include the perspective of the rights of minors regarding digital media while avoiding a vision of minimising risk or adopting an alarmist view. To this end, a balanced approach should be sought [13]. Similarly, other researchers have indicated a need to reinforce the idea of teaching children whom to befriend in social networks. For example, this would include choosing those who treat others well and ignoring those who treat other schoolmates with contempt. These efforts should be part of a wider attempt to create a secure online environment for minors [14]. In addition, it is necessary to remember that cyberbullying among equals is not the only risk that minors can face online. For example, minors may find themselves in situations of vulnerability and become trapped in illegal activity through contacts initiated online. Preventing such problems is part of the contemporary struggle to develop an international joint programme to protect minors [15]. Minors should also be educated on how technologies can be used for social change and be familiarised with how such change is being promoted through, for instance, the use of online platforms to protect the rights of young women [16].

1.2. Cyberbullying Does not Occur Alone, It Coexists with other Types of Violence

There is extensive literature dealing with cyberbullying among minors. The consequences of such bullying can be severe and in the worst cases, may disturb the happy and harmonious development of girls and boys, as shown by the number of suicides of young people linked to cyberbullying [17]. Therefore, several authors emphasise the importance of regarding cyberbullying as an issue that also affects health [18]. A study on children between the ages of 14 and 17 in six European countries found that 21.4% had suffered episodes of cyberbullying in the last twelve months. According to the same study, such experiences were more frequent among girls than boys (23.9% vs. 18.5%) [18]. Moreover, recent developments point to the need of seeing the whole picture of violence, since cyberbullying coexists with other types of violence (bullying, sexual harassment, etc.) and they need to be treated together [19,20]. In fact, cyberbullying includes different types of violent interactions (flaming, harassing, cyberstalking, spreading rumours, among others) [21]. In our study, we paid attention to all of them. All these types of violence share a same root; a socialisation on attractiveness linked to violence [22]. This type of socialisation occurs where social interactions (media, peers' group, family, school) generate a type of socialisation that links attractiveness to violence. Therefore, prevention programmes based on this contribution aim at promoting social interactions where attractiveness is not linked to violence. According to this contribution, the key factor for understanding the whole picture of violence is the type of socialisation that children are learning through their daily interactions [22].

1.3. Community Intervention and Interactions of All Agents Involved in Educational Centres

Several research teams have investigated digital citizenship training to address violent risks. For example, Jones and Mitchell [23] demonstrated how training that included instruction on respectful online behaviour and active online citizenship encouraged individuals to assume an attitude of active observer in harassment situations, i.e., not to remain passive.

In recent years, investigations emphasising the urgency of developing programmes that involve the wider social environment have emerged. This includes, not leaving child victims of cyberbullying to themselves but involving their entire social community to get to the root of why cyberbullying occurs [24,25]. Cyberbullying exists because of the aforementioned socialisation that links attractiveness to violence [22]. This outcome explains the tendency of cyberbullies to be the most popular members of their group [14]. As a form of social learning, this perception can be changed, and there are schools in which violence has been rejected by involving the entire community [9]. Therefore, strategies to prevent cyberbullying must go beyond the recommendation of parental supervision [26] and focus on the entire community. Prevention programmes should include all the relevant aspects of the problem: From school to families, the intervention of peers, and the use of information and communications technology (ICT) and social networks on the basis of preventive models, not only punitive ones [24,27]. In addition, the non-trivialization of violence and the active stance of the entire educational community are important [28]. This transversal endeavour known as "0 violence from 0 years old" [29] starts from early childhood. The development of empathy is basic to educate individuals into adopting an active and realistic position in the face of cyberbullying, yet it is one of the barriers found in the scientific literature [30]. Individuals must also learn how to act when confronted with cyberbullying [31]. In this sense, it is also necessary to note that cyberbullying prevention should consider the victims and those who defend them. The latter often suffer reprisals for their support, which in the scientific literature is known as second-order sexual harassment [32]. Other authors agree that the minors with greater social capital, that is, "wealth" in their social relations, are the ones who act with a more proactive attitude in response to cyberbullying. Within a group of equals, these minors can encourage a change of attitude in response to such events [33].

When minors know how to play the role of the observer in response to cyberbullying, their effect in curbing cyberbullying increases [34]. Other research describes the impact of involving young people in models of community collaboration to prevent cyberbullying and harassment. These interventions obtain greater results because they reduce the fear of bullying and increase the confidence of minors in the adults who surround them [35]. Other findings indicate the importance of training mentors for young people in the leadership of prevention programmes [36]. The need to belong and participate in the school improves children's health [37].

The role of adults is fundamental. According to one study, 60% of the victims of cyberbullying seek trustworthy adults when they report abuse [38]. Based on these results, programmes that incorporate an active role for adults in the community reduce episodes of cyberbullying. The action coordinated through a dialogical leadership model develops a more effective transformation [39]. In addition, the involvement of non-academic families is essential [40], especially non-academic women, whose participation is crucial. Their involvement is facilitated by creating dialogical participation spaces [41] as well as the promotion of communicative acts that ensure protective factors [42]. Finally, communication should be highlighted as a basic element. Minors require adult interlocutors who are able to create safe and reliable communication spaces in which minors can communicate the problems they face [43]. The literature review shows positive results on prevention of bullying and cyberbullying through the active role of observers [25,44,45]. Among these programmes, the Green Dot Bystander Intervention Program is highlighted, which was introduced in 26 secondary schools in Kentucky and has been shown to be effective in reducing sexual harassment and other types of violence in the community [45]. Through the *Cyber Friendly Schools* (*CFS*) in Canada, researchers noted that schools and teachers cannot prevent cyberbullying alone. Families, the minors and the community in general must jointly address this goal if cyberbullying is to be prevented both in- and outside the school [44]. Another example is the Medienhelden Programme from Germany, based on the link between cognitive and affective empathy and the prevention of cyberbullying. In this programme, 722 secondary schools with students between 11 and 17 years old were evaluated, finding that an intervention over time reduced the episodes of cyberbullying and increased the feeling of empathy [46].

The cyberbullying prevention programmes with the best results involve the entire educational community, encourage zero tolerance for any type of cyberbullying or other type of violent interactions and train minors, teachers and families to collaborate in the creation of spaces for dialogue. It is recommended that educational centres apply only programmes based on scientific evidence and establish a transversal line of action instead of teaching concrete, specific behaviour in the classroom.

Considering these previous contributions, the research questions addressed in this paper are: a) Does DMPRC foster an environment where children feel confident to denounce cases of cyberbullying? Does the coordination of adults (teachers and family) collaborating in a Zero Tolerance to Violence programme create a safer space? And last, does DMPRC reduce violent interactions while increasing active solidarity towards the victims and those who support them?

2. Materials and Methods

This research was based on a qualitative case study using the communicative methodology approach [47]. The aim of this methodology is to find those results that improve the living conditions of people, thus guaranteeing the social impact of the research [48]. The main characteristic of this type of methodology is the dialogic construction of knowledge. This means establishing dialogical interactions mediated by an egalitarian dialogue between the research team and the participants [49]. The aim is to contrast the scientific evidence with the life-world knowledge and the experience of the people interviewed, in order to grasp in depth, the social reality studied.

2.1. Selection of the Case Study

The selected case study was based on the qualitative analysis of the application of the dialogical model of prevention and resolution of conflicts. [9]. DMPRC, which is characterised by the involvement of the whole educational community (teachers, family, students and other social agents), has two main characteristics. On the one hand, coexistence agreements are reached in an assembly through a dialogic process that involves students, family members and teachers. On the other hand, spaces for dialogue are created with the aim to reject violence and promote interactions that construct a type of socialisation that links attractiveness with nonviolent models [5]. The school creates a coexistence commission that is composed by different community members (students, family, teachers), so they monitor the implementation of the agreement and contribute to the creation of a safer space for all. The model was applied in an educational centre for early and primary school education in Terrassa, a city in Catalonia (Spain). This school has implemented DMPRC since the school year 2014–2015. In this case study, the research focused on analysing the results of the application of this model in cyberbullying detection and prevention. The educational centre, that is a learning community, had been previously studied because of the positive results achieved in a collaboration between teachers and families, including its impact on improving the lives of neighbourhood residents [50]. However, this study provides the first results on cyberbullying prevention obtained in this school.

2.2. Data Collection

The educational centre had been implementing a successful educational programme involving DMPRC for four academic school years. The research team monitored the results of the programme in terms of improving coexistence during ten months in 2017. Among the various outcomes obtained, this article presents those results regarding action taken in response to cyberbullying that occurred in a specific class of the last key stage of primary school. The analysed data were collected using three research techniques: Documentary analysis of the data on the programme, communicative observation of coexistence commission and in-depth interviews. The documentary analysis included, basically, the documents related to the results obtained by the school, and the documentation related to the implementation of DMPRC. The communicative observation of the coexistence commission at the centre (N = 6), was conducted by one of the researchers, who participated in all of them. Five observed commissions were held at the educational centre and were attended by 18 people on average—students, teachers and family members. The sixth communicative observation was held on "Zero Violence" workshop, and 90 people attended. Students that participated in these gatherings explained how the coexistence agreement was being implemented and which were the problems that they had to face in order to guarantee an environment free of violence. Then, an open dialogue between students, teachers and family members was developed, in order to address the problems found. Finally, we developed in-depth interviews (N = 4) with members of the educational community directly involved in the follow-up on the cyberbullying case occurred. The communicative observations facilitated the analysis of the interactions between students, families and teachers at the coexistence commission. In these sessions, the most relevant problems were addressed and joint solutions were found. In one observation session, a case of cyberbullying emerged. This case is discussed in greater detail in this article. In-depth interviews were conducted with several people: The person responsible for promoting coexistence, the teacher of the class in which the cyberbullying case occurred, the centre's director and the mother of a student. The aim of the interviews was to increase our understanding of the different roles of responsibility adopted regarding the action taken, and the results that were achieved.

2.3. Ethical Issues

The case study was developed following the ethical criteria developed in the research "Saleacom. Overcoming Inequalities in Schools and Learning Communities: Innovative Education for a New Century" funded by the European Commission (Reference number: 645668).

3. Results

Our research results suggested three main achievements. The first was how the implementation of DMPRC helped break the silence in situations of harassment. In the specific episode of cyberbullying analysed, breaking the silence involved getting children to empower themselves and denounce the cyberbullying cases. The second achievement was the improved intervention by the adult community in response to cyberbullying, which fostered the creation of a safe environment where minors gained sufficient trust to bring up problems that occurred outside the school. The third achievement was active solidarity with the victims and the individuals who support them, thus succeeding at the prevention of re-victimisation.

3.1. From Silence to an Active Stance against Cyberbullying

The coexistence commission was mixed assemblies involving families, teachers and students. They addressed daily problems with respect to coexistence, how to act before such problems and how to prevent them. The coexistence commission can be described as the space for dialogue where the application of DMPRC is monitored. One goal supported by students, family members (who were primarily non-academics) and teachers was achieved; coexistence was improved in all areas since they began to apply DMPRC. Another highly important result was that both girls and boys had developed the confidence to report cyberbullying or other types of violent interactions. According to the researched participants, such reports had not occurred in the past. Therefore, the first research question is confirmed, since the dialogic model of prevention of conflict helped children denounce cyberbullying and feel more confident to do so. An example of this reporting was shared by the teacher of a class group in which cyberbullying was identified.

"One day, a child in my class tells me that he wants to talk to me and that he will come with another classmate. So, they tell me that there has been a situation of cyberbullying through the homework chat tool they have in class, and then, he tells me at three o'clock I'll bring the mobile and show it to you. (...). And yes, when they showed the conversation, some girls were insulting another saying that nobody could stand her, that she was ugly and stupid, and they kept laughing at her. And he intervened, saying, 'what you are doing is cyberbullying', and another answered that it was a lie; and since he saw that they did not stop, he decided to tell me about it.".

(Antonia)

As explained by the teacher in an interview, this student intervened in the WhatsApp group conversation because of the constant dialogue held in the school regarding such interactions and how to act in a courageous manner. According to his teacher, when asked why he was so determined to denounce the situation, the student answered, "because you are brave if you denounce, and if you do not do it, you're not" (Maria). This is an action that empowers the educational community to act, and that can improve the physical and emotional wellbeing of the victim and the people who support him. His teacher also added, "The victim is fine; the peers treat her well with respect. (...) in the case of the child who reported the cyberbullying case, the class has admired him" (Maria, teacher). According to the interviewee, in this manner, it has been possible to create a climate in the school where silence is not desired when cyberbullying or other types of violent interactions occur. On the contrary, instead of silence, actively facing harassment has become attractive. According to the interviewees, girls and boys who perceive this new climate feel empowered and dare to talk about cyberbullying or other aggressive interactions, something that did not occur in the school before DMPRC was implemented.

3.2. More Secure and Trusted Environments when Adults are Working in the Same Direction with Evidence

Regarding the question of whether or not the coordination of adults (teachers and family) collaborating in Zero Tolerance Violence creates a safer space, the answer is affirmative, in line with the scientific findings in this field. According to the data analysed, students feel secure at school, they treat coexistence problems as a community concern and the fact of seeing their families and teachers together increases their confidence. One of the contributions explained by the coordinator of the coexistence commission was that students also talk about the problems that they have outside school:

"You think that the increase in the security feeling is due to the fact that now they also turn to us with problems that occur with other children in the neighbourhood". Similarly, the centre's director highlighted the students' trust in the educational community: "The students feel that they have the support of the adults who care for them and protect them, an environment they can count on". In another example, the interviewed mother noted that, "ever since the problem of cyberbullying was discussed in the gathering, teachers, students, family members, children are much better".

(Hamida)

In this sense, the interviewees indicated that working together to eradicate violence creates a good atmosphere achieved in various domains within the school: In the coexistence commission, in the training of family members and teachers, and in the daily dialogues that occur in the school. The positive effect achieved in all these domains has been guided by scientific evidence that supports DMPRC and the validity of dialogic pedagogical gatherings. For the coexistence coordinator, the role played by this type of discussion was key to establishing harmony in the school's approach to preventing violence and teachers' actions according to this principle:

"(...) The process of reading is fundamental: Scientific evidence, reading and sharing, and implementing. Without that part of the training, we would not succeed because everyone would go with his or her own preconceived ideas, and we would not be so successful. (...)".

(Montserrat)

Therefore, one key to success was to address the problem using scientific evidence. Another one was to engage the entire community in dialogue to agree on common criteria for action, both in the family and at school.

3.3. Active Solidarity toward Victims and the Individuals who Support Them

Last, we highlight an important result regarding a change of attitude toward victims and the individuals who support them. Regarding the question of whether or not DMPRC reduces cyberbullying and increases active solidarity with the victims and those who support them, the answer is affirmative. According to the interviewees, in the past, when one student bullied another, other students that saw this behaviour chose to be quiet because they felt afraid of the consequences of supporting the victim, for instance being bullied too. Some students even decided to engage in the bullying in order to be more popular. Now, since the application of DMPRC, this behaviour has changed. One teacher explained an attack on a child who reported an episode of cyberbullying: "The day after denouncing the cyberbullying and making it public, one of the children was attacked; someone had written *rat* in his book" (Antonia). According to the teacher, in response, the class was stopped and the students discussed the problem. The class group demonstrated solidarity with the child who had denounced the cyberbullying case because the child had shown courage, and the student who wrote the insult was left without support. In this way, students learn to reject violent behaviour by practicing solidarity, and the bullies change more quickly because they do not find social recognition from their peers, from the families or the teachers. No one supported the violent behaviour, according to the interviewees.

4. Discussion

The literature review suggested that research needs to provide more evidence on successful programmes addressed to prevent cyberbullying cases in schools [7,8]. Recent findings suggested the need to focus on the components of intervention programmes which are most effective in reducing cyberbullying perpetration and victimisation [8]. This case study provided evidence that contributes to advances in this research field. The dialogic model of prevention and resolution of conflicts implemented the recommendation of involving the whole community (students, teachers and family) [24,25,45] and obtained excellent results.

This involvement is characterised by a dialogic process where members of the community reach agreements on coexistence and monitor the application of such agreements through the coexistence commission. In this commission, students have a prominent role supported by adults of the community (teachers and family) [9]. By seeing that their reference adults work together for eradicating all types of violence, children feel more confident to report cyberbullying episodes. The school or families did not prohibit the use of media; in fact, in this case students have a WhatsApp group for homework. It was in this group that the cyberbullying episode occurred. Nevertheless, adults do not leave students alone with those online interactions but apply the balance approach of children media use [13,14]. Adults accompany this use through dialogic intervention. For this reason, when one child saw the cyberbullying episode, he felt the courage to explain it to his teacher, because bystander attitudes [25,44,45] are encouraged by the community every day. However, one of the components that none of the programmes analysed in the literature review explained is the second characteristic of DMPRC. This second characteristic focuses on the promotion of interactions that reject violence, while promoting interactions that construct a type of socialisation that links attractiveness with nonviolent models [9].

This contribution overcomes one of the barriers found in the literature review; the fact that cyberbullies tend to be considered among the most popular members of their group of peers [14]. If children feel that being a cyberbully makes you more attractive and popular, the prevention programme will always fail. For this reason, one of the success components found in the application of this dialogic model of prevention and resolution of conflicts is that it addresses this problem by including interactions that promote attractiveness towards nonviolent attitudes. Thus, the scenario is reversed, and the brave and popular students are those who reject violence. An example of this can be seen in the fact that one of the students increased his attractiveness after rejecting the violence in the WhatsApp group and denouncing the cyberbullying case. One of the cyberbullies tried to attack him saying that he was a rat, but instead of being bullied by the other peers, the group faced this attack by supporting him and the victim of cyberbullying. Therefore, the solidarity attitude increased between peers, and the child who bullied learnt that he had no more peer support for his behaviour. This way is one of the most effective manners to change this behaviour according to the analysis of the literature review and the fieldwork done. This last contribution helps to advance the research of effectiveness of components on cyberbullying prevention programmes.

The limitation of this research relates to the fact that the in-depth interviews were conducted only with adults. Even though student voices were heard indirectly in the observations and interviews, future research should seek to gather students' opinions in a more direct manner, for instance through communicative discussion groups. This would allow gaining insight in their results' contribution of the dialogic model of prevention and resolution of conflicts that faces cyberbullying as well as other types of violent interactions.

5. Conclusions

Despite this limitation, the article contributed to the scientific literature by offering qualitative evidence of the impact of applying the dialogical model of prevention and resolution of conflicts. Without the programme, the girl who was cyberbullied in the WhatsApp group would continue suffering this violence today. Yet, now, she feels protected and has more friends willing to show their support. At the same time, the evidence contributed to the crucial role of bystanders, by showing that when their action is seen as brave and attractive, its effectiveness is increased. In addition, all the children in the school feel more confident in their adult environment than they did before. They do not hide what occurs, and they show trust. They know that to denounce it is to be brave and when facing a problem, they seek the support of their teachers and families in order to find a solution all together, as they stated in the interviews. Future research can examine more in depth the type of interactions that successfully achieve the eradication of all types of violence, including cyberbullying interactions.

Author Contributions: Investigation, L.d.B.; Conceptualization and Methodology, O.S.; Formal Analysis and Writing Original Draft, B.V.-C.; Formal Analysis, Writing, Review, C.M.P.

Funding: This research "Saleacom. Overcoming Inequalities in Schools and Learning Communities: Innovative Education for a New Century" was funded by the European Commission's Programme Marie Curie RISE. Horizon 2020 (2015–2017). Reference number: 645668.

Conflicts of Interest: The authors declare that they have no conflict of interest.

References

1. Machimbarrena, J.M.; Calvete, E.; Fernández-González, L.; Álvarez-Bardón, A.; Álvarez-Fernández, L.; González-Cabrera, J. Internet Risks: An overview of victimization in cyberbullying, cyber Dating abuse, sexting, online grooming and problematic internet use. *Int. J. Environ. Res. Public Health* **2018**, *15*, 2471. [CrossRef] [PubMed]
2. Urra Canales, M.; Acosta Oidor, C.; Salazar Baena, V.; Ruiz, J. Bullying. Description of the roles of victim, bully, peer group, school, family and society. *Int. J. Sociol. Educ.* **2018**, *7*, 278–299. [CrossRef]
3. UNESCO. School Violence and Bullying Global Status Report. Available online: http://unesdoc.unesco.org/images/0024/002469/246970e.pdf (accessed on 12 November 2018).
4. Athanasiou, K.; Melegkovits, E.; Andrie, E.K.; Magoulas, C.; Tzavara, C.K.; Richardson, C.; Greydanus, D.; Tsolia, M.; Tsitsika, A.K. Cross-national aspects of cyberbullying victimization among 14–17-year-old adolescents across seven European countries. *BMC Public Health* **2018**, *18*, 800. [CrossRef] [PubMed]

5. Baldry, A.C.; Farrington, D.P.; Sorrentino, A.; Blaya, C. Cyberbullying and cybervictimization. In *International Perspectives on Cyberbullying*; Palgrave Macmillan: Cham, Switzerland, 2018; pp. 3–23.
6. Palladino, B.E.; Menesini, E.; Nocentini, A.; Luik, P.; Naruskov, K.; Ucanok, Z.; Dogan, A.; Schultze-Krumbholz, A.; Hess, M.; Scheithauer, H. Perceived severity of cyberbullying: Differences and similarities across four countries. *Front. Psychol.* **2017**, *8*, 1524. [CrossRef] [PubMed]
7. Della Cioppa, V.; O'Neil, A.; Craig, W. Learning from traditional bullying interventions: A review of research on cyberbullying and best practice. *Aggress. Violent Behav.* **2015**, *23*, 61–68. [CrossRef]
8. Gaffney, H.; Farrington, D.P.; Espelage, D.L.; Ttofi, M.M. Are ciberbullying intervention and prevention programs effective? A systematic and meta-analytical review. *Aggress. Violent Behav.* **2018**, in press. [CrossRef]
9. Aiello, E.; Puigvert, L.; Schubert, T. Preventing violent radicalization of youth through dialogic evidence-based policies. *Int. Sociol.* **2018**, *33*, 435–453. [CrossRef]
10. European Commission. *Added Value of Research, Innovation and Science Portfolio. MEMO/11/520*; European Commission: Brussels, Belgium, 2011; Available online: http://europa.eu/rapid/press-release_MEMO-11-520_en.htm (accessed on 25 October 2018).
11. Aguaded, J.I. Desde la infoxicación al derecho a la comunicación. *Comunicar* **2014**, *XXI*, 7–8. [CrossRef]
12. Livingstone, S.; Ólafsson, K.; Helsper, E.J.; Lupiáñez-Villanueva, F.; Veltri, G.A.; Folkvord, F. Maximizing opportunities and minimizing risks for children online: The role of digital skills in emerging strategies of parental mediation. *J. Commun.* **2017**, *67*, 82–105. [CrossRef]
13. Livingstone, S.; Third, A. Children and young people's rights in the digital age: An emerging agenda. *New Media Soc.* **2017**, *19*, 657–670. [CrossRef]
14. Wegge, D.; Vandebosch, H.; Eggermont, S.; Walrave, M. The strong, the weak, and the unbalanced: The link Between tie strength and cyberaggression on a social network site. *Soc. Sci. Comput. Rev.* **2015**, *33*, 315–342. [CrossRef]
15. Limoncelli, S.A. The global development of contemporary anti-human trafficking advocacy. *Int. Sociol.* **2017**, *32*, 814–834. [CrossRef]
16. Matos, C. New Brazilian feminisms and online networks: Cyberfeminism, protest and the female 'Arab Spring'. *Int. Sociol.* **2017**, *32*, 417–434. [CrossRef]
17. Bauman, S.; Toomey, R.B.; Walker, J.L. Associations among bullying, cyberbullying, and suicide in high school students. *J. Adolesc.* **2013**, *36*, 341–350. [CrossRef] [PubMed]
18. Kowalski, R.M.; Limber, S.P. Psychological, physical, and academic correlates of cyberbullying and traditional bullying. *J. Adolesc. Health* **2013**, *53*, S13–S20. [CrossRef] [PubMed]
19. Mercer Kollar, L.M.; Leemis, R.W.; Davis, J.P.; Basile, K.C.; Espelage, D.L. Traditional and cyber bullying and sexual harassment: A longitudinal assessment of risk and protective factors. *Aggress. Behav.* **2018**, *45*, 181–192.
20. Hamby, S.; Taylor, E.; Jones, L.; Mitchell, K.J.; Turner, H.A.; Newlin, C. From poly-victimization to poly-strengths: Understanding the web of violence can transform research on youth violence and illuminate the path to prevention and resilience. *J. Interpers. Violence* **2018**, *33*, 719–739. [CrossRef]
21. Capurso, S.; Paradžik, L.; Čale Mratović, M. Cyberbullying among children and adolescents—An overview on epidemiological studies and effective preventive programs. *Kriminologija Socijalna Integracija* **2018**, *25*, 127–137. [CrossRef]
22. Puigvert, L. Preventive socialization of gender violence: Moving forward using the communicative methodology of research. *Qual. Inq.* **2014**, *20*, 839–843. [CrossRef]
23. Jones, L.M.; Mitchell, K.J. Defining and measuring youth digital citizenship. *New Media Soc.* **2016**, *18*, 2063–2079. [CrossRef]
24. Cassidy, W.; Faucher, C.; Jackson, M.; Jackson, M. Cyberbullying among youth: A comprehensive review of current international research and its implications and application to policy and practice. *Sch. Psychol. Int.* **2013**, *34*, 575–612. [CrossRef]
25. Storer, H.L.; Casey, E.A.; Herrenkohl, T.I. Developing "whole school" bystander interventions: The role of school-settings in influencing adolescents responses to dating violence and bullying. *Child. Youth Serv. Rev.* **2017**, *74*, 87–95. [CrossRef]
26. Khurana, A.; Bleakley, A.; Jordan, A.B.; Romer, D. The protective effects of parental monitoring and internet restriction on adolescents' risk of online harassment. *J. Youth Adolesc.* **2015**, *44*, 1039–1047. [CrossRef]

27. Ortega Barón, J.; Buelga, S.; Cava, M.J. Influencia del clima escolar y familiar en adolescentes, víctimas de ciberacoso. *Comunicar* **2016**, *24*, 57–65. [CrossRef]

28. Duque, E.; Teixidó, J. Bullying and gender. Prevention from school organization. *Multidiscip. J. Educ. Res.* **2016**, *6*, 176–204. [CrossRef]

29. Oliver, E. Zero Violence since early childhood: The dialogic recreation of knowledge. *Qual. Inq.* **2014**, *20*, 902–908. [CrossRef]

30. Nickerson, A.B.; Aloe, A.M.; Werth, J.M. The relation of empathy and defending in bullying: A meta-analytic investigation. *Sch. Psychol. Rev.* **2015**, *44*, 372–390. [CrossRef]

31. Nickerson, A.B.; Aloe, A.M.; Livingston, J.A.; Feeley, T.H. Measurement of the bystander intervention model for bullying and sexual harassment. *J. Adolesc.* **2014**, *37*, 391–400. [CrossRef] [PubMed]

32. Vidu, A.; Valls, R.; Puigvert, L.; Melgar, P.; Joanpere, M. Second order of sexual harassment—SOSH. *REMIE Multidiscip. J. Educ. Res.* **2017**, *7*, 1–26. [CrossRef]

33. Jenkins, L.N.; Fredrick, S.S. Social capital and bystander behavior in bullying: Internalizing problems as a barrier to prosocial intervention. *J. Youth Adolesc.* **2017**, *46*, 757–771. [CrossRef]

34. Brody, N.; Vangelisti, A.L. Bystander intervention in cyberbullying. *Commun. Monogr.* **2016**, *83*, 94–119. [CrossRef]

35. Gibson, J.E.; Flaspohler, P.D.; Watts, V. Engaging youth in bullying prevention through community-based participatory research. *Fam. Community Health* **2015**, *38*, 120–130. [CrossRef] [PubMed]

36. Patterson, L.J.; Allan, A.; Cross, D. Adolescent perceptions of bystanders' responses to cyberbullying. *New Media Soc.* **2017**, *19*, 366–383. [CrossRef]

37. Arslan, G. Understanding the association between school belonging and emotional health in adolescents. *Int. J. Educ. Psychol.* **2018**, *7*, 21–41. [CrossRef]

38. Jones, L.M.; Mitchell, K.J.; Turner, H.A. Victim reports of bystander reactions to in-person and online peer harassment: A national survey of adolescents. *J. Youth Adolesc.* **2015**, *44*, 2308–2320. [CrossRef] [PubMed]

39. Redondo, G. Dialogic Leadership and new alternative masculinities: Emerging synergies for social rransformation. *Masculinities Soc. Chang.* **2016**, *5*, 70. [CrossRef]

40. Vanderhoven, E.; Schellens, T.; Valcke, M. Decreasing risky behavior on social network sites: The impact of parental involvement in secondary education interventions. *J. Prim. Prev.* **2016**, *37*, 247–261. [CrossRef] [PubMed]

41. Tellado, I. Bridges between individuals and communities: Dialogic participation fueling meaningful social engagement. *Res. Ageing Soc. Policy* **2017**, *5*, 8–31. [CrossRef]

42. Rios-Gonzalez, O.; Peña Axt, J.C.; Duque Sanchez, E.; De Botton Fernández, L. The language of ethics and double standards in the affective and sexual socialization of youth. Communicative acts in the family environment as protective or risk factors of intimate partner violence. *Front. Sociol.* **2018**, *3*, 19. [CrossRef]

43. Larrañaga, E.; Yubero, S.; Ovejero, A.; Navarro, R. Loneliness, parent-child communication and cyberbullying victimization among Spanish youths. *Comput. Hum. Behav.* **2016**, *65*, 1–8. [CrossRef]

44. Cross, D.; Shaw, T.; Hadwen, K.; Cardoso, P.; Slee, P.; Roberts, C.; Thomas, L.; Barnes, A. Longitudinal impact of the Cyber Friendly Schools program on adolescents' cyberbullying behavior. *Aggress. Behav.* **2016**, *42*, 166–180. [CrossRef]

45. Coker, A.L.; Bush, H.M.; Cook-Craig, P.G.; DeGue, S.A.; Clear, E.R.; Brancato, C.J.; Fisher, B.S.; Recktenwald, E.A. RCT testing bystander effectiveness to reduce violence. *Am. J. Prev. Med.* **2017**, *52*, 566–578. [CrossRef] [PubMed]

46. Schultze-Krumbholz, A.; Schultze, M.; Zagorscak, P.; Wölfer, R.; Scheithauer, H. Feeling cybervictims' pain.-The effect of empathy training on cyberbullying. *Aggress. Behav.* **2016**, *42*, 147–156. [CrossRef] [PubMed]

47. Flecha, R.; Soler, M. Communicative Methodology: Successful actions and dialogic democracy. *Curr. Sociol.* **2014**, *62*, 232–242. [CrossRef]

48. Reale, E.; Avramov, D.; Canhial, K.; Donovan, C.; Flecha, R.; Holm, P.; Larkin, C.; Lepori, B.; Mosoni-Fried, J.; Oliver, E.; et al. A review of literature on evaluating the scientific, social and political impact of social sciences and humanities research. *Res. Eval.* **2017**, *27*, 298–308. [CrossRef]

49. Soler-Gallart, M. Dialogic relations and interactions as an alternative to power. In *Achieving Social Impact: Sociology in the Public Sphere*; Springer International Publishing: Cham, Switzerland, 2017; pp. 21–42, ISBN 978-3-319-60270-7.

50. Girbés-Peco, S.; Renta, A.I.; De Botton, L.; Álvarez, P. The Montserrat's neighbourhood dream: Involving Moroccan residents in a school-based community development process in urban Spain. *Soc. Cult. Geogr.* **2018**, 1–23. [CrossRef]

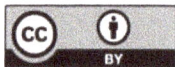

International Journal of
*Environmental Research
and Public Health*

MDPI

Article

Effectiveness of the TEI Program for Bullying and Cyberbullying Reduction and School Climate Improvement

Rosario Ferrer-Cascales [1], Natalia Albaladejo-Blázquez [1,*] , Miriam Sánchez-SanSegundo [1] ,
Irene Portilla-Tamarit [1], Oriol Lordan [2] and Nicolás Ruiz-Robledillo [1]

[1]   Department of Health Psychology, Faculty of Health Science, University of Alicante, 03690 Alicante, Spain;
       rosario.ferrer@ua.es (R.F.-C.); miriam.sanchez@ua.es (M.S.-S.S.); irene.portilla@ua.es (I.P.-T.);
       nicolas.ruiz@ua.es (N.R.-R.)
[2]   Management Department, Universitat Politècnica de Catalunya, 08222 Terrassa, Spain; oriol.lordan@upc.edu
*   Correspondence: natalia.albaladejo@ua.es; Tel.: +34-965-903-990

Received: 30 December 2018; Accepted: 14 February 2019; Published: 16 February 2019

Abstract: The increase in the prevalence of bullying and cyberbullying in recent years worldwide is undeniable. Although several intervention programs oriented towards the reduction of bullying and cyberbullying have been developed and implemented, significant disparities have been found regarding their efficacy. In most of the cases, the lack of the implementation of interventions involving all of the school community could be on the basis of this limited efficacy. The present study aimed to evaluate the effectiveness of the TEI Program, an intervention based on peer tutoring, in the reduction of bullying and cyberbullying, and in the improvement of school climate. The design of the study was quasi-experimental, in which 2057 Spanish students (aged 11 to 16 years) participated from 22 schools, and were randomly assigned to the experimental group (10 schools, 987 students) or the control group (12 schools, 1070 students). The obtained results showed a significant reduction in bullying behavior, peer victimization, fighting, cyberbullying and cybervictimization in the experimental group after the intervention implementation. Similarly, a significant improvement in factors of school climate was found only in this group. The obtained results demonstrated that the TEI program is effective in reducing bully and cyberbully behavior, and at the same time, improving the school climate.

Keywords: bullying; cyberbullying; school climate; intervention program

---

1. Introduction

Bullying and cyberbullying, as phenomena increasing in prevalence, are public health problems which entail severely negative consequences for health and quality of life, both for victims and perpetrators [1]. Researchers have found that between 40% and 55% of students in school are involved in some way of victimization (as victims, aggressors or observers), between 20% and 50% report experiences of verbal harassment and between 2% to 7% of students have been victims of a severe form of physical aggression [1,2]. Prevalence rates of bullying behaviors found in different countries vary widely depending on the ages of samples and the period of time over which information is requested [3]. For example, several studies have demonstrated that in Chinese societies school bullying behaviors varies widely according to samples of adolescents aged 10 to 18, which rank from 8% to 52% [4]. For cyberbullying, there are also variations in prevalence rates of self-reported victimization with rates of 55% in North America and Asia, 25% in Canada and 30% in Europe [3,5,6].

The global increase in prevalence in bullying and cyberbullying has supposed the basis of the development of a series of anti-bullying interventions, although some of them possess limited efficacy [7]. A recent meta-analysis has demonstrated that anti-bullying programs effectively reduce school-bullying perpetration by approximately 19–20%, and school-bullying victimization by approximately 15–16% [8]. Among the most significant protective factors against bullying and cyberbullying victimization, school climate, school safety and peer influence have been found to lower rates of victimization among peers [5]. School climate can be defined as the quality of the interactions between students, teachers, parents, and school staff, reflecting the norms, values, and goals that represent the educational and social missions of the school [9]. School and the relationships that adolescents establish in this context play an important role in socioemotional development during adolescence [10]. Some authors indicate that the promotion of safe schools through the improvement of school climate and those in which teachers, students and families are involved, with an active participation of the whole community should be part of the intervention programs oriented to the prevention and intervention of bullying [11,12]. However, these multicomponent programs have been less studied and the results to date are controversial [13]. Thus, while some studies have demonstrated positive results [12], other studies have failed to find a significant association. For example, in a metanalysis by Ttofi and Farrington [13], school-based interventions including work with peers did not demonstrate effectiveness in bullying reduction. The dichotomization of the analyzed variables and the lack of an exhaustive analysis of peer tutoring activities employed in the revised studies could explain these negative results [14]. Moreover, it is likely that this ambiguity in the obtained results is based on the specific characteristics of activities of peer tutoring programs, rather than the nature of the intervention. Given these controversial results, new studies are required to simultaneously identify the variables that could modulate this effectiveness, in which the school climate could play a main role [15].

In this study, we examined the effectiveness of the TEI program, a Spanish initiative for bullying and cyberbullying reduction based on the ecological model of peer tutoring in schools.

TEI Program "Peer Tutoring"

TEI program, acronyms that refer to the terms in Spanish *"Tutoría Entre Iguales"*, is a school-based intervention of peer-tutoring, oriented towards the prevention of school violence and cyberbullying, and designed for students of secondary education schooling. The main objective of this program is the improvement of the school climate and the promotion of a positive school coexistence through the development of adequate solving problem strategies and the integration of a culture of zero tolerance for violence as an identity school trait. The TEI program is based on an institutional intervention that entails the collaboration and commitment of the whole school community. It is designed on the basis of the Ecological Systems Theory of Bronfenbrenner [16], the principles of emotional intelligence theories from the studies of Salovey and Mayer [17] and Goleman [18]; and positive psychology [19]. The development and implementation of the intervention can be described as follows:

Stage 1: Dissemination and Awareness about the Intervention along the School Community

The beginning of the intervention program is based on the information about and dissemination of the principles of the program between all members of the school community (teachers, families and students). In this stage, the application of the intervention program is approved by the management team of the teaching center. During this stage, families receive information regarding the objectives and characteristics of the program by the TEI staff, a group of specialized education professionals involved in the development and implementation of TEI program in schools. Besides being informed, families are encouraged to be actively involved in the implementation of the program during the school year. Volunteer parents receive training on detection and action against harassment and victimization.

Stage 2: Teacher Training

The TEI staff develops an initial intensive training for teachers with a duration of 30 h (10 h in face-to-face format and 20 h in virtual format). During this educational training, teachers of the school create a TEI group of teachers and a coordinator is designated. This group is responsible for coordinating the implementation of the intervention in the school.

Stage 3: Student Tutors Training

Students tutors receive an initial training of 3 sessions lasting 1 h, based on the socioaffective method. The contents of this training are addressed to personal qualities of tutors, tutor functions, social abilities, prosocial behavior, empathy and problem-solving strategies. The TEI staff carry out 1 session of 1 h quarterly to follow up on the implementation of the intervention with student tutors. About 94% of students from all centers involved in the project were interested in participating as tutors. The rest of the students participated in the coordination by helping the teachers of the school involved in the program. The goal was that all students were involved in some way in the program.

Stage 4: Pairing Students

During this phase, the group of teachers who coordinate TEI implementation in the school created pairs of tutor-tutee, taking into account the age of the participants and the interpersonal skills. The maximus age difference between tutor and tutee was 2 years. Concerning to interpersonal skills, the students were classified by teachers on a likert scale of 1 to 3 (low, medium and high demand) points depending on the vulnerability or risk of harassment and the skills to help their peers. Students with high interpersonal skills were assigned as tutors of vulnerable younger students. Furthermore, an interview between tutors and tutees was conducted, and group dynamics during this session were developed to promote cooperativeness between them.

Stage 5: Intervention Development

This stage is based on the permanent training of the conformed pairs throughout three specific types of activities:

- Cohesion activities. The objective is to consolidate and facilitate the tutor-tutee relationship. 2 sessions are held per quarter during school hours.
- Tutorial activities. A formal tutoring is carried out each month between the tutor and tutee, as well as between tutors and program coordinators. In the same way, there are also informal tutorials that take place during recess, when leaving class, in the corridors, etc. The development of informal tutorials is highly promoted in the intervention program, taking into account that they are considered the main key to achieve the objectives of the intervention. The student tutor keeps a record of the informal tutorials carried out.
- Specific training activities. The program includes an intervention of 9 sessions lasting 1 h each, distributed throughout the academic year within the tutorial action plan. Each session is aimed towards the development of a specific skill. The methodology of the sessions is as follows: tutors present the skill to be worked and the specific activity to perform in class. Then, the activity is put into practice through specific tasks, and finally, tutors and tutees summarize the contents of the session by completing a mural or graphic poster in order to transfer the knowledge worked in the session to the whole school. The contents of the sessions are: emotional self-knowledge, emotional regulation, social competences and the positive use of ICTs.

Stage 6: Closing

A joint activity aimed to the diploma delivery accrediting participation in the TEI program to all involved agents (tutors, tutees, teaching staff and family volunteers) is performed at the end of the academic year.

Bearing all this in mind, the main aim of the present study is to evaluate the effectiveness of the TEI program reducing bullying and cyberbullying and promoting a positive school climate in schools. Following the results of the previous research regarding this issue, it has been hypothesized that the TEI program, based on peer tutoring, will be effective in the reduction of bullying and cyberbullying [12].

In the same way, it is expected that the application of this program in schools results in a school climate improvement [12].

2. Materials and Methods

2.1. Procedure

The sample was derived from a randomized small-scale trial of peer tutoring program in 22 public secondary education schools of Spain. The program and the battery of instruments used were presented and explained to the centers' management teams, who valued it positively. They presented it to each School Council as part of the Coexistence Project and Improvement Plan of the Educational Center who granted informed consent to participate in it. Secondary education schools were matched at baseline based on size and demographics to condition (i.e., intervention vs wait-list control). All procedures performed in the present study were in accordance with the ethical standards of the University of Alicante and the Educational Directive Committee from Schools involved in the study (Ref number: UA2015-1013).

The final sample included 2389 students who enrolled in the project in the fall of 2015. The inclusion criteria were: (1) presence in the classroom on the day of the survey; (2) ability to read and complete the questionnaires; (3) informed consent of parents and adolescents over 12 years of age before data collection. In total, 2057 students were included in the final analyses, since they had participated and completed phases T1 and T2 (86.1% of the initial sample) and their questionnaires could be correctly matched. The abandonment of just over three hundred and thirty-two students was mainly due to errors when completing the corresponding identification code that the students themselves had to create to guarantee their anonymity or absence on the day of data collection.

Students data collection was conducted in September-October 2015 (baseline, T1) using online surveys for the Experimental Group (EG) and Control Group (CG). Only students, teachers and families of the EG received the intervention. The second data collection (follow-up T2), took place after seven months, May-June 2016, a few weeks before the end of the same school year. Data for the CG were collected during the same period as for the EG.

2.2. Participants

Participants included 2057 students, of which 49.6 % (n = 1021) were female and 50.4 % (n = 1036) male. Participants ranged in age from 11 to 16 years at the beginning of the program, with a mean age of 13.08 (SD = 1.18). 987 students from 10 secondary education schools were assigned to the experimental group. A total of 496 students of third year of secondary education were tutors of 491 first year tutees; and 1070 students from 12 schools were assigned the control group. There were no significant differences between groups in gender (X^2 = 1.104, p = 0.29). However, in age, differences between groups were found (t = −2.962, p = 0.001). For that reason, age was controlled in the subsequent analyses as a covariate.

2.3. Measures

2.3.1. Bullying

The Illinois Bully Scale (20) is an 18 item, self-report measure that contains three subscales for measuring the frequency of fighting, peer victimization, and bully behavior. Students were asked to indicate how often in the past 30 days they have engaged in each behavior. Response options included "Never," "1 or 2 times," "3 or 4 times," "5 or 6 times," and "7 or more times." These response options allow the assessment of the persistence of the bullying. Higher scores indicate more self-reported bullying behaviors. The Spanish version of the Illinois Bully Scale in the present study was found to be a reliable and valid measure of bullying behavior showing a factor structure that fit indices in Spanish adolescents with a Kaiser-Meyer-Olkin index and Barlett sfericity (KMO = 0.906; χ^2 = 16,994.404;

gl = 153; p = 0.00) explaining the 58.01% of variance. While the confirmatory factor analysis obtains optimal adjustment indices χ^2 = 521.377; RMSEA = 0.041; SRMR = 0.029; CFI = 0.976; GFI = 0.973; NNFI = 0.968; and RFI = 0.959 according to Hu and Bentler [20]. Internal consistency (Cronbach's alpha) for each factor in the sample analyzed in this study was good: bully behavior (α = 0.89); peer victimization (α = 0.75) and frequency of fighting (α = 0.76).

2.3.2. Cyberbullying

Cyberbullying was evaluated employing the E-Victimization Scale (E-VS) and E-Bullying Scale (E-BS) [21]. These scales identify bullies and victims of bullying that use electronic devices and ICTs developed for youth. The E-VS includes 5 items, while the E-BS is composed of 6 items, all of them introduced by the sentence: "In the last 7 days ... " Students are asked to indicate the frequency (from 0 to 6 or more times) of which they have suffered (E-VS) or have inflicted (E-BS) certain behaviors via ICTs. Given this scale were not available for the wider Spanish population, we followed the international standards published by the International Test Commission, using the translation-back-translation process [22,23]. In the validation these scales show their suitability in the exploratory factor analysis with a Kaiser-Meyer-Olkin index and Barlett sfericity (KMO = 0.856; χ^2 = 9960.413; gl = 55; p = 0.001) explaining the 58.65% of variance. The confirmatory factor analysis obtains optimal adjustment indices χ^2 = 169.689; RMSEA = 0.039; SRMR = 0.024; CFI = 0.986; GFI = 0.985; NNFI = 0.981; and RFI = 0.975 according to Hu and Bentler [24]. Internal consistency (Cronbach's alpha) for each factor in the analyzed sample in this study was good: E-VS (α = 0.85) and E-BS (α = 0.80).

2.3.3. School Climate

The Spanish version of the school climate questionnaire has been previously validated for evaluating the quality of school climate in Spanish high-schools, showing adequate psychometric properties in this context [25]. The overall instrument is composed of 49 items, grouped into 10 subscales ranked on a 4-point Likert scale. In the present study we only included four subscales assessing Satisfaction with school (8 items), Sense of belonging (5 items), Cooperation (3 items), and Communication between family and school (6 items). These subscales have showed good reliability coefficients, with alpha Cronbach values ranking from α = 0.88 for Satisfaction; α = 0.75 for Sense of belonging; α = 0.76 for Cooperation; and α = 0.85 for Communication between family and school.

2.4. Data Analysis

For the analyses, scores of participants from the EG and CG in each of the evaluated variables were employed. First, T-test comparison between EG and CG were employed to analyse possible differences in baseline between groups. Effect size estimation was also computed for each pair of variables using Cohen's definitions (1988). ANCOVA of repeated measures of 'moment' (T1 pre-intervention vs T2 post-intervention) with 'group' (participants from the EG vs participants from the CG) as between-subject factor was performed to analyze the effectiveness of the intervention reducing bullying and cyberbullying, and improving school climate. For significant results, partial eta-squared (η^2) was reported as a measure of the effect size [26]. Furthermore, the percentage change between scores from T1 to T2 was calculated following this formula: [(T2 − T1/T1)]*100. As has been previously indicated, age was introduced in the analyses as a covariate. All statistical analyses were performed using SPSS (International Business Machines Corporation (IBM), Armonk, NY, USA), Statistics for Windows, Version 23.0, considering p < 0.05 to be significant. The descriptive values are expressed as mean and standard deviation (M and SD, respectively).

3. Results

3.1. Descriptive Statistics in T1 and T2 for the Both Groups (EG and CG) and Percentage Change for Bullying, Cyberbullying and School Climate

Regarding bullying and cyberbullying, the conducted analyses did not revealed significant differences between the EG and the CG in baseline scores (T1) for bully behavior (t = 1.57, p = 0.11; Cohen's d = 0.06), peer victimization (t = −0.55, p = 0.57; Cohen's d= 0.02), fighting (t = 0.68, p = 0.49; Cohen's d = 0.03), cyberbullying (t = 1.40, p = 0.16; Cohen's d = 0.06) or cybervictimization (t = 1.11, p = 0.26; Cohen's d = 0.04). With regard to school climate, no differences were found between groups in satisfaction (t = −1.21, p = 0.22; Cohen's d = −0.05), sense of belonging (t = 1.41, p = 0.15; Cohen's d = 0.06), cooperation (t = −1.33, p = 0.18; Cohen's d = −0.05) and communication between family and school (t = −1.12, p = 0.25; Cohen's d = − 0.04), measured at baseline (Table 1).

Table 1. Mean and Standard Deviation (T1-T2) and percentage change by groups.

Variable	Scale	Condition EG (*n* = 987) CG (*n* = 1070)	Mean (SD) T1	Mean (SD) T2	Percentage Change
Bullying	Bully behavior	EG	3.80 (5.76)	3.37 (4.68)	−11.31%
		CG	3.44 (4.51)	4.80 (5.92)	39.53%
	Peer victimization	EG	2.05 (2.93)	1.93 (2.84)	−5.85%
		CG	1.97 (2.94)	2.64 (3.50)	34.01%
	Fighting	EG	1.83 (2.89)	1.76 (2.84)	−3.82%
		CG	1.74 (2.81)	2.52 (3.62)	44.82%
Cyberbullying	Cyberbullying	EG	2.27 (3.10)	1.59 (3.80)	−29.95%
		CG	2.08 (3.13)	2.21 (4.48)	6.25%
	Cyber victimization	EG	3.19 (4.82)	1.94 (4.51)	−39.18%
		CG	2.95 (5.10)	2.70 (5.30)	−8.47%
School climate	Satisfaction	EG	17.20 (4.65)	18.08 (4.78)	5.11%
		CG	17.46 (4.98)	17.17 (4.68)	−1.66%
	Sense of belonging	EG	6.92 (2.50)	11 (2.82)	58.95%
		CG	6.76 (2.60)	8.94 (2.98)	32.24%
	Cooperation	EG	5.86 (2.)	7.51 (1.61)	28.32%
		CG	5.98 (1.99)	5.91 (2.06)	−1.66%
	Communication between family and school	EG	13.65 (3.47)	15.98 (2.45)	17.06%
		CG	13.82 (3.62)	13.12 (3.29)	−5.06%

The results regarding the impact of the TEI program on the prevalence of the different variables showed different percentage variations in CG and EG. Table 1 shows how the involvement in bully/victimization and cyberbullying/cybervictimization decreased over time only in EG; while the school climate subscales mostly increased in the students who participated in the peer tutoring program.

3.2. Effectiveness of the Intervention in Bullying Reduction

The obtained results show a significant effect of the interaction group*time for Bully behavior ($F_{(1, 20)}$ = 30.973; p = 0.00; η^2 = 0.015), Peer victimization ($F_{(1, 20)}$ = 15.299; p = 0.00; η^2 = 0.007) and Fighting ($F_{(1, 20)}$ = 19.552; p = 0.00; η^2 = 0.009). As previously indicated, age was introduced in the model as a covariate, but did not reach statistical significance for Bully behaviors ($F_{(1, 20)}$ = 9.389;

$p = 0.256$), Peer victimization ($F_{(1, 20)} = 0.2$; $p = 0.644$), Fighting ($F_{(1, 20)} = 0.318$; $p = 0.573$). The values of the Bully behavior, Peer victimization and Fighting subscales decreased significantly from T1 to T2 only in the students who participated in the TEI intervention program, finding statistically significant differences between the EG and CG in T2 ($p = 0.001$) (see Figures 1–3).

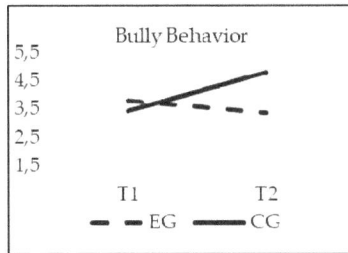

Figure 1. Interaction effects of group (EG-CG) and time (T1-T2) in Bully Behavior.

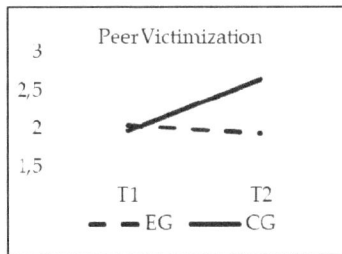

Figure 2. Interaction effects of group (EG-CG) and time (T1-T2) in Peer Victimization.

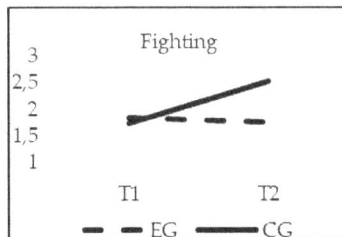

Figure 3. Interaction effects of group (EG-CG) and time (T1-T2) in Fighting.

3.3. Effectiveness of the Intervention in Cyberbullying Reduction

With respect to Cyberbullying, a significant interaction effect of group*time was found for Cyberbullying (E-Bullying Scale) ($F_{(1, 20)} = 12.382$; $p = 0.000$; $\eta^2 = 0.006$), and Cybervictimization (E-Victimization Scale) ($F_{(1, 20)} = 9.516$; $p = 0.002$; $\eta^2 = 0.005$). When age was introduced in the model as a covariate, no significant statistical effects of this variable were found for Cyberbullying ($F_{(1, 20)} = 2.733$; $p = 0.098$) or Cybervictimization ($F_{(1, 20)} = 0.435$; $p = 0.510$). As it can be seen in Figures 4 and 5, in the CG the scores were similar from T1 to T2 ($p > 0.05$). However, in the EG the scores were significantly lower in the T2 phase, finding statistically significant differences between the EG and the CG in T2 ($p = 0.001$).

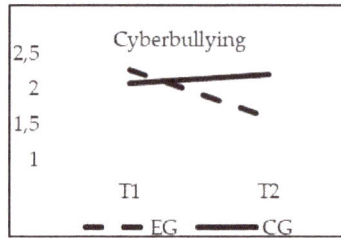

Figure 4. Interaction effects of group (EG-CG) and time (T1-T2) in Cyberbullying (E-Bullying Scale).

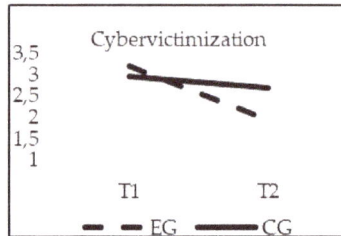

Figure 5. Interaction effects of group (EG-CG) and time (T1-T2) in Cybervictimization (E-Victimization Scale).

3.4. Effectiveness of the Intervention in School Climate Improvement

The analyses of differences regarding School Climate showed a significant effect of the interaction group*time in Satisfaction ($F_{(1, 20)}$ = 16.818; p = 0.000; η^2 = 0.008); Sense of belonging ($F_{(1, 20)}$ = 126.234; p = 0.00; η^2 = 0.058); Cooperation ($F_{(1, 20)}$ = 195.768; p = 0.00; η^2 = 0.089) and Communication between family and school ($F_{(1, 20)}$ = 233.528; p = 0.00; η^2 = 0.102). As in the previous cases, when age was introduced in the model as a covariate, this variable did not reach statistical significance in any of the variables of the School Climate: Satisfaction ($F_{(1, 20)}$ = 2.056; p = 0.152), Sense of belonging ($F_{(1, 20)}$ = 2.515; p = 0.113), Cooperation ($F_{(1, 20)}$ = 2.132; p = 0.4), and Communication between family and school ($F_{(1, 20)}$ = 1.853; p = 0.174). Although the EG and CG obtained similar scores in all of the subscales of the School Climate questionnaire in T1 (p > 0.05), only the experimental group significantly increased their scores in all variables of school climate in T2, finding statistically significant differences between groups at this moment (p = 0.001) (Figures 6–9).

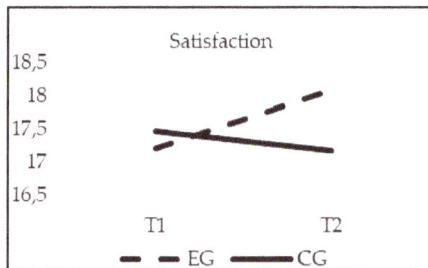

Figure 6. Interaction effects of group (EG-CG) and time (T1-T2) in Satisfaction.

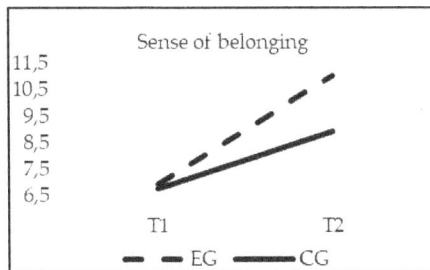

Figure 7. Interaction effects of group (EG-CG) and time (T1-T2) in Sense of belonging.

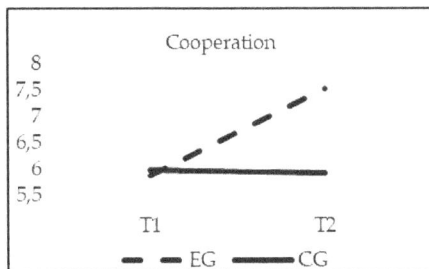

Figure 8. Interaction effects of group (EG-CG) and time (T1-T2) Cooperation.

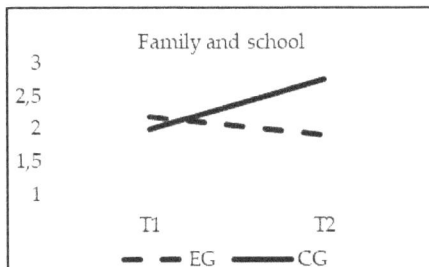

Figure 9. Interaction effects of group (EG-CG) and time (T1-T2) in Communication between family and school.

4. Discussion

The present study aimed at the evaluation the effectiveness of the TEI Program in the reduction of bullying and cyberbullying, and the improvement of school climate in a sample of adolescents. Our results suggest that the Spanish TEI program may be effective for improving school climate factors including satisfaction with the school, sense of belonging, cooperation and positive communication between family and school. These factors were positively related to low rates of fighting, bullying and cyberbullying victimization.

The TEI program is based on its highly organized proposal, the involvement of all members of the educational community in the intervention and the development of a set of specific materials and activities that could be adapted to the school needs and context. Different training activities are carried out, paying special attention to the formal and informal tutorials that the students will participate in with other students and with the coordinator. In this sense, as previously indicated, the program puts a lot of emphasis on informal tutorials, which are considered as the key element to achieve the objectives of the intervention by generating a real and informal support network between students. These actions generate an environment where cooperation, communication and negotiation are highly promoted, giving voice and space to the students and to the whole educational community. Thanks to this, members of the school community could manifest openly their personal needs, creating situations of social learning in the school environment. In this context, students listen to each other, detect possible situations of interpersonal conflict or harassment and empathize with peers in difficult situations. In this way, students are empowered in order to develop a feeling of coexistence in which violence has no place.

Contrary to previous research in which interventions based on peer tutoring did not demonstrate effectiveness in the reduction of bullying among schools [13], this research pointed out how programs created following this theoretical approach could be useful for this aim. As has been explained by Cowie and others [27,28], peer-tutoring could be an excellent tool for violence reduction in schools by promoting an increase of self-perception and introspection abilities in students, while interpersonal, social and conflict resolution skills are trained. The increase of befriending, mediation skills and active listening have been proposed as the main mechanisms that could be on the basis of violence reduction in schools communities which implement peer-tutoring interventions [27]. This fact entails the development of a caring school community in which violence has no place. Unlike other type of programs in which the intervention of teachers is more directive and invasive, peer-tutoring gives responsibility to students, an approach that ethological studies of conflict resolutions have demonstrated to be the best strategy [27]. Furthermore, this intervention approach has benefits for the whole community, but fundamentally, for tutors and tutees. In a classic study aimed to identify positive results of peer tutoring both for tutors and tutees, the author identified that after the peer tutoring intervention, tutors had more self-confidence, developed a higher grade of responsibility and experienced an increase of their feelings of belonging to the school community [29]. Furthermore, peer tutoring usually improved their self-esteem, as they assumed the responsibility of doing something that contributed to the improvement of their school environment. The reasons that they indicated for these changes were based on the interpersonal and prosocial behavior training that they received, mainly active listening. For tutees and possible victims, the program gives them the possibility of communicating what happens to them or having favorable interlocutors to transmit it, since tutors are peers that are willing to help and are usually in a better social position in the school [30]. Aggressors are also influenced by the intervention, because their performance and the environment generated by peer tutoring forces them to perceive, evaluate and become aware about the acts they carry out and the negative consequences of harming their peers. Witnesses of bullying are also affected, so the capacity of reflection regarding violence is fostered in the program, and they are more aware of every form of abuse, even those may be more hidden or unnoticed, adopting a more active behavior in situations of bullying and cyberbullying [30].

All of these results derived from peer tutoring interventions are clearly opposed to the development and maintenance of school violence, so they could be proposed as possible mechanisms explaining the effectiveness of the TEI program in violence reduction. Therefore, the development of prosocial and altruistic behaviors, the instruction regarding problems solving strategies such as active listening and the promotion of empathy towards peers could be on the basis of the effectiveness of peer tutoring programs. However, this type of interventions is oriented towards the whole school community, and for that reason, other complementary explanations should be addressed, putting the focus on global variables, such as school climate. The improvement of school climate could be one of the underlying mechanisms of the positive obtained results regarding the efficacy of TEI program on bullying and cyberbullying. In this sense, significant improvements have been found in all of the variables that characterized this construct. Probably, one of the main mechanisms explaining the effectiveness of the proposed intervention program could be based on the demonstrated improvement of the school climate in the experimental group. Recent research has demonstrated that school climate has direct impacts on bullying. A school in which student feels safe, comfortable and engaged with the community will probably show lower rates of bullying, as demonstrated in previous research [15]. In our study, the students who received the intervention exhibited significant improvements in general satisfaction with the school, as a significant increase of engagement feelings, cooperation between students and communication between families and the school. It is likely that the intervention program could promote a better school climate characterized by the promotion of better school connectedness. Defined as the sense of belonging, attachment, and bonding, a school climate in which students receive positive social support from their peers and teachers increases their academic engagement and could reduce their risk of violent behaviors, such as bullying [15]. The perception of school connection and caring relationships with peers, teachers and school staff, feeling socially connected and supported, could prevent the phenomenon of peer violence in school.

Although the present study entails a significant advance in the comprehension of the effectiveness of anti-bullying interventions based on peer-tutoring in the bullying and cyberbullying reduction, some limitations of the research should be pointed out. First, the use of self-report measures, with the inherent bias of social desirability, is a limitation of the study. Future studies should include hetero-report measures in which parents and teachers discuss adolescent attitudes and behaviors and/or observational techniques to assess and ratify the program's effects. Second, the procedure of the study covered only two assessment times, pre and post-intervention. Due to the controversial results obtained in previous research regarding the long-term effects of school-based interventions for bullying reduction, it would be recommendable to have a longitudinal follow up after the end of the program. This fact will be addressed by future studies, throughout the evaluation of the long-term effectiveness of the TEI program. Moreover, participants of the present study are students from a specific location in Spain, which could be a limitation for the generalization of the obtained results. Future studies should address this issue by replicating the present study internationally. In any case, despite the aforementioned limitations, the design of the study was quasi-experimental, with a randomized sample, which has been identified as the best procedure to explore the effectiveness of school-based interventions. Furthermore, the sample is large in both groups, and the main types of school violence have been evaluated, bullying and cyberbullying, demonstrating the effectiveness of TEI program for the reduction of both, and for the improvement of school climate.

5. Conclusions

The peer tutoring program analyzed in this research has an institutional character that involves the entire educational community, generating a creation of a culture of peaceful coexistence and non-violence in schools, fostering greater emotional education and more satisfactory relations between peers. In this way, the prevention, detection and intervention of situations of violence between peers by students is highly promoted, as is the main objective of the intervention program. Recalling that bullying and cyberbullying are one of the main public health problems affecting adolescents and their families, the necessity of developing and implementing effective interventions in schools is extremely urgent. To our knowledge, this is the first study seeking to analyze the effectiveness of TEI program reducing bullying and cyberbullying and improving school climate among Spanish students. In this regard, the present research demonstrates that the TEI program is an effective and useful intervention program to be applied in schools, in order to prevent and reduce school violence. This fact highlights the importance of implementing interventions based on peer tutoring programs, as its efficacy has been widely demonstrated in previous research [14,31,32]. In this sense, the TEI program could be a useful tool for educators and clinicians who work in school environments and for professionals in need of validated and efficient intervention strategies for the reduction of all forms of school violence.

Author Contributions: Conceived and designed the experiments: R.F.-C., N.R.-R., N.A-B., M.S.-S.; Analyzed the data: N.A-B., O.L., R.F.-C., I.P.-T. Wrote the paper: R.F.-C., N.R.-R., N.A-B., I.P.-T., M.S.-S.; Data interpretation and critical revision of manuscript: R.F.-C., N.R.-R., N.A-B., I.P.-T., M.S.-S.; and all authors reviewed and approved the manuscript.

Funding: This study was funded by the Office of the Vice President of Research and Knowledge Transfer of the University of Alicante (GRE-16-32).

Acknowledgments: We want to thank the TEI Program Team from the University of Barcelona and especially Andrés González Bellido, coordinator and author of the program. Additionally, we want to thank all the students, trainers, and school staff for their involvement in this study.

Conflicts of Interest: The authors declare no conflict of interest.

References

1. Menesini, E.; Salmivalli, C. Bullying in schools: The state of knowledge and effective interventions. *Psychol. Health Med.* **2017**, *22*, 240–253. [CrossRef] [PubMed]
2. Chan, H.C.; Wong, D.S.W. Traditional school bullying and cyberbullying in Chinese societies: Prevalence and a review of the whole-school intervention approach. *Aggress. Violent Behav.* **2015**, *23*, 98–108. [CrossRef]
3. Garaigordobil, M. Prevalencia y consecuencias del cyberbullying: Una revisión. *Int. J. Psychol. Psychol. Ther.* **2011**, *11*, 233–254.
4. Chan, H.C.; Wong, D.S.W. Traditional school bullying and cyberbullying perpetration: Examining the psychosocial characteristics of Hong Kong male and female adolescents. *Youth Soc.* **2019**, *51*, 3–29. [CrossRef]
5. Zych, I.; Farrington, D.P.; Llorent, V.J.; Ttofi, M.M. *Protecting children against bullying and its consequences*; Springer: Basel, Switzerland, 2017.
6. Wong, D.S.W.; Chan, H.C.O.; Cheng, C.H.K. Cyberbullying perpetration and victimization among adolescents in Hong Kong. *Child Youth Serv. Rev.* **2014**, *36*, 133–140. [CrossRef]
7. Cantone, E.; Piras, A.P.; Vellante, M.; Preti, A.; Daníelsdóttir, S.; D'Aloja, E.; Lesinskiene, S.; Angermeyer, M.C.; Carta, M.G.; Bhugra, D. Interventions on bullying and cyberbullying in schools: A systematic review. *Clin. Pract. Epidemiol. Ment. Health* **2015**, *11*, 58–76. [PubMed]
8. Gaffney, H.; Ttofi, M.M.; Farrington, D.P. Evaluating the effectiveness of school-bullying prevention programs: An updated meta-analytical review. *Aggress. Violent Behav.* **2018**. [CrossRef]
9. Wang, M.-T.; Degol, J.L. School Climate: A Review of the construct, measurement, and impact on student outcomes. *Educ. Psychol. Rev.* **2016**, *28*, 315–352. [CrossRef]
10. Kidger, J.; Araya, R.; Donovan, J.; Gunnell, D. The effect of the school environment on the emotional health of adolescents: A systematic review. *Pediatrics* **2012**, *129*, 925–949. [CrossRef]
11. Silva, J.L.D.; Oliveira, W.A.; Mello, F.C.M.; Andrade, L.S.; Bazon, M.R.; Silva, M.A.I. Anti-bullying interventions in schools: A systematic literature review. *Cienc Saude Coletiva* **2017**, *22*, 2329–2340. [CrossRef]
12. Cowie, H.; Smith, P. Peer support as a means of improving school safety and reducing bullying and violence. In *Handbook of Youth Prevention Science*; Routledge: New York, NY, USA, 2010.
13. Ttofi, M.M.; Farrington, D.P. Effectiveness of school-based programs to reduce bullying: A systematic and meta-analytic review. *J. Exp. Criminol.* **2011**, *7*, 27–56. [CrossRef]
14. Smith, P.K.; Salmivalli, C.; Cowie, H. Effectiveness of school-based programs to reduce bullying: A commentary. *J. Exp. Criminol.* **2012**, *8*, 433–441. [CrossRef]
15. Hong, J.S.; Espelage, D.L.; Lee, J.M. School climate and bullying prevention programs. In *The Wiley Handbook on Violence*; Education John Wiley & Sons, Ltd.: Hoboken, NJ, USA, 2018.
16. Bronfenbrenner, U. Contexts of child rearing: Problems and prospects. *Am. Psychol.* **1979**, *34*, 844–850. [CrossRef]
17. Salovey, P.; Mayer, J.D. Emotional intelligence. *Imagin. Cogn. Personal* **1990**, *9*, 185–211. [CrossRef]
18. Goleman, D. *Emotional Intelligence: Why It Can Matter More Than IQ for Character, Health and Lifelong Achievement*; Bantam Books: New York, NY, USA, 1995.
19. Seligman, M.E.; Csikszentmihalyi, M. Positive psychology: An introduction. *Am. Psychol.* **2000**, *55*, 5–14. [CrossRef]
20. Hu, L.; Bentler, P.M. Cutoff criteria for fit indexes in covariance structure analysis: Conventional criteria versus new alternatives. *Struct. Equ. Model Multidiscip. J.* **1999**, *6*, 1–55. [CrossRef]
21. Lam, L.T.; Li, Y. The validation of the E-Victimisation Scale (E-VS) and the E-Bullying Scale (E-BS) for adolescents. *Comput. Hum. Behav.* **2013**, *29*, 3–7. [CrossRef]
22. Hambleton, R.K.; Merenda, P.F.; Spielberger, C.D. *Adapting educational and psychological tests for Cross-Cultural Assessment*; Psychology Press: Mahwah, NJ, USA, 2005.
23. Muñiz, J.; Elosua, P.; Hambleton, R.K. International test commission guidelines for test translation and adaptation: Second edition. *Psicothema* **2013**, *25*, 151–157. [PubMed]

24. Espelage, D.L.; Holt, M.K. Bullying and victimization during early adolescence. *J. Emot. Abuse* **2001**, *2*, 123–142. [CrossRef]

25. Diaz-Aguado, M.J.; Martínez-Arias, R.; Martín-Babarro, J. Observatorio estatal de la violencia escolar. Estudio estatal sobre la convivencia escolar en la educación secundaria obligatoria. [State study on school coexistence in compulsory secondary education]. Spanish Ministry of Education, 2010. Available online: https://sede.educacion.gob.es/publiventa/d/13567/19/0 (accessed on 30 December 2018).

26. Richardson, J.T.E. Eta squared and partial eta squared as measures of effect size in educational research. *Educ. Res. Rev.* **2011**, *6*, 135–137. [CrossRef]

27. Cowie, H. Peer support as an intervention to counteract school bullying: Listen to the children: Bullying: The moral and social orders at play. *Child Soc.* **2011**, *25*, 287–292. [CrossRef]

28. Smith, P.K.; Watson, D. *An Evaluation of the Childline in Partnership with Schools (CHIPS) Programme*; DfES publications: London, UK, 2004.

29. Cowie, H. Perspectives of teachers and pupils on the experience of peer support against bullying. *Educ. Res. Eval.* **1998**, *4*, 108–125. [CrossRef]

30. Cowie, H.; Oztug, O. Pupils' perceptions of safety at school. *Pastor. Care Educ.* **2008**, *26*, 59–67. [CrossRef]

31. Ortega, R.; Lera, M.-J. The Seville anti-bullying in school project. *Aggress. Behav.* **2000**, *26*, 113–123. [CrossRef]

32. Cartwright, N. Setting up and sustaining peer support systems in a range of schools over 20 years. *Pastor. Care Educ.* **2005**, *23*, 45–50. [CrossRef]

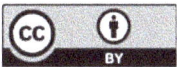

International Journal of
*Environmental Research
and Public Health*

MDPI

Article

Effects of Intervention Program Prev@cib on Traditional Bullying and Cyberbullying

Jessica Ortega-Barón [1,*], Sofía Buelga [2], Ester Ayllón [3], Belén Martínez-Ferrer [4] and María-Jesús Cava [2]

[1] Faculty of Education, Department of Psychology of Education and Psychobiology, International University of la Rioja (UNIR), Avenida de la Paz, 137, 26006 Logroño, Spain
[2] Faculty of Psychology, Department Social Psychology, University of Valencia, Avda Blasco Ibañez, 21, 46010 Valencia, Spain; sofia.buelga@uv.es (S.B.); Maria.J.Cava@uv.es (M.-J.C.)
[3] Faculty of Human Sciences and Education, Department of Psychology and Sociology, University of Zaragoza, Valentín Carderera, 4, 22003 Huesca, Spain; eayllon@unizar.es
[4] Faculty of Social Sciences, Department of Education and Social Psychology, University Pablo Olavide, 41013 Sevilla, Spain; bmarfer2@upo.es
* Correspondence: jessica.ortega@unir.net; Tel.: +34-96-386-45-75

Received: 27 December 2018; Accepted: 11 February 2019; Published: 13 February 2019

Abstract: Due to the negative consequences of being bullied and the increase in cyberbullying among adolescents, there is a need for evidence-based programs to prevent and intervene in these types of peer violence. The aim of this study was to evaluate the effectiveness of the Prev@cib bullying and cyberbullying program, drawing on three theoretical frameworks: the ecological model, empowerment theory, and the model of personal and social responsibility. The Prev@cib program was evaluated using a repeated-measures pre-post-test design with an experimental group and a control group. The sample consisted of 660 adolescents between 12 and 17 years old ($M = 13.58$, $SD = 1.26$), randomly assigned to the experimental and control groups. Repeated-measures ANOVA of pre-post-test scores were conducted. Results showed a significant decrease in bullying and victimization and cyberbullying and cybervictimization in the experimental group, compared to the control group, indicating that the Prev@cib program is effective in reducing bullying and cyberbullying. Taking into account the harmful effects of these types of violence, the results have important implications in the prevention of these behaviors because they provide scientific evidence of the program's effectiveness.

Keywords: bullying; cyberbullying; prevention program; Prev@cib; adolescents

1. Introduction

1.1. Bullying and Cyberbullying

Information and communication technologies have many advantages for adolescents, allowing them to have unlimited access to all types of information and fostering interactions with peers at any place and time [1,2]. However, these tools have enabled new forms of violence, such as cyberbullying, to emerge [3,4]. Cyberbullying is defined as intentional and aggressive behavior repeated frequently over a period of time through the use (by an individual or group) of electronic devices against a victim who cannot easily defend him/herself [5].

Bullying and cyberbullying have some features in common, such as the imbalance of power between the victim and the aggressor and the intentionality and repetition of the violent behavior [6,7]. These similarities lead some authors to consider cyberbullying to be a modality of traditional bullying [8–10]. In fact, numerous studies have found continuity between school bullying and cyberbullying [11–13], justified by the connection between the offline and online environments [14]. Thus, the study by Hinduja & Patchin (2010) [15] showed that over 60% of adolescents were involved in both forms of bullying. Therefore, it is common for aggressors emerging in the classroom to continue this behavior elsewhere through the smartphone and Internet.

This continued bullying in offline and online settings seems to produce a high level of psychological distress and behavior problems in the victim [10,16], as well as strong feelings of anxiety, depression, fear, nervousness, irritability, somatizations, sleep disorders, and concentration difficulties [17,18]. Victims of bullying and cyberbullying are more likely to have suicidal ideations and make suicide attempts [15,19], which also negatively affect the family and social environment [20–22]. Bullies and cyberbullies also experience negative consequences that can persist in adult life. Different studies have shown that bullying and/or cyberbullying aggressors have greater depression symptoms, break the rules more, consume more drugs, have a more negative attitude toward authority figures, and participate more in violent and criminal behaviors in other areas of their lives [23,24]. Additionally, increased awareness and reporting of mental health problems that may stem from bullying justify the importance of designing and implementing anti-bullying programs during adolescence [25].

1.2. Intervention Programs in Bullying and Cyberbullying

Due to the social concern about bullying and cyberbullying, numerous programs have been developed to prevent and intervene in these two modalities of peer violence [26–28]. Most of these programs have focused specifically on bullying or cyberbullying. For example, the Olweus Bullying Prevention Program [29] and Social Skills Training [30] are designed to reduce and prevent bullying and victimization. In addition, some antibullying interventions have included other psychosocial variables, such as empathy, self-esteem, or sensitivity towards the victims [31,32], which are understood as resources that prevent and reduce school bullying. Other antibullying programs have been designed to reduce bullying, but were also found to be useful for reducing cyberbullying, such as the Kiva program [33] and the ViSC Social Competence Program [34].

In general, previous meta-analyses and systematic reviews have provided little scientific evidence about the effectiveness of bullying and cyberbullying interventions [35–37]. In fact, compared to bullying programs, few programs that focus specifically on cyberbullying have been experimentally assessed. Some programs that have shown positive effects in preventing and reducing cyberbullying are the Tabby Improved Program [38] and the Cyber Friendly Schools Project [39]. The majority of the programs focused on cyberbullying work on both types of bullying, for example, The Media Heroes Cyberbullying Prevention Program [40] and the Cyberprogram 2.0 [41]. The authors of these programs consider cyberbullying and bullying to be closely linked, making it crucial to address these two problems together.

In sum, due to the great social relevance that cyberbullying is acquiring worldwide, it is fundamental to develop anti-cyber(bullying) programs that are clearly grounded in theoretical frameworks and experimentally tested.

1.3. Prev@cib Program

Prev@cib is based on three theoretical frameworks: the ecological model [42], empowerment theory [43], and the personal and social responsibility model by Hellison (1995) [44]. First, regarding the ecological model, several individual, microsocial, and contextual risk and protection factors related to traditional bullying and cyberbullying were taken into account [42]. Although the Prev@cib program is focused on students, we conducted a course to train teachers in how to implement the program. In this context, we took the teachers' opinions and comments into account throughout the implementation of the Prev@cib program. Second, in order to offer adolescents tools and resources to use when facing this type of problem, this program also draws on empowerment theory [43]. According to this theory, individual, group, and community resources are strengthened as a basic strategy to allow adolescents to control their lives in both the virtual and school environments. In this regard, the

Prev@cib program offers different resources and coping strategies to better deal with the problem of bullying and cyberbullying. Third, this program is also based on the personal and social responsibility model by Hellison (1995) [44], which argues that responsible behaviors can be taught and generalized to other contexts in life. This theory is used to encourage the idea of shared responsibility in the problems of bullying and cyberbullying, in order to achieve adolescents' greater involvement in their prevention and reduction. Based on this theory, in Module 3, the Prev@cib program focuses on the importance of involving all the students in solving and impeding peer bullying and cyberbullying.

Grounded in this theoretical foundation, the Prev@cib consists of 10 one-hour sessions distributed in three modules: information, awareness, and involvement (Table 1).

- Module 1. Information about risk and prevention factors in the bullying and cyberbullying problem. This module also includes information about sexting and grooming. In fact, some studies have found evidence of a relationship between cyberbullying and sexting and cybergrooming [16,45]. The module consists of four sessions designed to provide adolescents with information about the characteristics, types, and risk factors associated with these problems. In this way, the adolescents increase their awareness and detection of the existing dangers, especially in the virtual world. They are also taught strategies to protect themselves on the Internet and avoid becoming involved in potential cyberbullying problems.
- Module 2. Awareness and sensitization about cyberbullying. This consists of two sessions designed to make the participants aware of and sensitive to the harm and negative consequences of peer violence, both in school and through technologies. It is important for adolescents to understand the harmful consequences of school and cybernetic violence, in order to foster changes at cognitive, behavioral, and attitudinal levels and prevent and reduce this peer abuse at school and online.
- Module 3. Involvement in and commitment to prevention and intervention in cyberbullying. This module is composed of four sessions designed to encourage students' involvement in and commitment to preventing and acting on this problem. In this regard, an emphasis is placed on the role of all the students in stopping and preventing the appearance and continuance of bullying. Thus, in the classroom, a climate of respect is fostered, so that no type of violence is tolerated among the adolescents in the school or virtual environment.

Table 1. Sessions of the Prev@cib program.

	Modules	Sessions
	Module 1. Information	Session 1. My life is a display window Session 2. Bullying and cyberbullying Session 3. Sexting and grooming Session 4. Cyber-protection
	Module 2. Awareness	Session 5. Consequences and we are all responsible Session 6. What if you were the victim?
	Module 3. Involvement	Session 7. What to do when faced with bullying? Session 8. (Cyber)helpers Session 9. I like myself, I like you Session 10. No more bullying

In addition to these 10 intervention sessions, the program contains two other one-hour sessions to experimentally evaluate the effects of the program (pre-test and post-test).

To implement this program, the recommendations of Garaigordobil and Martínez-Valderrey (2014) [41] were followed, regarding: inter-session constancy (the same interval between one session and another); time-space constancy (all the sessions held at the same time and in the same classroom, whenever possible); constancy in the person who implements the program (the same person administers all the sessions); and constancy in the session structure (same session structure, even though the contents and activities carried out may differ).

Taking into account the need for evaluations of programs focused on bullying and cyberbullying prevention, the main aim of the present study is to evaluate and test the effectiveness of the Prev@cib program on (cyber)bullying and (cyber)victimization among adolescent students. Specifically, the hypotheses are: (1) after the program, the intervention group will obtain lower scores on violent school behavior than the control group; (2) the intervention group will obtain lower scores on school victimization than the control group; (3) the intervention group will obtain lower scores on cyberbullying than the control group; and (4) the intervention group will obtain lower scores on cybervictimization than the control group.

2. Materials and Methods

2.1. Study Design and Participants

To evaluate the effects of the Prev@cib program, a repeated-measures (pre-test and post-test) quasi-experimental design was used with an experimental group and a control group. Initially, the sample was composed of 692 adolescents. Thirty-two participants were eliminated (4.63% of the sample) because they did not correctly fill out the questionnaires or because they missed more than one session of the Prev@cib program.

The final participants in the Prev@cib program were 660 adolescents (53.2% girls and 46.8% boys) between 12 and 17 years old ($M = 13.58$, $SD = 1.26$). The participants belonged to 35 classes from four high schools (compulsory secondary education) in Valencia (Spain). Of them, 28.8 percent were in 7th grade, 32 percent were in 8th grade, 21.5 percent were 9th grade, and 17.5 percent were in 10th grade.

As Table 2 shows, 434 students (24 classes) participated in the experimental group, and 236 students (11 classes) in the control group. The average number of students per class was 23. For gender, age, and grade in school, no significant differences were found between experimental and control participants, so that both groups were similar in terms of age ($t = -2.10$; $p = 0.361$), gender ($\chi^2(1) = 0.33$; $p = 0.568$), and grade in school ($\chi^2(1) = 0.01$; $p = 0.919$).

Table 2. Sample characteristics and group differences by condition: frequency and percentage.

Variables	Experimental Group (n = 434)	Control Group (n = 236)	p
Age M (DT)	13.50 (1.29)	13.72 (1.21)	0.361
Sex			0.568
Boys	229 (34.7%)	122 (18.5%)	
Girls	195 (29.5%)	114 (17.3%)	
Grade in secondary education			0.919
Grade 7	136 (20.6%)	54 (8.2%)	
Grade 8	121 (18.3%)	92 (13.8%)	
Grade 9	88 (13.4%)	52 (7.9%)	
Grade 10	77 (11.7%)	40 (6.1%)	

Note: Age (*t* test), gender, and grade in school (Chi squared).

2.2. Procedure

Various informative meetings were held with the selected schools to explain the objectives and methodology of the Prev@cib program. The high schools were selected through non-probability convenience sampling based on their accessibility and previous interest in participating in this study. After obtaining parent permission and authorization, the researchers randomly assigned the adolescents to one of two groups: (1) an experimental group, where the Prev@cib program was implemented; (2) a control group, where the program was not implemented.

To evaluate the short-term effects of this pilot program, all the adolescents (experimental and control group) filled out a structured pen-and-paper questionnaire in their classrooms. Under the supervision of a least one of the researchers, this self-report questionnaire took approximately one hour to complete. When the questionnaires were administered, the adolescents were told that their participation would be voluntary and anonymous.

The Prev@cib program, which lasted 9 months, was implemented in the experimental group during their homeroom schedule. A pre-test was carried out in September 2016; a post-test in May 2017. The intervention took place from October through April 2017. The experimental and control groups filled out a battery of instruments in the pre and post-test phases. The Prev@cib program was administered by 13 teachers and four researchers previously trained by one of the investigators in this study.

Parental consent for participation was received from all participants. Furthermore, all the adolescents gave their informed consent before they participated in this study. This study followed the ethical values established in the 1964 Declaration of Helsinki and its later amendments, and the UNESCO Universal Declaration of Human Rights. In addition, all the procedures performed in the study were approved by the Ethics Committee of the University of Valencia, Spain (Project identification code: H1456762885511).

2.3. Measurement Variables and Instruments

Scale of Peer Victimization at School [46,47]. This instrument is composed of 12 items that evaluate the degree of victimization at school in the past school year (e.g., "A classmate hit or punched me" or "A classmate separated me from my group of friends"). Responses are given on a Likert-type scale ranging from 1 to 5 (never, only once, a few times in the past month, many times in the past month, and this happens to me quite often). Cronbach's alphas for this scale in this study were 0.88 (pre-test) and 0.90 (post-test).

Scale of School Aggression [48,49]. This Likert-type scale is composed of 12 items with a response range from 1 to 5 (never, seldom, sometimes, often, and always). This scale evaluates aggressive behaviors toward peers in the school context in the past 12 months (e.g., "I am someone who hits, kicks, and punches others"). Cronbach's alphas for this scale in this study were 0.72 (pre-test) and 0.79 (post-test).

Scale of Victimization through the Cell Phone and Internet [50]. The CYBVIC scale is composed of 15 items that measure the adolescent's experience as a victim of cyberbullying through the cell phone or Internet in the past 12 months (e.g., "I have been insulted or ridiculed through social networks, Internet, or cell phone"). From the victim's perspective, this scale measures cybernetic behaviors of harassment, persecution, belittlement, invasion of privacy, social exclusion, and identity theft. The items were responded to using a Likert-type scale with five response options (never, seldom, sometimes, often, quite often). Cronbach's alphas for this scale in this study were 0.88 (pre-test) and 0.89 (post-test).

Scale of Aggression through the Cell phone and Internet [50]. The CYB-AGRESS scale is composed of 15 items that measure the frequency with which the respondent has participated in aggressive behaviors through new technologies in the past 12 months (e.g., "I have insulted or made fun of someone through social networks, Internet, or cell phone"). From the aggressor's perspective, the scale measures cybernetic behaviors of harassment, persecution, belittlement, invasion of privacy, social exclusion, and identity theft. The items are answered on a Likert-type scale with five response options (never, seldom, sometimes, often, and a lot). Cronbach's alphas for this scale in this study were 0.80 (pre-test) and 0.90 (post-test).

Prior to administration, the definitions of bullying and cyberbullying were provided for all scales, and adolescents responded with this type of behavior in mind. In addition, on these scales, the adolescents were asked about the duration of the episodes and the frequency and persistence of bullying and cyberbullying.

2.4. Statistical Analysis

Data analysis was carried out using the SPSS statistical package (version 22, SPSS Inc., Chicago, IL, USA). To evaluate the effects of the program on each of the study variables, several 2 x 2 mixed factorial ANOVAs were used, with a between-subjects factor (experimental group and control group) and a within-subjects factor (before and after the program: pre-test and post-test). The use of this analysis is recommended when the groups selected are natural and not equal in the initial situation [51]. The interaction term in the mixed factorial ANOVA describes the effect of the program and is equivalent to t-tests on difference scores (post-test pre-test). The eta-square (η^2) value is used as an indicator of the size of the effect. Cohen (1988) suggested that $\eta^2 \leq 0.06$ can be considered a 'small' effect size, $0.07 \leq \eta^2 \leq 0.14$ represents a 'medium' effect size, and >0.14 is a 'large' effect size [52].

3. Results

3.1. Effects of Intervention Program Prev@cib on Traditional Bullying

Regarding bullying, a significant group x time interaction effect was found $F(1, 658) = 6.67, p < 0.01$, with a medium effect size, $\eta^2 = 0.09$. As Table 3 and Figure 1 show, although bullying decreased in both the experimental and control groups, this decrease was significantly more pronounced in the experimental group. The same pattern was obtained for victimization, $F(1, 658) = 7.80, p < 0.01$, with a medium effect size, $\eta^2 = 0.10$; victimization at post-test was lower than at pre-test, especially in the experimental group.

Table 3. Between-group effects and repeated-measures analysis of variance (ANOVA 2 × 2) in bullying.

Variables		M (DT)			F (p)			η^2
	Group	Pre-test	Post-test	Time Effect	Group Effect	Interaction Effect	
Bullying	Experimental	3.87 (0.92)	3.48 (1.07)	48.95 ***	8.40 **	6.67 *	0.09
	Control	3.96 (0.96)	3.78 (0.93)				
Victimization (bullying)	Experimental	4.97 (1.89)	4.27 (1.67)	36.26 ***	7.80 **	5.75 *	0.10
	Control	5.12 (2.02)	4.82 (1.90)				

Note: η^2 = Eta squared effect size; $0.07 \leq \eta^2 \leq 0.14$ = medium size; * $p < 0.05$; ** $p < 0.01$; *** $p < 0.001$.

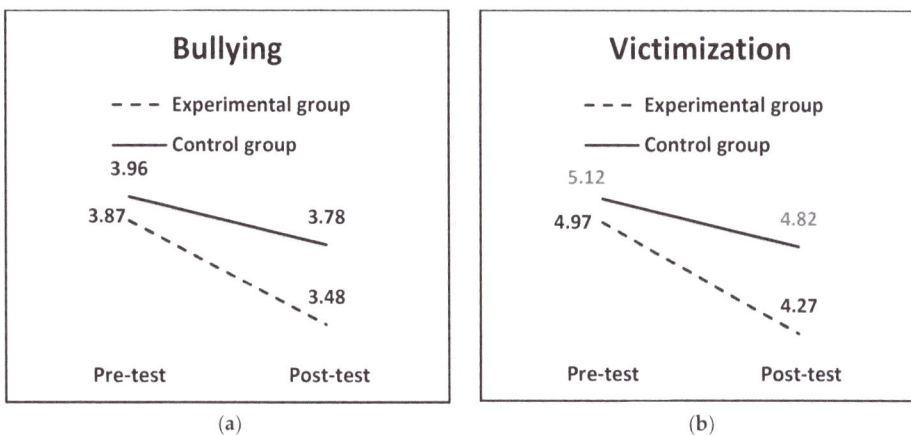

Figure 1. Means obtained by the groups (experimental and control) on bullying (**a**) and victimization (**b**).

3.2. Effects of Prev@cib Intervention Program on Cyberbullying

For cyberbullying, results yielded a significant group ×time effect, F (1, 658) = 7.03, $p < 0.01$, with a small effect size η^2 = 0.05. Findings indicated that cyberbullying remained stable in the control group, whereas it decreased in the experimental group (see Table 4 and Figure 2). A significant group × time effect was also obtained for cybervictimization F (1, 658) = 11.63; $p < 0.001$, with a small effect size, η^2 = 0.04. As Table 4 and Figure 2 show, cybervictimization increased slightly in the control group, whereas it decreased in the experimental group.

Table 4. Between-group effects and repeated-measures analysis of variance (ANOVA 2 × 2) in cyberbullying.

Variables		*M (DT)*		*F (p)*			η^2
	Group	Pre-test	Post-test	Time Effect	Group Effect	Interaction Effect	
Cyberbullying	Experimental	1.21 (0.28)	1.14 (0.32)	7.39 **	7.03 **	4.67 *	0.05
	Control	1.24 (0.34)	1.23 (0.41)				
Cyber Victimization	Experimental	1.27 (0.41)	1.20 (0.32)	1.16	6.38 *	11.63 ***	0.04
	Control	1.28 (0.39)	1.32 (0.47)				

Note: η^2 = Eta squared effect size; $\eta^2 \leq 0.06$ = small size; * $p < 0.05$; ** $p < 0.01$; *** $p < 0.001$.

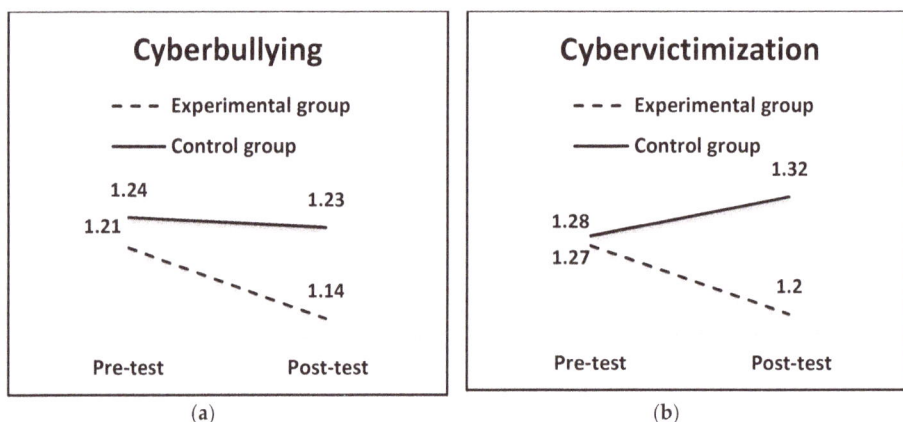

Figure 2. Means obtained by the groups (experimental and control) on cyberbullying (**a**) and cybervictimization (**b**).

4. Discussion

The main objective of this study was to experimentally assess the effects of the Prev@cib Program. Specifically, the short-term impact of the Prev@cib Program was shown on bullying and cyberbullying perpetration and victimization among adolescents.

The Prev@cib program is based on three theories that support the contents of the program. This theoretical framework provides a solid and rigorous basis for this novel and necessary proposal in this area of research. Thus, the Prev@cib program is based on the ecological model [42] because it emphasizes the protector factors and personal, microsocial, and contextual risk factors associated with bullying and cyberbullying. Second, it also contains principles and theoretical constructs of empowerment theory [43], related to resources and strategies for controlling and exercising self-determination over one's life. In this case, these resources help adolescents to improve life at school with peers and avoid poor use of new technologies. For example, the program contains activities about cybernetic security measures or the legal consequences of violence perpetration, both "face to face" and virtual. Third, the Prev@cib program is based on the model of personal and social responsibility [44]. Thus, it addresses the need for adolescents to accept shared responsibility in bullying and cyberbullying problems, in order to involve them in preventing and reducing these forms of violence. Thus, adolescents are made aware that, through their silence, they contribute to maintaining the situation of peer abuse.

The findings emphasize the effectiveness of the Prev@cib intervention program for both bullying and cyberbullying. Specifically, in the experimental group, a reduction was observed in the involvement in bullying and cyberbullying as aggressors and victims, compared to the control group. This decrease in bullying and cyberbullying in the experimental group could be explained by the variety and suitability of the contents. The positive results of Prev@cib are consistent with other programs that have also shown their experimental effectiveness [27,28,37].

Consequently, all the hypotheses proposed in our study were confirmed. Regarding the hypotheses related to "face to face" bullying, other programs also obtained positive effects in reducing victimization and perpetration of this type of violence, for example, the Olweus Bullying Prevention Program [29] or the ViSC Social Competence Program [34]. Previous studies emphasized the importance of the school environment in reducing the rates of bullying [53,54]. In this regard, the Prev@cib program was designed to reduce and prevent aggressiveness through activities involving cooperative learning, understanding, and shared responsibility in the school. Thus, the school climate is fostered as a protector factor, rather than a risk factor, in the manifestation of aggressive behaviors. This intervention is fundamental because adolescents who exhibit aggressive behaviors toward their classmates have been found to present other violent behaviors outside the classroom [24,55]. The Cyberprogram 2.0 also shares this focus by emphasizing conflict resolution strategies in the school context in order to reduce impulsive and premeditated aggressiveness in other social settings [41]. Future research should study the effects of the Prev@cib program on reducing these two types of aggressiveness, premeditated and impulsive, in order to more closely examine these expressions of violence toward peers.

In addition, the Prev@cib Program significantly reduced school victimization. The implications of these positive results are important for the victims of school bullying, who usually experience feelings of anxiety, depression, psycho-somatizations, suicidal ideation, and problems in school as a result of the continued abuse [17,56]. These negative effects of bullying increase even more when the victim is not only bullied in the school context, but also through new technologies [20,57]. Along these lines, in the Media Heroes Cyberbullying Prevention Program [40], the most positive effects of the program were obtained in victims who experienced bullying and cyberbullying at the same time, by significantly reducing their psychological distress. It is important for adolescents to be aware of the seriousness of the problem and become sensitive to the suffering of the victims in order to eradicate or reduce these types of violence [58,59]. From this perspective, the Prev@cib program specifically addresses this question in an awareness module through, for example, the activity "What if you were the victim?"

Moreover, other main objectives of the Prev@cib program related to the last two study hypotheses also showed effective results in reducing cyberbullying. Whereas in the intervention group, cyberbullying decreased in the post-test phase, in the control group, these behaviors did not decline, and instead remained constant over time. These results are congruent with those from other programs that obtained positive effects on reducing cyberaggression, such as The Brief Internet Cyberbullying Prevention Program [60] or Tabby Improved program [38]. An interesting question related to cyberbullying behaviors involves victims of traditional bullying who use the Internet to get revenge. Indeed, the impunity offered by the anonymity of the Internet has led some bullying victims to view the virtual space as the ideal way to punish their aggressors [61]. The Arizona program focuses on this issue, producing a reduction in revenge by victims after the intervention [62]. One of the future challenges of intervention programs, including ours, is to try to eradicate these types of vengeful behaviors where bullying victims become cyberbullies in the virtual space.

In the case of cybervictimization, the results of the Prev@cib program also confirmed the hypothesis of a decline in cybervictimization in the intervention group, compared to their baseline and the control group. Thus, whereas cybervictimization decreased in the intervention group, it increased in the control group. Along these lines, other programs such as the Cyber Friendly Schools Project [39] or Surf-Fair [63] also obtained positive effects on reducing cybervictimization in the participants. Taking into account that (cyber)victimization causes several types of present and future psychosocial damage in targets of this type of violence [64], it is important to join forces to protect our children and adolescents. Furthermore, as other studies have suggested, if we do not intervene in this problem, we run the risk of cyberbullying becoming normalized in adolescence, thus affecting adolescents' wellbeing and development, as well as peaceful co-existence in high schools [15,65].

In sum, the Prev@cib program has been shown to have positive effects on reducing bullying and cyberbullying, and also aggression and victimization. However, the effect size of the program is smaller for cyberbullying than bullying. This result is consistent with those obtained by different authors [66]. It has been pointed out that cyberbullying program effects are often limited to increasing Internet safety knowledge [67]. Future research interventions should provide some online sessions to foster interpersonal connectivity through the Internet.

The results support the idea that adolescents involved in traditional bullying are also usually involved in cyberbullying [11,68]. Based on this assumption of continuity between traditional bullying and cyberbullying, the Prev@cib program, like programs by other researchers, includes activities to address both problems with the participants [27,36].

This study has some limitations that should be taken into account when interpreting the conclusions of this study. The first limitation is related to the representativity of the sample. Although the sample of participants is large because it is a classroom intervention, the generalization of the results to the adolescent population must be carried out with caution. Future studies could implement the Prev@cib program in other samples of adolescents from other countries. A longitudinal study should also be carried out to test the stability of the long-term changes observed in the intervention group. It would also be interesting to include other variables, such as school climate, to observe how it changes during the program. In this regard, some authors suggested that cyberbullying victims do not perceive the teacher as a source of authority who helps to solve their bullying problems with peers [24,58]. This lack of confidence in teachers indicates not only that they should be included in intervention programs, but also that teachers' support should be evaluated after the program. In addition, another limitation is the small effect size of the Prev@cib program on cyberbullying. According to some meta-analyses and review studies [27,36], in general, the effect sizes of bullying and cyberbullying intervention programs are usually small. Another limitation is that students are nested within 35 classes from four schools, which may lead to low independence in the data. Although groups were randomly assigned to ensure their equivalence [69], it was impractical to randomize participants at an individual level, due to the risk of social threats to validity [70]. Future research should take this limitation into account by considering class-level and school-level analysis and conducting a multilevel or hierarchical analysis. Finally, another limitation of this manuscript could be the use of self-reports as the only assessment instruments in the study. Even so, previous studies highlight the acceptable reliability and validity levels of adolescent self-reports to measure risk behaviors [71,72].

In spite of the limitations, this study provides a novel program to prevent bullying and cyberbullying in adolescence, based on scientific evidence. Prev@cib is a theoretically-based program that has been shown to have positive effects on reducing bullying and cyberbullying perpetration and victimization.

5. Conclusions

This study presents the experimental validation of the effects of the Prev@cib program, which has the objective of preventing and reducing bullying and cyberbullying among adolescents. Specifically, this program is based on three theoretical frameworks: the ecological model, empowerment theory, and the personal and social responsibility model. Regarding the contents, the Prev@cib program consists of ten sessions distributed in three modules: (1) Information; (2) Awareness and sensitization; and (3) Involvement and commitment. To evaluate the effectiveness of the Prev@cib program, a quasi-experimental repeated-measures pre-test and post-test design was used with an experimental group and a control group.

The results of the present study showed the efficacy of the Prev@cib program. The program had positive effects on reducing bullying in the participants. Specifically, the findings show that in the experimental group, compared to the control group, school perpetration and victimization behaviors declined significantly. These positive effects were also observed for cyberbullying in the experimental group.

In summary, our results present scientific evidence that the Prev@cib program is effective in reducing and preventing bullying and cyberbullying in the adolescent population.

Author Contributions: J.O.-B. and S.B. conducted the research project and delivered the program; E.A. and B.M.-F. collected and analyzed the data; M.-J.C. reviewed the theoretical framework and revised the references and the formal issues. All authors wrote the paper and read and approved the final manuscript.

Funding: This research was financed by the project ACIF/2014/110 "Prevention of the harassment in adolescents through the New Technologies of Information and Communication: Prev Program@cib", funded by Consellería de Educació, Cultura i Esport (Generalitat Valenciana, Programa VALi+d).

Acknowledgments: We thank the students, professors, school counselors, and directors of the participating schools.

Conflicts of Interest: The authors declare no conflicts of interest.

References

1. Mishna, F.; Saini, M.; Solomon, S. Ongoing and online: Children and youth's perceptions of cyber bullying. *Child. Youth Serv. Rev.* **2009**, *31*, 1222–1228. [CrossRef]
2. Yubero, S.; Larrañaga, E.; Villora, B.; Navarro, R. Negative peer relationships on piracy behavior: A cross-sectional study of the associations between cyberbullying involvement and digital piracy. *Int. J. Environ. Res. Public Health* **2017**, *14*, 1180. [CrossRef]
3. Moreno–Ruiz, D.; Martínez–Ferrer, B.; García–Bacete, F. Parenting styles, cyberaggression, and cybervictimization among adolescents. *Comput. Hum. Behav.* **2019**, *93*, 252–259. [CrossRef]
4. Aboujaoude, E.; Savage, M.W.; Starcevic, V.; Salame, W.O. Cyberbullying: Review of an old problem gone viral. *J. Adolesc. Heal.* **2015**, *57*, 10–18. [CrossRef]
5. Smith, P.K.; Mahdavi, J.; Carvalho, M.; Fisher, S.; Russell, S.; Tippett, N. Cyberbullying: Its nature and impact in secondary school pupils. *J. Child Psychol. Psychiatry Allied Discip.* **2008**, *49*, 376–385. [CrossRef]
6. Waasdorp, T.E.; Bradshaw, C.P. The overlap between cyberbullying and traditional bullying. *J. Adolesc. Heal.* **2015**, *56*, 483–488. [CrossRef]
7. Navarro, R.; Yubero, S.; Larrañaga, E. Psychosocial risk factors for involvement in bullying behaviors: Empirical comparison between cyberbullying and social bullying victims and bullies. *Sch. Ment. Health* **2015**, *7*, 235–248. [CrossRef]
8. Erdur-Baker, Ö. Cyberbullying and its correlation to traditional bullying, gender and frequent and risky usage of internet-mediated communication tools. *New Media Soc.* **2010**, *12*, 109–125. [CrossRef]
9. Li, Q. New bottle but old wine: A research of cyberbullying in schools. *Comput. Hum. Behav.* **2007**, *23*, 1777–1791. [CrossRef]
10. Slonje, R.; Smith, P.K.; Frisén, A. Perceived reasons for the negative impact of cyberbullying and traditional bullying. *Eur. J. Dev. Psychol.* **2017**, *14*, 295–310. [CrossRef]
11. Lazuras, L.; Barkoukis, V.; Tsorbatzoudis, H. Face-to-face bullying and cyberbullying in adolescents: Trans-contextual effects and role overlap. *Technol. Soc.* **2017**, *48*, 97–101. [CrossRef]
12. Olweus, D. School bullying: Development and some important challenges. *Annu. Rev. Clin. Psychol.* **2013**, *9*, 1–30. [CrossRef]
13. Kowalski, R.M.; Morgan, C.A.; Limber, S.P. Traditional bullying as a potential warning sign of cyberbullying. *Sch. Psychol. Int.* **2012**, *33*, 505–519. [CrossRef]

14. Martínez-Ferrer, B.; Moreno, D.; Musitu, G. Are adolescents engaged in the problematic use of social networking sites more involved in peer aggression and victimization? *Front. Psychol.* **2018**, *9*, 1–13. [CrossRef]
15. Hinduja, S.; Patchin, J.W. Bullying, cyberbullying, and suicide. *Arch. Suicide Res.* **2010**, *14*, 206–221. [CrossRef]
16. Machimbarrena, J.M.; Calvete, E.; Fernández-González, L.; Álvarez-Bardón, A.; Álvarez-Fernández, L.; González-Cabrera, J. Internet risks: An overview of victimization in cyberbullying, cyber dating abuse, sexting, online grooming and problematic internet use. *Int. J. Environ. Res. Public Health* **2018**, *15*, 2471. [CrossRef]
17. Campbell, M.; Spears, B.; Slee, P.; Butler, D.; Kift, S. Victims' perceptions of traditional and cyberbullying, and the psychosocial correlates of their victimisation. *Emot. Behav. Difficulties* **2012**, *17*, 389–401. [CrossRef]
18. Pham, T.; Adesman, A. Teen victimization: Prevalence and consequences of traditional and cyberbullying. *Curr. Opin. Pediatr.* **2015**, *27*, 748–756. [CrossRef]
19. Iranzo, B.; Buelga, S.; Cava, M.J.; Ortega-Barón, J. Cyberbullying, psychosocial adjustment and suicide ideation in adolescence. *Psychosoc. Interv.* **2019**, in press.
20. Buelga, S.; Martínez–Ferrer, B.; Cava, M.J. Differences in family climate and family communication among cyberbullies, cybervictims, and cyber bully–victims in adolescents. *Comput. Hum. Behav.* **2017**, *76*, 164–173. [CrossRef]
21. Bevilacqua, L.; Shackleton, N.; Hale, D.; Allen, E.; Bond, L.; Christie, D.; Elbourne, D.; Fitzgerald-Yau, N.; Fletcher, A.; Jones, R.; et al. The role of family and school-level factors in bullying and cyberbullying: A cross-sectional study. *BMC Pediatr.* **2017**, *17*, 1–10. [CrossRef]
22. Festl, R.; Quandt, T. Social relations and cyberbullying: The influence of individual and structural attributes on victimization and perpetration via the internet. *Hum. Commun. Res.* **2013**, *39*, 101–126. [CrossRef]
23. Mitchell, K.J.; Jones, L.M. Cyberbullying and bullying must be studied within a broader peer victimization framework. *J. Adolesc. Heal.* **2015**, *56*, 473–474. [CrossRef]
24. Ortega-Baron, J.; Buelga, S.; Cava, M.J.; Torralba, E. School violence and attitude toward authority of student perpetrators of cyberbullying. *J. Psychodidactics* **2017**, *22*, 23–28.
25. Rigby, K.; Smith, P.K. Is school bullying really on the rise? *Soc. Psychol. Educ.* **2011**, *14*, 441–455. [CrossRef]
26. Couvillon, M.A.; Ilieva, V. Recommended practices: A review of schoolwide preventative programs and strategies on cyberbullying. *Prev. Sch. Fail. Altern. Educ. Child. Youth* **2011**, *55*, 96–101. [CrossRef]
27. Della Cioppa, V.; O'Neil, A.; Craig, W. Learning from traditional bullying interventions: A review of research on cyberbullying and best practice. *Aggress. Violent Behav.* **2015**, *23*, 61–68. [CrossRef]
28. Smith, J.D.; Schneider, B.H.; Smith, P.K.; Ananiadou, K. The effectiveness of whole-school antibullying programs: A synthesis of evaluation research. *Sch. Psych. Rev.* **2004**, *33*, 547–560.
29. Olweus, D.; Limber, S.P. Bullying in school: Evaluation and dissemination of the Olweus bullying prevention program. *Am. J. Orthopsychiatry* **2010**, *1*, 124–134. [CrossRef]
30. Fox, C.L.; Boulton, M.J. Evaluating the effectiveness of a social skills training (SST) programme for victims of bullying. *Educ. Res.* **2003**, *45*, 231–247. [CrossRef]
31. Menesini, E.; Codecasa, E.; Benelli, B.; Cowie, H. Enhancing children's responsibility to take action against bullying: Evaluation of a Be Friending intervention in italian middle schools. *Aggress. Behav.* **2003**, *29*, 1–14. [CrossRef]
32. Şahin, M. An investigation into the efficiency of empathy training program on preventing bullying in primary schools. *Child. Youth Serv. Rev.* **2012**, *34*, 1325–1330. [CrossRef]
33. Williford, A.; Elledge, L.C.; Boulton, A.J.; DePaolis, K.J.; Little, T.D.; Salmivalli, C. Effects of the KiVa antibullying program on cyberbullying and cybervictimization frequency among finnish youth. *J. Clin. Child Adolesc. Psychol.* **2013**, *42*, 820–833. [CrossRef]
34. Gradinger, P.; Yanagida, T.; Strohmeier, D.; Spiel, C. Prevention of cyberbullying and cyber victimization: Evaluation of the ViSC Social Competence Program. *J. Sch. Violence* **2015**, *14*, 87–110. [CrossRef]
35. Pearce, N.; Cross, D.; Monks, H.; Waters, S.; Falconer, S. Current evidence of best practice in whole-school bullying intervention and its potential to inform cyberbullying interventions. *Aust. J. Guid. Couns.* **2011**, *21*, 1–21. [CrossRef]
36. Cantone, E.; Piras, A.P.; Vellante, M.; Preti, A.; Daníelsdóttir, S.; D'Aloja, E.; Lesinskiene, S.; Angermeyer, M.C.; Carta, M.G.; Bhugra, D. Interventions on bullying and cyberbullying in schools: A systematic review. *Clin. Pract. Epidemiol. Ment. Heal.* **2015**, *11*, 58–76.

37. Gaffney, H.; Farrington, D.P.; Espelage, D.L.; Ttofi, M.M. Are cyberbullying intervention and prevention programs effective? A systematic and meta-analytical review. *Aggress. Violent Behav.* **2018**, in press. [CrossRef]

38. Sorrentino, A.; Baldry, A.; Farrington, D. The efficacy of the Tabby improved prevention and intervention program in reducing cyberbullying and cybervictimization among students. *Int. J. Environ. Res. Public Health* **2018**, *15*, 2536. [CrossRef]

39. Cross, D.; Shaw, T.; Hadwen, K.; Cardoso, P.; Slee, P.; Roberts, C.; Thomas, L.; Barnes, A. Longitudinal impact of the Cyber Friendly Schools program on adolescents' cyberbullying behavior. *Aggress. Behav.* **2016**, *42*, 166–180. [CrossRef]

40. Chaux, E.; Velásquez, A.M.; Schultze-Krumbholz, A.; Scheithauer, H. Effects of the cyberbullying prevention program media heroes (Medienhelden) on traditional bullying. *Aggress. Behav.* **2016**, *42*, 157–165. [CrossRef]

41. Garaigordobil, M.; Martínez-Valderrey, V. Effect of Cyberprogram 2.0 on reducing victimization and improving social competence in adolescence. *J. Psychodidactics* **2014**, *19*, 289–306. [CrossRef]

42. Bronfenbrenner, U. *The Ecology of Human Development: Experiments by Nature and Design*; Harvard University: Cambrigde, MA, USA, 1981; ISBN 18340806.

43. Zimmerman, M.A. Empowerment Theory. In *Handbook of Community Psychology*; Rappaport, J., Seidman, E., Eds.; Springer US: New York, NY, USA, 2000; pp. 43–64.

44. Hellison, D. *Teaching Responsibility through Physical Activity*; Human Kinetics: Champaign, IL, USA, 1995.

45. Gámez-Guadix, M.; Mateos-Pérez, E. Longitudinal and reciprocal relationships between sexting, online sexual solicitations, and cyberbullying among minors. *Comput. Hum. Behav.* **2019**, *94*, 70–76. [CrossRef]

46. Mynard, H.; Joseph, S. Development of the multidimensional peer-victimization scale. *Aggress. Behav.* **2000**, *26*, 169–178. [CrossRef]

47. Cava, M.J.; Buelga, S. Propiedades psicométricas de la escala de victimización escolar entre iguales (VE-I). *Rev. Evaluar* **2018**, *18*, 40–53.

48. Torregosa, M.; Inglés, C.; Estévez, E.; Musitu, G.; García-Fernández, J.M. Evaluación de la conducta violenta en la adolescencia: Revisión de cuestionarios, inventarios, y escalas en población española. *Aula Abierta* **2011**, *39*, 37–50.

49. Little, T.D.; Henrich, C.C.; Jones, S.M.; Hawley, P.H. Disentangling the "whys" from the "whats" of aggressive behaviour. *Int. J. Behav. Dev.* **2003**, *27*, 122–133. [CrossRef]

50. Buelga, S.; Ortega-Baron, J.; Torralba, E. Psychometric propierties of revised scales of cyberbullying (CybVic_R, CybAG_R). In Proceedings of the II Congreso Internacional de la Sociedad Científica Española de Psicología Social, Elche, Spain, 20–22 October 2016.

51. Weinfurt, K.P. The anova to mixed model transition. In *Reading and Understanding MORE Multivariate Statistics*; Grimm, L.G., Yarnold, P.R., Eds.; Elsevier Ltd.: Washington, DC, USA, 2000; pp. 317–361.

52. Cohen, J. *Statistical Power Analysis for the Behavioral Sciences*, 2nd ed.; Lawrence Erlbaum Associates: Hillsdale, NJ, USA, 1988.

53. Olsson, G.; Brolin, S.; Bitte, M. School collective efficacy and bullying behaviour: A multilevel study. *Int. J. Environ. Res. Public Health* **2017**, *14*, 1607. [CrossRef]

54. Wachs, S.; Bilz, L.; Fischer, S.; Schubarth, W.; Wright, M. Students' willingness to intervene in bullying: Direct and indirect associations with classroom cohesion and self-efficacy. *Int. J. Environ. Res. Public Health* **2018**, *15*, 2577. [CrossRef]

55. Vandebosch, H.; van Cleemput, K. Cyberbullying among youngsters: Profiles of bullies and victims. *New Media Soc.* **2009**, *11*, 1349–1371. [CrossRef]

56. Bauman, S.; Toomey, R.B.; Walker, J.L. Associations among bullying, cyberbullying, and suicide in high school students. *J. Adolesc.* **2013**, *36*, 341–350. [CrossRef]

57. Quintana-Orts, C.; Rey, L. Traditional bullying, cyberbullying and mental health in early adolescents: Forgiveness as a protective factor of peer victimisation. *Int. J. Environ. Res. Public Health* **2018**, *15*. [CrossRef]

58. Houndoumadi, A.; Pateraki, L. Bullying and bullies in Greek elementary schools: pupils' attitudes and teachers'/parents' awareness. *Educ. Rev.* **2001**, *53*, 19–26. [CrossRef]

59. Buelga, S.; Martínez-Ferrer, B.; Musitu, G. Family relationships and cyberbullying. In *Cyberbullying across the Globe: Gender, Family and mental Health*; Springer International Publishing: Basel, Switzeland, 2015; pp. 99–114.

60. Doane, A.N.; Kelley, M.L.; Pearson, M.R. Reducing cyberbullying: A theory of reasoned action-based video prevention program for college students. *Aggress. Behav.* **2016**, *42*, 136–146. [CrossRef] [PubMed]

61. Barlett, C.; Chamberlin, K.; Witkower, Z. Predicting cyberbullying perpetration in emerging adults: A theoretical test of the Barlett Gentile Cyberbullying Model. *Aggress. Behav.* **2017**, *43*, 147–154. [CrossRef] [PubMed]

62. Roberto, A.J.; Eden, J.; Savage, M.W.; Ramos-Salazar, L.; Deiss, D.M. Outcome evaluation results of school-based cybersafety promotion and cyberbullying prevention intervention for middle school students. *Health Commun.* **2014**, *29*, 1029–1042. [CrossRef] [PubMed]

63. Pieschl, S.; Kourteva, P.; Stauf, L. Challenges in the evaluation of cyberbullying prevention insights from two case studies. *Int. J. Dev. Sci.* **2017**, *11*, 45–54. [CrossRef]

64. Tomşa, R.; Jenaro, C.; Campbell, M.; Neacşu, D. Student's experiences with traditional bullying and cyberbullying: Findings from a romanian sample. *Procedia—Soc. Behav. Sci.* **2013**, *78*, 586–590. [CrossRef]

65. Cassidy, W.; Jackson, M.; Brown, K.N. Sticks and stones can break my bones, but how can pixels hurt me?: students' experiences with cyber-bullying. *Sch. Psychol. Int.* **2009**, *30*, 383–402. [CrossRef]

66. Mishna, F.; Cook, C.; Saini, M.; Wu, M.J.; MacFadden, R. Interventions to prevent and reduce cyber abuse of youth: A systematic review. *Res. Soc. Work Pract.* **2011**, *21*, 5–14. [CrossRef]

67. Polanin, J.; Espelage, D.; Pigott, T. A meta-analysis of school-based bullying prevention programs' effects on bystander intervention behavior. *Sch. Psychol. Rev.* **2012**, *41*, 47–65.

68. Kubiszewski, V.; Fontaine, R.; Potard, C.; Auzoult, L. Does cyberbullying overlap with school bullying when taking modality of involvement into account? *Comput. Hum. Behav.* **2015**, *43*, 49–57. [CrossRef]

69. Huck, S.W. *Reading Statistics and Research*; Pearson: New York, NY, USA, 2000; ISBN 13 978-0-205-51067-2.

70. Portney, L.; Watkins, M.P. Foundations of clinical research: Applications to practice. In *Foundations of Clinical Research: Applications to Practice*; Prentice Hall: Upper Saddle River, NJ, USA, 2009; pp. 619–658. ISBN 9780803646575.

71. Flisher, A.J.; Evans, J.; Muller, M.; Lombard, C. Brief report: Test-retest reliability of self-reported adolescent risk behaviour. *J. Adolesc.* **2004**, *27*, 207–212. [CrossRef] [PubMed]

72. Ansel, L.L.; Barry, C.T.; Gillen, C.T.A.; Herrington, L.L. An analysis of four self-report measures of adolescent callous-unemotional traits: Exploring unique prediction of delinquency, aggression, and conduct problems. *J. Psychopathol. Behav. Assess.* **2015**, *37*, 207–216. [CrossRef]

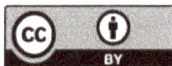

International Journal of
Environmental Research and Public Health

MDPI

Article

Asegúrate: An Intervention Program against Cyberbullying Based on Teachers' Commitment and on Design of Its Instructional Materials

Rosario Del Rey [1,*], **Rosario Ortega-Ruiz** [2] and **José Antonio Casas** [2]

[1] Department of Educational and Developmental Psychology, Universidad de Sevilla, 41019 Seville, Spain
[2] Department of Psychology, Universidad de Córdoba, 41013 Córdoba, Spain; ortegaruiz@uco.es (R.O.-R.);
jacasas@uco.es (J.A.C.)
* Correspondence: delrey@us.es

Received: 16 December 2018; Accepted: 29 January 2019; Published: 2 February 2019

Abstract: This article presents the impact on cyberbullying of the Asegúrate program. This educational program is based on the theory of normative social behavior, self-regulation skills, and the beliefs held by adolescents and consists in a whole package of strategies and resources to help teachers to include in the ordinary curricula. The evaluation of Asegúrate was carried out with a sample of 4779 students (48.9% girls) in 5th and 6th grade in primary education and compulsory secondary education (M = 12.76; SD = 1.67) through a quasi-experimental methodology, with two measures over time. The instrument used was the European Cyberbullying Intervention Project Questionnaire. The results show that the involvement in cyberbullying as cyber-victim, cyber-aggressor, and cyber-bully-victim increase without intervention, whereas it diminishes when intervention is carried out by the teachers who have received specific training and have used the didactic Asegúrate package. Additionally, the impact of the intervention on the different types of behaviors was analyzed, and the results show that Asegúrate is more effective with some forms than with others. Consequently, the Asegúrate program is effective for decreasing the prevalence of cyberbullying, but some modifications need to be made to impact on all the different forms it can take.

Keywords: Asegúrate program; cyberbullying; cyber-victim; cyber-aggressor

1. Introduction

In recent years, there has been increased awareness among both teachers and school counsellors that interpersonal relationships between pupils, and the classroom atmosphere in general, are complex processes that are heavily influenced by the social microculture of that particular school and the educational and the pedagogical style of the teaching staff [1]. Until the 1970s, very little attention was paid to certain interpersonal processes, such as the existence of bullying [2]. The increased recognition of this phenomenon has helped to draw more attention to the importance of interpersonal relationships between pupils and how these affect the classroom atmosphere in general [3,4]. The publication and wider circulation of the findings of this research into bullying, and later cyberbullying, has led ordinary school teachers, school counselors, and school staff in general to give more thought to the socio-affective atmosphere in schools, which should be seen as a crucial part of a school's culture [5]. Over the past thirty years or so, considerable advances have been made in our knowledge of bullying in terms of its prevalence, associated factors, risk indicators, intervention programs, and educational policies [6], and although we cannot yet affirm that all teachers and school counsellors fully comprehend how widespread the problem is, it is clear that they are becoming increasingly aware of its relevance as a factor which harms the healthy balance of welfare and social harmony in schools.

However, since the arrival of internet and, above all, mobile digital technology and social networks accessed via smartphones, social interaction among children and adolescents has become far more complex [7]. Despite the fact that this technological revolution has brought huge benefits in the quality of life of people in many areas of life, such as improved processes of teaching and learning [8], it has also given rise to new problems, such as the evolution of traditional bullying into cyberbullying [9,10]. This poses new challenges to schools, whose job it is to detect and try to prevent this new type of bullying, which while sharing many of the same characteristics as traditional bullying, has other specific features of its own, such as the difficulty for teachers to gain access to these interactions without disturbing the fully justifiable right to intimacy of these children.

Cyberbullying has been studied from a number of different angles [11], but the most common approach is to deal with it as an extension of traditional bullying "in which the aggression occurs through modern technological devices, and specifically mobile phones or the internet" [12]. This lends it some particular characteristics which are specific to virtual environments and which set it apart it from traditional forms of bullying [13]. Among the features which clearly differentiate traditional bullying from cyberbullying are the possibility that the harassment can take place at any time—24/7, as the well-known phrase goes [14]—and the fact that they are not limited solely to the context of school [15]. Some of the main characteristics of traditional bullying, such as repetition, the power imbalance, and being intentional, are also manifested in slightly different ways in cyberbullying [16]. In cyberbullying, repetition can occur from a single act of aggression if a message or image is sent to many people or forwarded to others [12]. In cyberbullying, the imbalance of power is no longer purely face to face: it can lie in the perpetrator's greater technological expertise or even to the anonymity afforded to them by virtual environments [17]. Conversely, the idea of intentionality, of knowingly doing harm to others, may not be a factor in some cases of cyberbullying, as many children may be unaware of the negative consequences of sending or forwarding their messages [18].

The prevalence rates of cyberbullying vary considerably from one study to another [19]. According to a recent systematic review including 66 meta-analysis studies and systematic reviews, at least 1 in every 5–7 children is involved in cyberbullying [20]. Similarly, a meta-analysis summarizing 80 studies showed an average rate of involvement of 16% for cyber-aggression and 15% for cyber-victimization, although no figure was given for the dual role of bully/victim [21]. Prevalence rates also appear to vary significantly depending on the way cyberbullying is evaluated and the types of aggression which are included [22–25]. The few existing longitudinal studies show that the prevalence of cyberbullying is on the rise. It is clear, therefore, that action must be taken against this growing problem, which is producing such serious consequences [26].

This scientific evidence about the existence and consequences of cyberbullying, together with alarming stories of cyber-victims, which appear in the media and its close links with traditional bullying [27–29] have led to the measures and programs previously used against bullying being adapted to educate children against cyberbullying, to try and stamp it out or, at least, alleviate its effects [30]. The ViSC Social Competence Program [31], for instance, was originally designed to counter traditional bullying and has been shown to have some effect on cyberbullying, although the authors themselves have admitted that a greater impact would be achieved if specifically designed programs were used. Some programs to prevent and counter cyberbullying have in fact already been designed and evaluated positively. In all, eight programs have been evaluated to date; however, they all seem to be more effective against cyber-victimization than cyberbullying [32] and specific training processes are required which demand an extremely high degree of involvement on the part of the teaching staff, even before the intervention program with the pupils takes place [33].

It has been shown that the teaching staff play a vital role in the effective implementation of programs against traditional bullying [34], and the knowledge and experience they have in dealing with past cases of bullying are particularly valuable [35]. We therefore consider it crucial that teachers gain direct, hands-on experience in introducing anti-cyberbullying programs, which also allows the programs to reach a greater number of people in the educational community and, as a result, obtain more effective results [36]. In the same way, the more directly teachers are involved in analyzing cyberbullying and devising strategies to cope with it, the better grasp they will have of the phenomenon [37], thus responding to the need for teachers to feel better informed and more professionally prepared for this task [38]. In fact, teachers and school principals already consider themselves key players in the prevention and management of all types of cyberbullying [39], despite the fact that their knowledge may be limited to its more widely-known forms [40].

Unlike other research projects in which teaching staff have been trained intensively or extensively to participate in implementing programs against cyberbullying [41], the Asegúrate program has been designed for use by teachers without the need to take part in costly training processes [42]. The training of teachers is of course extremely important in any area of action, but it is also our aim that every school, regardless of its means, has the chance to run a program against cyberbullying. We hope, therefore, that the Asegúrate teaching material will serve as a useful tool for schools, which lack the necessary resources to run specific training courses. The Asegúrate teaching materials consist of a Teacher's Manual, worksheets for presenting the program in the classroom, and a guide to working together with the children's families, which uses materials designed to raise awareness.

The Teacher's Manual: A Key Component of the Asegúrate Program

The Asegúrate program rests on three theoretical pillars: the theory of normative social behavior, the principles of constructivist methodologies, and the development of self-regulation skills. The first of these highlights how social behavior is significantly influenced by three normative mechanisms: group identity, expectations, and recognized legal norms. It upholds the notion that our behavior is likely driven by what is perceived as socially acceptable, normal, and legal [43,44]. The constructivism principles are concreted on the fact that each session starts with the exploration of young people's own ideas and beliefs [45]. As regards the development of self-regulation skills, Asegúrate includes reflective activities aimed at enhancing metacognitive skills to develop strategic learning among students [46]. Further details can be obtained by reading Del Rey et al. [47].

The complete program consists of eight sessions on cyberbullying and other related factors, including the ways people communicate on social networks and their implications; anomalies in online behavior; criteria for establishing safe online friendships; cybergossip; sexting; the abuse of the Internet and social networks, and the norms of cyber-etiquette. Detailed instructions are given as to how to conduct the tasks for each of the eight sessions in the program. Each session contains a specific activity that ensures that the requirements of the Asegúrate methodology are fully complied with. Each teacher is therefore given a full description of the steps to follow with their pupils, and extra resources and explanations are included. Finally, there is a self-access reference section including a glossary of terms, a resource bank (such as descriptions of the most popular YouTubers), links to further reading, etc. Another section provides the answer keys and instructions for evaluating each session and the Asegúrate program as a whole. Apart from the manual, the Asegúrate program also features audio-visual material for each of the sessions for teachers to use with the pupils and their families, as well as awareness-raising publicity resources such as posters, stickers, or bookmarks. The idea is for the teachers to use this complete range of resources to help them tackle the problem of cyberbullying with their pupils.

The Teacher's Manual fulfils the basic requirements as a useful teaching guide for professional adults to learn autonomously and provides both general guidelines and detailed procedures, including thorough instructions for the tasks and roles, self-help, and specifically targeted orientation [48]. The orientation consists of clear, concise information about the current situation of cyberbullying, a description of the program, and a summary of the methodology used, which is one of the key features of the program. All the Asegúrate presentation sessions are designed with a similar sequence of learning stages, planned in such a way that all participants can work together to understand the key issues. This sequence of activities is made up of five stages, named in the following way, to echo the activities which young people perform on social networks: (a) "Trending topic" explores the current ideas held by the participants; (b) "My profile" encourages the participants to reflect on any of their own activities on the social networks which might be described as "not normal"; (c) "Stop to think" focuses on analyzing the reasons which lead us, or others, to behave in certain ways when using social networks; (d) "Like/Don't like" identifies the possible consequences of their own (and others') positive or negative behavior on social networks; and (e) "I share" allows each session to end with a conclusion and an individual and/or collective declaration of commitment.

Taking all of the above into account, the aim of this study was to evaluate the effectiveness of the Asegúrate program in counterbalancing, through education, the involvement of schoolchildren in cyberbullying, whether in the roles of victim, aggressor, or in the dual role of cyberbully/victim, as well as stemming the increase in cyber-victimization and cyber-aggression both in general and specific cases of aggression.

2. Materials and Methods

This study has a longitudinal, quasi-experimental design. There are two study groups—a quasi-experimental group and a quasi-control group—and two data collection points—a pre-test before the program and a post-test at the end of the program.

2.1. Participants

A total of 4779 pupils (48.9% girls) took part in this study, from the 5th year of Spanish primary education (average age: 10–11) to the 4th year of Spanish secondary education (average age: 15–16 or higher), from 18 different schools. The ages ranged from 10 to 18 years old (M = 12.76, SD = 1.77). The experimental group consisted of 2316 pupils (50.4% girls) from 18 schools, and the control group contained 2463 pupils (47.5% girls) from 10 schools. The sampling was incidental: access was through invitations issued to schools to participate in the program, and the schools could agree whether to accept or not.

2.2. Questionnaire

The European Cyberbullying Intervention Project Questionnaire (ECIPQ) was used to assess the level of involvement in cyberbullying [49]. This scale was composed of 22 items and contained two different dimensions, assessing the frequency of cyber-victimization and cyber-aggression over the last two months. The responses were Likert-type (0 = No, 1 = Yes, once or twice, 2 = Yes, once or twice a month, 3 = Yes, about once a week, 4 = Yes, more than once a week). Examples of the items for cyber-victimization included the following: *Someone has posted threatening messages against me on Internet, social networks, or WhatsApp*. Examples for cyberbullying included the following: *I have insulted someone through social networks or WhatsApp*. The reliability of the scale for the present study was α = 0.80 (α = 0.76 for cyber-victimization and α = 0.73 for cyberbullying).

2.3. Process

The schools were contacted by phone and asked if they would like to take part in the study. An appointment was arranged for those schools which agreed, and the schedules and the classes which would participate in the study were decided. With the agreement of the teaching staff, the questionnaires were administered during class time by staff in training, who were specially instructed for this task. Before answering the questionnaires, the participants were fully briefed about the voluntary nature of participating in the study, the anonymity and confidentiality of the data, and the importance of giving truthful answers.

After the data was collected in February 2017, the Asegúrate program was carried out in the quasi-experimental groups, but not in the control groups. After the program was completed, the questionnaires were repeated, at least three months after they were first answered, June 2017 at the latest. Those schools where the program was not carried out were offered the chance to take part in it once the study was completed.

The research was carried out following the ethical standards agreed on by each schools' Parents' Association, and was approved by the Andalusia Biomedical Research Ethics Coordination Committee (0568-N-14), which adheres to the guidelines of the International Conference of Good Clinical Practice. All the materials and questionnaires that made up the project were presented and explained to the school management, which gave it their approval in all cases. They, in turn, discussed it with the School Council, as part of the schools' Projects for Peaceful Coexistence and School Improvement Plans; again, full approval was given for the schools to take part in the study.

2.4. Analysis of Results

The first step in analyzing the results of this research was to check the response frequencies for the different types of behavior evaluated by the questionnaire. Next, the prevalence of involvement was calculated following the criteria proposed by the authors of the scales used [49]: pupils were considered "victims" if they answered *"once or twice a month"* or more to any of the questions about victimization behavior and simultaneously answered *"no"* or *"once or twice"* to questions regarding all behavior related to aggression. To calculate the level of aggression, pupils were considered "bullies" if they stated that they had harassed someone *"once or twice a month"* or *"more frequently"* for any type of behavior classed as cyberbullying and simultaneously answered *"no"* or *"once or twice"* for types of behavior linked to cyber-victimization. In the same way, pupils were labeled "bully/victims" if they answered *"once or twice a month"* or more for behavior linked to victimization and aggression.

The percentage variation was then calculated for each of the groups (control group and quasi-experimental group). This variation shows the difference in prevalence between the values shown in the pre-test and those in the post-test. The following formula was used to calculate this variation: [(PrevalenceT2 − PrevalenceT1)/PrevalenceT1] × 100.

Finally, to evaluate the effectiveness of the program for the different types of behavior in the study, the linear mixed model or repeated measures MANOVA was calculated.

3. Results

Firstly, the descriptive results were calculated by examining the frequency of responses in both groups (experimental and control) for the different types of behavior measured by the questionnaire, in order to evaluate involvement in cyberbullying in the pre-test (see Table 1). The most important finding was that the most prevalent type of behavior in both groups, both for victimization and for aggression, was that which was most similar to traditional bullying (insults, threats, social exclusion, and spreading rumors). On the other hand, the types of behavior found more commonly in virtual environments, such as identity theft or re-editing images or videos, were much less frequent (see Table 1).

Table 1. Descriptive results calculated by groups experimental and control.

Items	0: No		1: Yes, Once or Twice		2: Yes, Once a Month		3: Yes, Once a Week		4: Yes, More Times a Week	
	% Exp	% Contr	% Exp	% Contr	% Exp	% Contr	% Exp	% Contr	% Exp	% Contr
Someone said nasty things to me or called me names using Internet, social networks, or WhatsApp.	72.6	79.9	22.2	16.3	2.7	2.4	0.7	0.6	1.7	0.9
Someone said nasty things about me to others using Internet, social networks, or WhatsApp.	78.7	84.2	17	12.6	2.3	1.9	0.8	0.6	1.3	0.7
Someone threatened me through texts or online messages.	88.1	92.5	10.1	6.5	0.9	0.7	0.3	0.2	0.6	0.1
Someone hacked into my account and stole personal information (e.g., through email or social networking accounts).	94.2	96	5.3	3.7	0.2	0.1	0.1	0.1	0.2	0.1
Someone hacked into my account and pretended to be me (e.g., through instant messaging or social networking accounts).	93.7	95.7	5.7	3.4	0.2	0.5	0.2	0	0.1	0
Someone created a fake account, pretending to be me (e.g., through instant messaging or social networking accounts).	95.1	96.3	4.4	3.3	0.2	0.3	0.1	0	0.2	0
Someone posted personal information about me online.	93.6	94.2	5.5	5.5	0.4	0.1	0.2	0	0.3	0.2
Someone posted embarrassing videos or pictures of me online.	90.9	93	7.4	5.9	0.7	0.6	0.5	0.3	0.5	0.3
Someone altered pictures or videos of me that I had posted online.	93.1	95.1	6.1	4.3	0.6	0.3	0.1	0.1	0.2	0.1
I was excluded or ignored by others in a social networking site or Internet.	80.6	86.6	16.5	12.1	1.5	0.9	0.4	0.2	0.9	0.2
Someone spread rumors about me on the Internet.	85.4	88.6	12.2	9.7	1.3	1.2	0.5	0.1	0.6	0.3
I said nasty things to someone or called them names using Internet, social networks, or WhatsApp.	79	83.6	17.9	14	1.6	1.7	0.9	0.3	0.7	0.4
I said nasty things about someone to other people using Internet, social networks, or WhatsApp.	82.6	85.5	14.6	12.3	1.4	1.4	0.8	0.5	0.7	0.4
I threatened someone through texts or online messages.	94.4	97.1	4.7	2.3	0.5	0.3	0.1	0.2	0.3	0
I hacked into someone's account and stole personal information (e.g., through email or social networking accounts).	97.8	98.9	1.7	1.1	0.3	0	0	0	0.2	0
I hacked into someone's account and pretended to be them (e.g., through instant messaging or social networking accounts).	98.2	98.8	1.4	1.1	0	0	0.1	0	0.3	0.1
I created a fake account, pretending to be someone else (e.g., through instant messaging or social networking accounts).	97	97.5	2.7	2.1	0.1	0.2	0.2	0.1	0.1	0
I posted personal information about someone online.	97.9	98.4	1.7	1.3	0.3	0.1	0.2	0.1	0	0
I posted embarrassing videos or pictures of someone online.	96.5	96.6	2.8	3	0.3	0.2	0.2	0.1	0.2	0.1
I altered pictures or videos of another person that had been posted online.	95.2	96.3	4.4	3.1	0.2	0.2	0.2	0.2	0.1	0.1
I excluded or ignored someone in a social networking site or Internet.	85.8	90.4	12	8.5	1	0.7	0.2	0.1	1	0.2
I spread rumors about someone on the Internet.	93.9	95	5.1	4.3	0.3	0.4	0.3	0.2	0.3	0

Next, we calculated the percentages of involvement in the different roles of cyberbullying (victims, aggressors and bully/victims), for both the experimental and control groups at both the pre-test and post-test stages (see Table 2). Here, the roles of victimization, aggression, and bully/victim were notably lower in the experimental group, compared with a slight decrease in number of victims and aggressors and a marked increase in the number of bully/victims in the control group.

Table 2. Percentages of involvement in the different roles of cyberbullying.

	% Not Involved	% Victims	% Aggressors	% Bully-Victims
PreExperimental	83.9	7.9	4.5	3.7
PostExperimental	87.5	6.0	3.1	3.4
PreControl	88.1	6.4	3.0	2.5
PostControl	88.5	6.0	2.5	3.0
%Experimental Change	4.29	−24.05	−31.11	−8.10
%Control Change	0.45	−6.25	−16.66	20

Finally, the repeated measures MANOVA was calculated for each of the 11 items of victimization and aggressive behavior measured in the cyberbullying questionnaire at the two stages when these were carried out (see Table 3). These results show significant overall differences in the level of victimization, with a clear decrease in the experimental group and no changes in the control group ($F_{(1, 4507)} = 12.63$, $p < 0.01$, d = 0.29). The same pattern could be observed for the level of aggression, where the control group score remained the same, while there was a significant fall in the score in the experimental group after the program was carried out ($F_{(1, 4526)} = 6.66$, $p < 0.01$, d = 0.25).

As regards the specific behavior of victimization, after the program was carried out, direct insults ($F_{(1, 4507)} = 4.05$, $p < 0.05$, d = 0.20), posting insults about the victim ($F_{(1, 4507)} = 5.16$, $p < 0.05$, d = 0.21), threats ($F_{(1, 4507)} = 5.25$, $p < 0.05$, d = 0.21), exclusion ($F_{(1, 4507)} = 15.75$, $p < 0.01$, d = 0.30), and spreading rumors ($F_{(1, 4507)} = 9.42$, $p < 0.01$, d = 0.25) decreased clearly in the experimental group compared to the control group, which showed either no changes or a slight fall.

As regards aggressive behavior, the scores for insults ($F_{(1, 4526)} = 14.66$, $p < 0.01$, d = 0.30), threats ($F_{(1, 4526)} = 5.87$, $p < 0.01$, d = 0.22), and exclusion ($F_{(1, 4526)} = 7.21$, $p < 0.01$, d = 0.23) decreased significantly in the experimental group compared to the control group, which saw hardly any changes or even a slight increase.

Table 3. Multivariate analysis of variance (MANOVA) results.

Items	Group	M (SD) Pre	M (SD) Post	Lambda de Wilks F	p
General Victimization	Exper	0.15 (0.25)	0.12 (0.25)	12.63	>0.01 *
	Control	0.10 (0.19)	0.10 (0.22)		
General Aggression	Exper	0.09 (0.18)	0.06 (0.19)	6.66	0.01 *
	Control	0.06 (0.15)	0.06 (0.16)		
Someone said nasty things to me or called me names using Internet, social networks, or WhatsApp.	Exper	0.37 (0.73)	0.33 (0.67)	4.05	0.04 *
	Control	0.26 (0.61)	0.26 (0.62)		
Someone said nasty things about me to others using Internet, social networks, or WhatsApp.	Exper	0.29 (0.67)	0.25 (0.60)	5.16	0.02 *
	Control	0.21 (0.56)	0.21 (0.56)		
Someone threatened me through texts or online messages.	Exper	0.15 (0.48)	0.13 (0.46)	5.25	0.02 *
	Control	0.09 (0.34)	0.10 (0.41)		
Someone hacked into my account and stole personal information (e.g., through email or social networking accounts).	Exper	0.07 (0.31)	0.07 (0.36)	1.17	0.29
	Control	0.05 (26)	0.06 (0.30)		
Someone hacked into my account and pretended to be me (e.g., through instant messaging or social networking accounts).	Exper	0.07 (31)	0.07 (0.37)	0.57	0.56
	Control	0.05 (0.23)	0.05 (0.29)		
Someone created a fake account, pretending to be me (e.g., through instant messaging or social networking accounts).	Exper	0.06 (0.29)	0.06 (0.31)	0.80	0.36
	Control	0.04 (0.22)	0.05 (0.26)		
Someone posted personal information about me online.	Exper	0.08 (0.36)	0.07 (0.32)	0.35	0.55
	Control	0.07 (0.29)	0.06 (0.30)		
Someone posted embarrassing videos or pictures of me online.	Exper	0.12 (0.45)	0.09 (0.38)	0.77	0.38
	Control	0.09 (0.38)	0.07 (0.33)		
Someone altered pictures or videos of me that I had posted online.	Exper	0.08 (0.33)	0.07 (0.32)	0.52	0.47
	Control	0.06 (0.28)	0.05 (0.27)		
I was excluded or ignored by others in a social networking site or Internet.	Exper	0.25 (0.59)	0.16 (0.48)	15.75	>0.01 *
	Control	0.15 (0.43)	0.13 (0.43)		
Someone spread rumors about me on the Internet.	Exper	0.19 (0.52)	0.12 (0.42)	9.42	>0.01 *
	Control	0.14 (0.43)	0.12 (0.45)		
I said nasty things to someone or called them names Internet, social networks, or WhatsApp.	Exper	0.27 (0.61)	0.19 (0.53)	14.66	0.00 *
	Control	0.20 (0.51)	0.19 (0.52)		
I said nasty things about someone to other people using Internet, social networks, or WhatsApp.	Exper	0.23 (0.57)	0.17 (0.52)	1.4	0.23
	Control	0.18 (0.49)	0.14 (0.44)		
I threatened someone through texts or online messages.	Exper	0.07 (0.34)	0.05 (0.28)	5.87	0.01 *
	Control	0.04 (0.24)	0.05 (0.29)		
I hacked into someone's account and stole personal information (e.g., through email or social networking accounts).	Exper	0.03 (0.24)	0.03 (0.24)	3.76	0.05
	Control	0.01 (0.14)	0.03 (0.25)		
I hacked into someone's account and pretended to be them (e.g., through instant messaging or social networking accounts).	Exper	0.03 (0.25)	0.02 (0.21)	2.2	0.13
	Control	0.02 (0.17)	0.03 (0.23)		
I created a fake account, pretending to be someone else (e.g., through instant messaging or social networking accounts).	Exper	0.04 (0.25)	0.05 (0.28)	1.21	0.27
	Control	0.03 (0.21)	0.03 (0.23)		
I posted personal information about someone online.	Exper	0.03 (0.21)	0.03 (0.25)	0.01	0.96
	Control	0.02 (0.16)	0.03 (0.19)		
I posted embarrassing videos or pictures of someone online.	Exper	0.05 (0.30)	0.04 (0.26)	0.01	0.99
	Control	0.04 (0.24)	0.04 (0.25)		
I altered pictures or videos of another person that had been posted online.	Exper	0.05 (0.27)	0.04 (0.24)	0.93	0.33
	Control	0.05 (0.27)	0.04 (0.26)		
I excluded or ignored someone in a social networking site or Internet.	Exper	0.19 (0.55)	0.11 (0.42)	7.21	>0.01 *
	Control	0.11 (0.38)	0.08 (0.33)		
I spread rumors about someone on the Internet.	Exper	0.08 (0.37)	0.07 (0.37)	0.10	0.75
	Control	0.06 (0.26)	0.05 (28)		

Notes: * $p < 0.05$

4. Discussion

The aim of this study was to assess the impact of Asegúrate, an educational program specifically designed to prevent, reduce, or alleviate cyberbullying, in which teachers were given a purpose-written self-training manual (Asegúrate) to use autonomously. This educational material focuses on cyberbullying and on the social behavior teenage boys and girls display online when using virtual social networks. The Asegúrate program assumes that teachers are sufficiently aware that this behavior can disrupt the social climate and well-being of their pupils and that they will carry out self-training and acquire suitable levels of professional competence to intervene when such behavior occurs. We also assumed that, if teachers increased their competence in this way by using the materials available to them including the Asegúrate manual, then the levels of cyberbullying in the classroom would improve, as measured by self-administered questionnaires given to the schoolchildren themselves, as is the norm in studies of bullying and cyberbullying [50]. This system of pre/post evaluation has enabled us to note any improvements in prevalence for the different aspects of cyberbullying/cyber-victimization evaluated with the questionnaires, and to rank the results in order of highest to lowest prevalence of the different types of cyberbullying.

This has allowed us to observe that verbal cyberbullying, which is close to traditional forms of bullying, such as insults, threats, social exclusion, and spreading rumors, is the most frequent type in both groups, both in victimization and aggression: in other words, the commonest form of cyberbullying is still very similar to traditional bullying. By this, we can deduce that the new forms of cyberbullying introduced by technology, such as identity theft or manipulating multimedia, images, or videos with the intention of offending or hurting the victim, are less widespread among the adolescent population, at least in the cross section of pupils who participated in this study. These results also seem to show that the main aspect that is transferred to the online context is traditional aggressive behavior, to a far greater degree than the actual use of technology. We feel this is a relevant discovery, since it supports the idea that rather than the digital platforms opening the floodgates to new kinds of bullying [51], cyberbullying mainly consists of simply adapting the usual offensive roles of bullying one's peers to the conditions provided by the current technology [27].

In addition, the secondary objective of this work was to evaluate the effectiveness and suitability of the self-training manuals written by our scientific team and made available to the teachers who took part in the study (the experimental group) to use as they saw fit. The Asegúrate teaching manual, interpreted and used autonomously by teachers in the schools involved in the study, has led to significant changes in the pupils' involvement in the program. The experimental group obtained extremely positive results in improving the situation regarding victimization, aggression, and the number of bully/victims. Some improvement was also noted in the control schools, but to a lesser extent than in those involved in the experiment. The most notable result was the clear decrease in victimization, aggression, and bully/victims in the experimental group, compared to the very slight fall for the control group in victims and aggressors and the sharp rise in bully/victims [52]. If these results are interpreted correctly, there is a higher risk of becoming bully/victims in those schools where no intervention program (i.e., Asegúrate) is applied. In other words, the rise in aggressiveness and victimization was the greatest risk in cases where the teachers did not specifically take part in self-training and become aware of how they could use their own professional skills to prevent the problem. When comparing the post-tests for the control group, the findings show an increased level of conflict from bully/victims.

The role of bully/victim, in which pupils are not only victimized by their peers, but are also aggressors at the same time, has been described as one which involves far greater problems of psychological adjustment [53]. Although there are few existing longitudinal studies on the subject, the Asegúrate program has proved effective in dealing with the phenomenon where cyberbullying leads to a higher incidence of this double role of involvement [54]. It has been shown that, when no action is taken—apart from other insignificant, circumstantial changes that cannot be measured objectively—the number of pupils who adopt both roles increases. The increased number of pupils involved in this controversial mixed role (bullying others as well as being a victim of bullying) could be considered as an underlying, often unnoticed, result of not acting against cyberbullying. We could say that, if the problem is ignored, and no action is taken, it results in a greater, indiscriminate risk of increased conflict, aggression, and victimization, which is possibly the most confusing and chaotic scenario produced by bullying and victimization.

When both experiences decrease (cyber-victimization and cyberbullying), the involvement of teachers can become an extremely relevant factor for change, since the phenomenon of cyberbullying is mutualistic, in that bullying is both given and received. Teachers who make it a priority in the course of their professional activity to focus on specific problems of bullying and deal with them effectively, guided by their own convictions, appear to exercise a strong influence against the spread of cyberbullying [55]. The Asegúrate program prioritizes professional autonomy and effective management, and the results obtained show good efficacy in terms of reducing cyber-victimization and cyberbullying. After the program was introduced, direct insults, abuse, or verbal aggression against the victim, threats, social exclusion, and rumor-spreading all diminished significantly. This clearly shows that, in groups where the teachers implemented the program, the incidence of threatening, insulting, and socially excluding behavior fell sharply. In particular, the repeated measures results for each of the 11 items of behavior of cyber-victimization and cyberbullying showed that the Asegúrate program proved particularly effective against the kinds of virtual bullying and victimization, which are most similar to face-to-face bullying: verbal abuse, and social and psychological exclusion. Bullying involving insulting and humiliating decreased in those schools which took part in the study, while it remained the same in the control schools. This decrease was significantly greater in the schools taking part in the study than in the control schools for bullying involving verbal abuse, victimization, and social exclusion. This program therefore seems to have fulfilled its primary objective, which was to offer teachers the necessary resources to take a stand against cyberbullying in their schools, a demand that has been so widely called for by the scientific community [56].

After the initial self-training, the teaching staff who put the Asegúrate program into practice made special efforts to combine activities specially designed by experts with their own interpretation and self-planned techniques, which they adapted to the social context of their own pupils. This illustrates the importance of the teaching staff as a key element in the intervention against cyberbullying [39]. Just as happens in traditional bullying, schoolchildren see the degree of teacher involvement as a highly relevant factor in reducing or facilitating their involvement [57]. It has also become clear that the extent to which pupils perceive that their teachers are involved in managing interpersonal relationships in the classroom has a high predictive value for cyberbullying. This reinforces the idea that, when the pupils themselves recognize high quality teaching, it includes the notion that this high quality both helps to prevent cyberbullying as well as improve the general atmosphere of the class [58].

The Asegúrate program has been effective against all the types of behavior, which are associated with involvement in cyberbullying, which represents such a problematic phenomenon for schools. In fact, the indicators which show a reduction of involvement in both roles reveal highly significant changes. Not only does the specific behavior of cyberbullying and cyber-victimization decrease, but also a large number of the boys and girls who were previously noted as "involved in cyberbullying phenomena" in the pre-test were classified in the post-test in the "not-involved" or "bystanders" group. In fact, there was a significant increase in the number of "bystanders" in the post-test in the experimental group compared with the control group, with around a 25% decrease in the number of cyber-victims and a fall of over 30% in the number of cyberbullies.

It should also be noted that the evaluation of the Asegúrate program has certain limitations. The use of self-reports has its obvious shortcomings, but perhaps the most relevant is that the Asegúrate program could be improved further with more specific training to deal with the specific behavior of schoolchildren when using digital devices. Although this type of behavior does not appear to be extremely widespread, the harmful, dangerous behavior it involves did not decrease in adolescents even after the program was carried out. It therefore seems essential to include a study of the dynamics of how adolescents use digital devices, as well as materials and training to help make the program more effective in this respect. Likewise, other variables that are impossible to measure in this type of research could be related to the changes found in other activities in the school, additional teacher training, etc.

5. Conclusions

The results we obtained are in line with the different articles in the scientific literature about the prevention of cyberbullying, which show that the teaching staff are one of the key factors in reducing and alleviating the problem [16,20,59]. However, our results go one step further: they show how effective material, designed by researchers who have thorough knowledge of the prevalence and characteristics of cyberbullying, used autonomously by teachers who know their pupils well and spend long periods of time in the classroom with them, is a highly effective and beneficial combination, because it does not disturb the normal daily life of the classroom. When intervention programs such as the one proposed in this research are put into practice, the autonomy and initiative of the teaching staff is viewed by the pupils in a positive light, as a vital means of support. Each teacher may adapt the material to suit the needs of their school and any particular class, but the practice of using common guidelines, such as those provided by the Asegúrate teaching material, has been widely accepted. This does not mean that external training processes are no longer necessary: on the contrary, this external support for their teaching helps the autonomous training provided by each teacher to be both more effective and better appreciated by the schoolchildren.

Although cyberbullying occurs in a virtual environment, where some teachers feel less comfortable or reluctant to explore because of their lack of prior experience [60], our results show that the most common behaviors are those more like traditional bullying ones. These types of behaviors through electronic device have been the most reduced by teachers, perhaps because they have previous experience in carrying out anti-bullying programs.

For this reason, our results emphasize that it is not essential that teachers immerse themselves or have an expert domain of virtual environments, social networks, or cross-platform applications to improve how their students behave online. The useful work that has been carried out over a long period of time against traditional harassment [61], which promotes values such as empathy and respect for colleagues, can be developed and transferred to the context of virtual environments, with the help of high quality teaching materials, such as those provided by the Asegúrate program.

Author Contributions: R.D.R. conducted the research project; R.D.R. and J.A.C. delivered the program and analyzed the data; R.D.R., J.A.C. and R.O.-R. wrote jointly the paper.

Funding: This research was funded by the Government of Spain—R+D plan—grant number "PSI2017-86723-R" and "PSI2016-74871-R".

Conflicts of Interest: The authors declare no conflict of interest.

References

1. Oberle, E.; Domitrovich, C.E.; Meyers, D.C.; Weissberg, R.P. Establishing systemic social and emotional learning approaches in schools: A framework for schoolwide implementation. *Camb. J. Educ.* **2016**, *46*, 277–297. [CrossRef]

2. Olweus, D. *Aggression in the Schools: Bullies and Whipping Boys*; Hemisphere Publishing Corporation: Washington, DC, USA, 1978; ISBN 0470993618.

3. Solberg, M.E.; Olweus, D.; Endresen, I.M. Bullies and victims at school: Are they the same pupils? *Br. J. Educ. Psychol.* **2007**, *77*, 441–464. [CrossRef] [PubMed]

4. Van Ryzin, M.J.; Roseth, C.J. Cooperative learning in Middle School: A means to improve peer relations and reduce victimization, bullying, and related outcomes. *J. Educ. Psychol.* **2018**, *110*, 1192–1201. [CrossRef]

5. Menesini, E.; Salmivalli, C. Bullying in schools: The state of knowledge and effective interventions. *Psychol. Health Med.* **2017**, *22*, 240–253. [CrossRef] [PubMed]

6.   Nocito Muñoz, G. Investigaciones sobre el acoso escolar en España: Implicacines psicoeducativas//Research on bullying in Spain: Psicho-educational implications. *Revista Española de Orientación y Psicopedagogía* **2017**, *28*, 104–118. [CrossRef]

7.   Garmendia, M.; Jiménez, E.; Casado, M.A.; Mascheroni, G. *Net Children Go Mobile: Riesgos y Oportunidades en Internet y el Uso de Dispositivos Móviles Entre Menores Españoles (2010–2015)*; Red.es/Universidad del País Vasco/Euskal Herriko Unibertsitatea: Madrid, Spain, 2016.

8.   Ertmer, P.A.; Ottenbreit-Leftwich, A.T. Teacher technology change: How knowledge, confidence, beliefs, and culture intersect. *J. Res. Technol. Educ.* **2010**, *42*, 255–284. [CrossRef]

9.   Kowalski, R.M.; Giumetti, G.W.; Schroeder, A.N.; Lattanner, M.R. Bullying in the digital age: A critical review and meta-analysis of cyberbullying research among youth. *Psychol. Bull.* **2014**, *140*, 1073–1137. [CrossRef]

10. Tokunaga, R.S. Following you home from school: A critical review and synthesis of research on cyberbullying victimization. *Comput. Hum. Behav.* **2010**, *26*, 277–287. [CrossRef]

11. Baldry, A.C.; Blaya, C.; Farrington, D.P. *International Perspectives on Cyberbullying: Prevalence, Risk Factors and Interventions*; Palgrave MacMillan: London, UK, 2018; ISBN 9783319732626.

12. Slonje, R.; Smith, P.K. Cyberbullying: Another main type of bullying? *Scand. J. Psychol.* **2008**, *49*, 147–154. [CrossRef]

13. Betts, L.R. *Cyberbullying: Approaches, Consequences and Interventions*; Palgrave Macmillan: Nottingham, UK, 2016; ISBN 9781137500090.

14. Willard, N. Flame retardant: Cyberbullies torment their victims 24/7: Here's how to stop the abuse. *Sch. Libr. J.* **2006**, *52*, 54.

15. Ovejero, A.; Smith, P.K.; Yubero, S. *El Acoso Escolar y su Prevención: Perspectivas Internacionales*; Biblioteca Nueva: Madrid, Spain, 2013; ISBN 8499405800.

16. Slonje, R.; Smith, P.K.; Frisén, A. The nature of cyberbullying, and strategies for prevention. *Comput. Hum. Behav.* **2013**, *29*, 26–32. [CrossRef]

17. Vandebosch, H.; Van Cleemput, K. Defining Cyberbullying: A Qualitative Research into the Perceptions of Youngsters. *CyberPsychol. Behav.* **2008**, *11*, 499–503. [CrossRef] [PubMed]

18. Curtichs, J.; Fuentes, M.A.; García, Y.; Toca, A. *Sentido Social: La Comunicación y el Sentido Común en la Era de la Internet*; Profit: Barcelona, España, 2011; ISBN 8492956275.

19. Athanasiou, K.; Melegkovits, E.; Andrie, E.K.; Magoulas, C.; Tzavara, C.K.; Richardson, C.; Greydanus, D.; Tsolia, M.; Tsitsika, A.K. Cross-national aspects of cyberbullying victimization among 14–17-year-old adolescents across seven European countries. *BMC Public Health* **2018**, *18*, 800. [CrossRef] [PubMed]

20. Zych, I.; Ortega-Ruiz, R.; Del Rey, R. Scientific research on bullying and cyberbullying: Where have we been and where are we going. *Aggress. Violent Behav.* **2015**, *24*, 188–198. [CrossRef]

21. Modecki, K.L.; Minchin, J.; Harbaugh, A.G.; Guerra, N.G.; Runions, K.C. Bullying prevalence across contexts: A meta-analysis measuring cyber and traditional bullying. *J. Adolesc. Health* **2014**, *55*, 602–611. [CrossRef]

22. Ybarra, M.L.; Boyd, D.; Korchmaros, J.D.; Oppenheim, J. (Koby) Defining and measuring cyberbullying within the larger context of bullying victimization. *J. Adolesc. Health* **2012**, *51*, 53–58. [CrossRef]

23. Cappadocia, M.C.; Pepler, D.; Cummings, J.G.; Craig, W. Individual motivations and characteristics associated with bystander intervention during bullying episodes among children and youth. *Can. J. Sch. Psychol.* **2012**, *27*, 201–216. [CrossRef]

24. Brochado, S.; Soares, S.; Fraga, S. A scoping review on studies of cyberbullying prevalence among adolescents. *Trauma Violence Abus.* **2017**, *18*, 523–531. [CrossRef]

25. Gámez-Guadix, M.; Orue, I.; Smith, P.K.; Calvete, E. Longitudinal and reciprocal relations of cyberbullying with depression, substance use, and problematic internet use among adolescents. *J. Adolesc. Health* **2013**, *53*, 446–452. [CrossRef]

26. Ang, R.P.; Goh, D.H. Cyberbullying among adolescents: The role of affective and cognitive empathy, and gender. *Child Psychiatry Hum. Dev.* **2010**, *41*, 387–397. [CrossRef]

27. Olweus, D. Cyberbullying: An overrated phenomenon? *Eur. J. Dev. Psychol.* **2012**, *9*, 520–538. [CrossRef]

28. Rachoene, M.; Oyedemi, T. From self-expression to social aggression: Cyberbullying culture among South African youth on Facebook. *Communicatio* **2015**, *41*, 302–319. [CrossRef]

29. Waasdorp, T.E.; Bradshaw, C.P. The overlap between cyberbullying and traditional bullying. *J. Adolesc. Health* **2015**, *56*, 483–488. [CrossRef] [PubMed]

30. Della Cioppa, V.; O'Neil, A.; Craig, W. Learning from traditional bullying interventions: A review of research on cyberbullying and best practice. *Aggress. Violent Behav.* **2015**, *23*, 61–68. [CrossRef]

31. Gradinger, P.; Yanagida, T.; Strohmeier, D.; Spiel, C. Prevention of cyberbullying and cyber victimization: evaluation of the visc social competence program. *J. Sch. Violence* **2015**, *14*, 87–110. [CrossRef]

32. Gaffney, H.; Farrington, D.P.; Espelage, D.L.; Ttofi, M.M. Are cyberbullying intervention and prevention programs effective? A systematic and meta-analytical review. *Aggress. Violent Behav.* **2018**. [CrossRef]

33. Cross, D.; Shaw, T.; Hadwen, K.; Cardoso, P.; Slee, P.; Roberts, C.; Thomas, L.; Barnes, A. Longitudinal impact of the cyber friendly schools program on adolescents' cyberbullying behavior. *Aggress. Behav.* **2016**, *42*, 166–180. [CrossRef]

34. Burger, C.; Strohmeier, D.; Spröber, N.; Bauman, S.; Rigby, K. How teachers respond to school bullying: An examination of self-reported intervention strategy use, moderator effects, and concurrent use of multiple strategies. *Teach. Teach. Educ.* **2015**, *51*, 191–202. [CrossRef]

35. Sakellariou, T.; Carroll, A.; Houghton, S. Rates of cyber victimization and bullying among male Australian primary and high school students. *Sch. Psychol. Int.* **2012**, *33*, 533–549. [CrossRef]

36. Cross, D.; Barnes, A.; Papageorgiou, A.; Hadwen, K.; Hearn, L.; Lester, L. A social–ecological framework for understanding and reducing cyberbullying behaviors. *Aggress. Violent Behav.* **2015**, *23*, 109–117. [CrossRef]

37. Barlett, C.P.; Gentile, D.A.; Dongdong, L.; Khoo, A. Predicting cyberbullying behavior from attitudes. *J. Media Psychol.* **2017**, 1–11. [CrossRef]

38. Macaulay, P.J.R.; Betts, L.R.; Stiller, J.; Kellezi, B. Perceptions and responses towards cyberbullying: A systematic review of teachers in the education system. *Aggress. Violent Behav.* **2018**, *43*, 1–12. [CrossRef]

39. Green, V.A.; Johnston, M.; Mattioni, L.; Prior, T.; Harcourt, S.; Lynch, T. Who is responsible for addressing cyberbullying? Perspectives from teachers and senior managers. *Int. J. Sch. Educ. Psychol.* **2017**, *5*, 100–114. [CrossRef]

40. Styron, R.A.; Bonner, J.L.; Styron, J.L.; Bridgeforth, J.; James, M.; Martin, C. Are teacher and principal candidates prepared to address student cyberbullying? *J. At-Risk Issues* **2016**, *19*, 19–28.

41. Schultze-Krumbholz, A.; Schultze, M.; Zagorscak, P.; Wölfer, R.; Scheithauer, H. Feeling cybervictims' pain—The effect of empathy training on cyberbullying. *Aggress. Behav.* **2016**, *42*, 147–156. [CrossRef] [PubMed]

42. Boulton, M.J. Teachers' self-efficacy, perceived effectiveness beliefs, and reported use of cognitive-behavioral approaches to bullying among pupils: Effects of in-service training with the I DECIDE program. *Behav. Ther.* **2014**, *45*, 328–343. [CrossRef]

43. Del Rey, R.; Casas, J.A.; Ortega, R. Impact of the ConRed program on different cyberbulling roles. *Aggress. Behav.* **2016**, *42*, 123–135. [CrossRef]

44. Rimal, R.N.; Lapinski, M.K. A re-explication of social norms, ten years later. *Commun. Theory* **2015**, *25*, 393–409. [CrossRef]

45. Powell, K.C.; Kalina, C.J. Cognitive and social constructivism: Developing tools for an effective classroom. *Education* **2009**, *130*, 241–250.

46. Joseph, N. Metacognition needed: Teaching middle and high school students to develop strategic learning skills. *Prev. Sch. Fail. Altern. Educ. Child. Youth* **2009**, *54*, 99–103. [CrossRef]

47. Del-Rey-Alamillo, R.; Mora-Merchán, J.A.; Casas, J.-A.; Ortega-Ruiz, R.; Elipe, P. "Asegúrate" Program: Effects on cyber-aggression and its risk factors. *Comunicar* **2018**, *26*, 39–48. [CrossRef]

48. García Hernández, I.; de la Cruz Blanco, G. Las guías didácticas: Recursos necesarios para el aprendizaje autónomo. *Edumecentro* **2014**, *6*, 162–175.

49. Del Rey, R.; Casas, J.A.; Ortega-Ruiz, R.; Schultze-Krumbholz, A.; Scheithauer, H.; Smith, P.; Thompson, F.; Barkoukis, V.; Tsorbatzoudis, H.; Brighi, A.; et al. Structural validation and cross-cultural robustness of the European cyberbullying intervention project questionnaire. *Comput. Hum. Behav.* **2015**, *50*, 141–147. [CrossRef]

50. Dehue, F. Cyberbullying research: New perspectives and alternative methodologies. Introduction to the Special Issue. *J. Community Appl. Soc. Psychol.* **2013**, *23*, 1–6. [CrossRef]

51. Dehue, F.; Bolman, C.; Völlink, T. Cyberbullying: Youngsters' experiences and parental perception. *CyberPsychol. Behav.* **2008**, *11*, 217–223. [CrossRef] [PubMed]

52. Pouwels, J.L.; van Noorden, T.H.J.; Lansu, T.A.M.; Cillessen, A.H.N. The participant roles of bullying in different grades: Prevalence and social status profiles. *Soc. Dev.* **2018**, *27*, 732–747. [CrossRef]

53. Gámez-Guadix, M.; Gini, G.; Calvete, E. Stability of cyberbullying victimization among adolescents: Prevalence and association with bully–victim status and psychosocial adjustment. *Comput. Hum. Behav.* **2015**, *53*, 140–148. [CrossRef]

54. Cappadocia, M.C.; Craig, W.M.; Pepler, D. Cyberbullying: Prevalence, Stability, and risk factors during adolescence. *Can. J. Sch. Psychol.* **2013**, *28*, 171–192. [CrossRef]

55. Cassidy, W.; Faucher, C.; Jackson, M. Cyberbullying among youth: A comprehensive review of current international research and its implications and application to policy and practice. *Sch. Psychol. Int.* **2013**, *34*, 575–612. [CrossRef]

56. Tangen, D.; Campbell, M. Cyberbullying prevention: One primary school's approach. *J. Psychol. Couns. Sch.* **2010**, *20*, 225–234. [CrossRef]

57. Casas, J.A.; Ortega-Ruiz, R.; Del Rey, R. Bullying: The impact of teacher management and trait emotional intelligence. *Br. J. Educ. Psychol.* **2015**, *85*, 407–423. [CrossRef] [PubMed]

58. Aldridge, J.M.; Fraser, B.J. Teachers' views of their school climate and its relationship with teacher self-efficacy and job satisfaction. *Learn. Environ. Res.* **2016**, *19*, 291–307. [CrossRef]

59. Hutson, E.; Kelly, S.; Militello, L.K. Systematic review of cyberbullying interventions for youth and parents with implications for evidence-based practice. *Worldviews Evid.-Based Nurs.* **2018**, *15*, 72–79. [CrossRef] [PubMed]

60. Patchin, J.W.; Hinduja, S. *Cyberbullying Prevention and Response: Expert Perspectives*; Taylor and Francis: New York, NY, USA, 2012; ISBN 9780203818312.

61. Zych, I.; Farrington, D.P.; Ttofi, M.M. Bullying and cyberbullying: Protective factors and effective interventions. *Aggress. Violent Behav.* **2018**. [CrossRef]

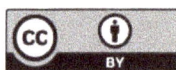

International Journal of
Environmental Research and Public Health

MDPI

Article

The Efficacy of the "Dat-e Adolescence" Prevention Program in the Reduction of Dating Violence and Bullying

Noelia Muñoz-Fernández [1], Javier Ortega-Rivera [2], Annalaura Nocentini [3], Ersilia Menesini [3] and Virginia Sánchez-Jiménez [2,*]

[1] Universidad Loyola Andalucía, 41014 Seville, Spain; nmunoz2@us.es
[2] Department of Developmental and Educational Psychology, University of Sevilla, 41807 Seville, Spain; javortega@us.es
[3] Department of Education, Languages, Intercultures, Literatures and Psychology, University of Florence, 50135 Florence, Italy; annalaura.nocentini@unifi.it (A.N.); ersilia.menesini@unifi.it (E.M.)
* Correspondence: virsan@us.es; Tel.:+34-95-455-7650

Received: 30 December 2018; Accepted: 23 January 2019; Published: 31 January 2019

Abstract: *Background*: The aim of this study was to assess the efficacy of the school-based "Dat-e Adolescence" prevention program in the reduction of dating aggression and victimization and bullying in adolescents. *Method*: a RCT design with three waves (pre-test, post-test and follow-up six months apart) and two groups (an experimental group and a control group) were used. One thousand four hundred and twenty three (1423) adolescents, mean age 14.98 (557 in the experimental group) participated in the study. *Results*: Efficacy evaluation was analyzed using Multiple-group latent growth models and showed that the Dat-e Adolescence program was effective in reducing sexual and severe physical dating violence and bullying victimization. *Conclusions*: The results suggest that dating violence prevention programs could be an effective approach for tackling different behavioral problems in adolescence given the protective and risk factors shared between dating violence and bullying.

Keywords: dating violence; bullying; prevention program; Dat-e Adolescence

1. Introduction

Dating violence is considered a subtype of intimate partner violence, which occurs in relationships that are more or less stable or lasting and encompasses aggressive behavior, be it psychological, physical, sexual, or via new technologies [1]. Although prevalence rates continue to be inconsistent, international studies have shown that psychological violence is the most frequent type, with percentages ranging from 20% to 80% [2,3], followed by physical forms at around 20%, and sexual violence at around 9% [4]. More recently, measures of online dating violence have yielded rates that vary from 2% to 50%, depending on the severity of the behavior under analysis [5]. Its consequences for adolescent development and health have also been highlighted, such as heavy episodic drinking, depressive symptomatology, suicidal ideation, smoking, and engaging in other antisocial behaviors [6]. Moreover, being involved in teen dating violence is associated with other behavioral problems such as bullying and sexual harassment. In this respect, studies have shown that bullying is a strong predictor of sexual harassment and dating violence in adolescence [7–10]. This association between dating violence and other forms of aggression has had various explanations. First, similar risk profiles for bullying and dating violence have been observed, such as attitudes towards violence and substance consumption [9]. Second, it has been hypothesized that the lessons learned in the peer relationship domain would be transferred to new contexts, such as romantic relationships [9,10], contributing to the internalization of an aggressive relational pattern [8–10]. In short, the prevalence and consequences of dating violence and its link to other behavioral problems have led us to define this phenomenon as a public health problem [1], which calls for preventive intervention to address these behaviors. Recognizing and considering its association with other, different behavioral problems would help to design ecological prevention programs that could improve their impact on adolescents' social networks [1].

In recent decades there has been a growing number of evidence-based dating violence prevention programs, of which we can mention the Safe Dates program [11]; the Fourth-R [12] and Shifting Boundaries [13], among others. Recent systematic reviews and meta-analyses [14–17] have concluded that dating violence prevention programs are promising for changing attitudes toward violence and for increasing adolescents' knowledge about the problem. However, the efficacy of these programs for reducing aggressive behavior has received less support and the results remain inconclusive. Research that has focused on synthetizing the available published literature has drawn two main conclusions: (1) few programs have shown positive effects in reducing dating aggression and victimization; and (2) not all forms of dating violence are sensitive to the treatment effects at the same level. In particular, three programs have reported changes in physical and/or sexual violence [13,18,19], whereas only one program has reported changes in psychological violence, namely the Safe Dates program [11,20]. Lastly, three studies [21–23] have identified changes in composite measures of different forms of abuse where psychological, physical and/or sexual violence were covered within the same measure. However, the absence of measure specificity makes it difficult to determine which outcome was responsible for the program's efficacy. In general terms, research suggests that the majority of programs appear to reduce severe and less frequent forms of violence, such as physical and sexual violence. In contrast, the results are less consistent when it comes to more frequent forms of violence, as is the case of psychological violence.

Some other available programs have tried to prevent aggressive behavior in adolescence in a more general way, attending to the reduction of bullying, dating violence or other forms of violence such as sexual harassment [12,13,24]. These studies acknowledge that dating violence and bullying share protective and risk factors, such as attitudes toward violence, feelings of anger, poor communication skills, and high levels of conflict [25]. The intervention on these factors could impact on these different aggressive behaviors at the same time. From this perspective, these programs may be considered cross-cutting in nature because a single program endeavors to prevent multiple problem behaviors, promoting the skills and strategies that young people need to tackle different forms of violence. As for their efficacy, some of these programs have failed to observe a significant reduction in dating violence and bullying [24]; others have observed decreased physical dating aggression but no decrease in peer aggression [12]; and others have reported a reduction in sexual dating violence, sexual harassment, and peer sexual violence [13]. Although these programs are promising from a cost-benefit analysis standpoint, the controversial results obtained thus far prevent us from concluding on the impact that dating violence prevention programs could have on other forms of interpersonal violence.

Considering the high variability found in terms of the efficacy of dating violence prevention programs, reviews and meta-analyses have identified some key aspects of the intervention design that appear able to be translated with greater success. Intervening during early adolescence (around age 13), when romantic relationships begin to show their importance in young people's lives and violent behavior, for the most part, has not yet surfaced, is recommended [26]. Other authors see the benefits of starting even earlier, intervening on predictors of dating violence such as bullying and sexual harassment [9,10]. Research also suggests the need to act upon the mediating variables to change behaviors—that is, on those variables that longitudinal studies have identified as precursors of dating violence [26]. In contrast, other authors [27] have concluded that violence prevention in young couples should not only focus on specific risk factors but also adopt a positive framework to promote the development of social and emotional skills. Intervention duration is also another relevant component. Short, 90-minute, single-session programs showed moderate results compared to longer programs whose effects were more robust over time [28,29]. It is also crucial to design comprehensive interventions of high methodological quality and rigor. Interventions applied to more than one context (e.g., school, family, teaching, and community settings), which incorporate randomized controlled trials (hereafter RCT) reported greater efficacy than other evaluation trials [15,28].

In Europe and specifically in Spain, there are no dating violence prevention programs that have been developed with high methodological quality using random assignment methods and whose design and procedure allow us to verify their efficacy in a reliable way [2]. This scenario is surprising when compared to the evidence-based programs available in Europe and Spain to address the prevention of school bullying and cyberbullying, as is the case of KiVa in Finland [30]; NoTrap! in Italy [31] and ConRed in Spain [32], among others. Specifically, Spanish dating violence prevention programs have shown low methodological quality characterized by participant selection through intentional sampling [33] and the use of quasi-experimental designs [34–36]. Most of these programs included a very small number of participants which makes it difficult to draw generalizable conclusions [33,35,36]. Considerable variability was also found in relation to efficacy analysis; while some programs intervened and assessed their effectiveness in attitudinal changes, beliefs and knowledge, others focused on behavioral changes. Specifically, those programs whose objective was to modify attitudes, beliefs and knowledge toward violence were effective [33–35]. On the other hand, only two programs have evaluated the program's effectiveness in relation to dating violence outcomes [35,36]. DaViPop [36] has been the only one to find positive results in the reduction of dating violence. This program also intervenes in romantic relationship quality, yielding positive results for support and future expectations. Within this framework, Dat-e Adolescence [37] has emerged as a response to the need for developing programs with high methodological quality and inspired by an evidence-based approach in the area of dating violence prevention in Spain. The aim of the present study was to examine the efficacy of the Dat-e Adolescence program (First Edition) in relation to reducing dating violence and bullying at follow-up measurement, that is, in the longer term as compared to the intervention implementation.

1.1. Theoretical Background of Dat-e Adolescence

Dating violence boasts specific characteristics that need to be taken into account. It is primarily mutual and bidirectional and related to conflicts in the dyad [17,38,39]. Studies have shown that this aggressive behavior is more common and less severe than other forms of violence in romantic relationships in adolescence, as gender-violence is, but it is clearly related [17]. At this respect, some of the risk factors that explain dating violence has an important role in gender- based violence. This is the case of peer context, which is not only crucial to the onset and maintenance of first romantic relationships [40], but also to violence in romantic relationships. Bullying and sexual harassment have been described as a stepping-stone to dating violence [9,10,41,42]. It has been observed that young people exposed to peer group violence tend to internalize acceptance of violence norms and develop a maladjusted perception of the consequences of violence on the victims, which poses a greater risk to violent behavior involvement in other relational contexts, including romantic relationships [43].

These characteristics are key aspects of the Dynamic Developmental Systems Model [44]. From a developmental and ecological perspective, this model acknowledges that dating violence is a complex problem associated with multiple risk factors [17]. It integrates different risk factors that contribute to violence among young couples (for a review of risk/protective factors, see [45,46]). Within this framework, abusive practices in the romantic relationship are seen as a consequence of the interaction that takes place among biological variables (e.g., genetic influences); individual variables (e.g., antisocial behavior); contextual factors (e.g., parental divorce); and the behaviors, beliefs and attitudes that each partner has acquired from socialization in different contexts (e.g., family, peers) throughout their life. Furthermore, in order to understand violence from this perspective, it is important to address not only the risk factors corresponding to each member of the couple, but also the relationship they develop and maintain; that is, their relational interactions and characteristics.

Accordingly, violence is seen as a consequence of jealousy, gender beliefs and attitudes about violence; of an insecure and/or avoidant attachment with the partner; of low levels of support and intimacy in the relationship; and lack of skills and strategies for tackling the misunderstandings and conflicts that often arise in the couple. Because of this dynamic, violence becomes stable within the romantic relationship, since abusive practices are consolidated as relational forms within couples [17,47].

This main risk factors addressed by DDS Model are considered in Dat-e Adolescence program. From our point of view, if boys and girls reflect about violence, gender norms, how the peer network influences their behavior, and they develop socio-emotional skills to be confident within their romantic relationships, they will be capable to build healthy relationships free of dating violence and gender-based violence. This comprehensive approach seems to be promising for prevention programs when working at universal level in community samples because permits to deep on the different expressions of violence that can occur within the couple, their nature, causes and how to deal with it [12,26].

1.2. The Dat-e Adolescence Program

Dat-e Adolescence is a school-based universal and multi-component prevention program designed for adolescents aged 12 to 19 years. It comprises seven 1-hour long sessions that can be implemented during school hours. In general terms, the program adopts a constructivist and experiential approach that encourages content learning through different teaching and learning experiences. It includes researcher- and peer-led training:

Researcher-led training. The first five sessions are administered by researchers during school hours. The main aims of these lessons are to (a) raise awareness of the concepts of love, myths about romantic love, and healthy behaviors in relationships; (b) encourage greater recognition, expression, and emotional regulation; and (c) promote enhanced self-esteem. In terms of couple dynamics, the program aims to (d) improve communication skills; and (e) promote the recognition of violent behavior in both traditional and online forms of violence. These lessons comprise discussions, role-playing, debates, and watching videos to promote socio-emotional skills and increase knowledge about romantic relationships and abuse. They consist of classroom and web-based activities, the latter via the program's online platform.

Peer-led training. The last two sessions are administered by peers during school hours. In the fifth session, two students from each class (one boy and one girl) volunteer to be the implementers of these final two sessions. These assistant students received four hours' training (two for each session) prior to the peer sessions. Presenting a conflictive or abusive context, these peer-led sessions aim to (a) raise awareness and promote coping strategies when aggression occurs and conflict-resolution strategies; and (b) raise awareness of the peer group and bystander's influence in the face of dating violence. These lessons comprise decision-making games and group dynamic exercises.

School session. A final activity is organized by the participating schools covering the main contents and lessons learned during the intervention.

The efficacy of Dat-e Adolescence has been assessed over two large RCT waves [37]. The program significantly modified beliefs towards violence, specifically on myths about romantic love (Cohen's *d* from −0.56 to −0.94); enhanced self-esteem (*d* = −0.15); and emotion regulation (*d* = −0.19) among participants. However, no significant effects were found for dating violence at post-test.

The present study tests the program's medium-term effect on moderate physical dating violence, severe physical dating violence and sexual dating violence as a primary outcome, and on bullying as a secondary outcome. It builds on the knowledge about the effectiveness of Dat-e Adolescence in comparison to previous assessments [37], examining the program's effects at follow-up (6 months apart) and assessing its efficacy on other behavioral outcomes. This research seeks to contribute to the debate on the efficacy of dating violence programs and to test their effects on preventing other related forms of interpersonal violence, for example, bullying. We hypothesized that the Dat-e Adolescence program would yield substantial reductions in primary and secondary outcomes at follow-up. This hypothesis is based on previous research that addressed the fact that prevention programs failed to find positive reduction of dating aggression and victimization at post-test despite some effects have been found at medium term. In this respect, De la Rue et al. [48] concluded that the impact of these programs on changing aggressive behavior would require not only changing attitudes and knowledge of violence, but the development of adolescents' socio-emotional skills that promote behavioral change when facing conflicts and disagreements with their partners. This skill-building training could help students to move to more healthy relationships, and later in time, to more positive and non-aggressive dating relationships. Since the program showed significant impact on improving emotional competence skills, such as students' emotion regulation, and changing attitudes towards violence at post-test, we might expect some kind of delayed effects on dating violence at medium-term. Moreover, considering that poor anger regulation [25] and low self-esteem [49–51] are risk factors involved in other behavioral problems, such as bullying, we also expect the program to have an effect on this form of interpersonal violence.

2. Materials and Methods

2.1. Participants

A total of 2050 adolescents participated in the study. For the main purpose of the study, they were selected based on having had romantic experience (n = 1423); 51.8% were male (n = 734), with ages ranging from 11 to 19 years (M = 14.98; SD = 1.39). 48.6% were in the first two-year cycle of high-school education (n = 691) and 51.4% in the second two-year cycle (n = 732). 830 participants studied in the province of Seville (58.3%) while 593 studied in the province of Córdoba (41.7%). Regarding romantic experience at Wave 1, 684 students had been in a relationship more than two months ago (48.1%); 305 had dated somebody in the last two months (21.4%); and 434 participants were in a current relationship (30.5%). 95.8% identified themselves as heterosexual or straight (n = 1357); 1% as gay or lesbian (n = 14); 1.6% as bisexual (n = 23); 0.2% as pansexual or demisexual (n = 3); and 1.3% did not know (n = 19). Around 95% of participants were born in Spain (n = 1357). The experimental group comprised 557 adolescents (53.8% male; age M = 14.88; SD = 1.30) from four high schools. The control group comprised 866 students (50.5% male; age M = 15.04; SD = 1.49) from three high schools. No differences in gender, $X^2(1)$ = 1.486; p = 0.231; CC = 0.03, or age, $F(1, 1415)$ = 3.121; p = 0.077; eta^2 = 0.002, were found between the control and experimental groups.

2.2. Attrition Analysis

Regarding attrition, 17% of participants completed the pre-test measure only (n = 242); 52.9% completed the pre-test and post-test measures (n = 753); and 30.1% of participants completed the pre-test, post-test, and follow-up measures (n = 428). Similar attrition rates were found for both groups, $X^2(2)$ = 1.932; p = 0.381. Specifically, 17.9% vs. 15.6% of control and experimental group participants, respectively, completed the pre-test measure; 53.1% vs. 52.6% of control and experimental group participants, respectively, completed the pre-test and post-test measures; and 29% vs. 31.8% of control and experimental group participants, respectively, completed all three waves. The high attrition rates observed at follow-up were due to four out of seven schools (experimental group = two schools, control group = two schools) choosing not to participate at follow-up (see flowchart, Figure 1). To establish similarities and differences between schools with follow-up and schools without follow-up, we compared the outcomes and sociodemographic variables at baseline level for both groups. No baseline differences for outcomes and sociodemographic variables were found between schools that participated at post-test and schools that participated at follow-up (see Table 1). For this reason, we decided to analyze intervention efficacy across all seven schools.

We explored pre-test differences in outcomes and sociodemographic variables among participants with different attrition characteristics (pre-test only, pre-test and post-test, and all three waves; see Table 1). No gender differences were found between attrition groups, $X^2(2)$ = 3.342; p = 0.188; CC = 0.05, nor for control group attrition, $X^2(2) = 4.103$; $p = 0.129$; CC = 0.07, or for experimental group attrition, $X^2(2) = 4.979$; $p = 0.083$; CC = 0.09. Univariate general linear models (GLM) were estimated to analyze the association between age, baseline outcomes, treatment condition, and attrition type. Baseline outcomes and age were identified as the dependent variables, whereas treatment condition and attrition type were the fixed factors. Differences were observed in age, $F(2, 1415) = 12.006$; $p = 0.000$; $eta^2 = 0.017$, moderate physical aggression, $F(2, 1368) = 7.355$; $p = 0.001$; $eta^2 = 0.011$, moderate physical victimization, $F(2, 1374) = 4.690$; $p = 0.009$; $eta^2 = 0.007$, severe physical aggression, $F(2, 1366) = 6.550$; $p = 0.001$; $eta^2 = 0.010$, bullying aggression, $F(2, 1396) = 5.891$; $p = 0.003$; $eta^2 = 0.008$, and bullying victimization, $F(2, 1402) = 4.867$; $p = 0.008$; $eta^2 = 0.007$, between pre-test measure only, post-test, and follow-up participants.

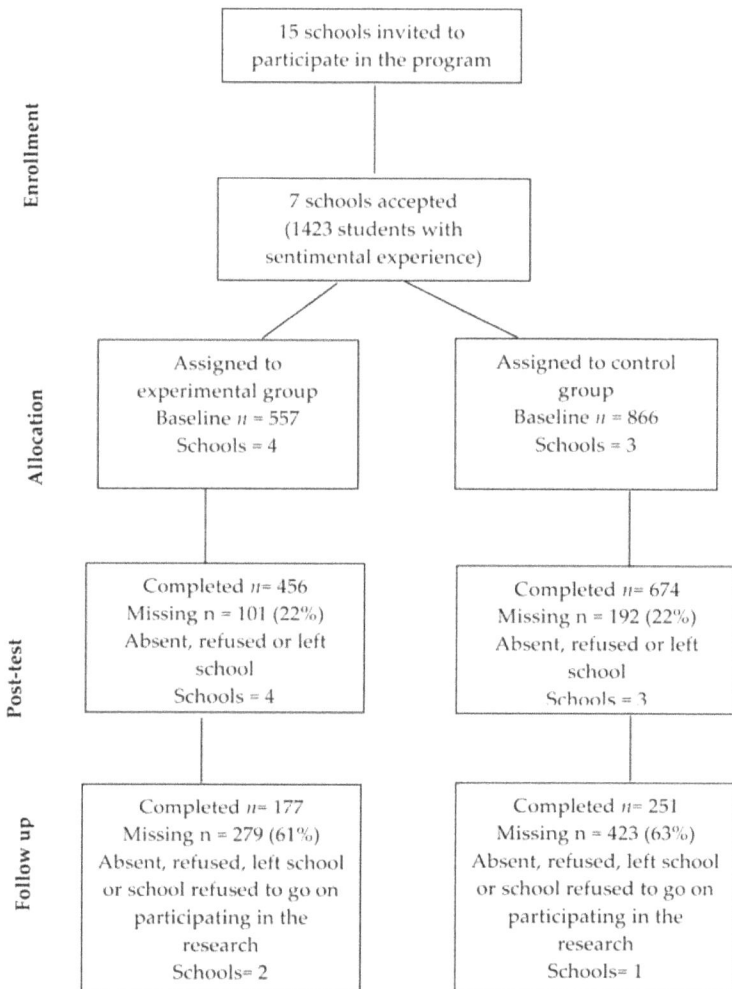

Figure 1. Flowchart of the recruitment and retention of participants in the evaluation.

Table 1. Attrition analysis. Comparison effects of attrition at school level and at participant level.

Outcomes	Comparison Effect of Attrition for Schools			Comparison Effect of Treatment Condition and Attrition for Participants								
	Schools at Post-Test (7 Schools)	Schools at Follow-Up (3 Schools)	Diff.	Participants with Only Pre-Test			Participants with Pre-Test and Post-Test			Participants with Three Waves		
				CG	EG	Total	CG	EG	Total	CG	EG	Total
Moderate Physical dating aggression	0.063 (0.235)	0.057 (0.214)	$T(1366) = -10.027$; $p = 0.304$; $d = -0.06$	0.096 (0.309)	0.097 (0.287)	0.096 (0.301)	0.069 (0.232)	0.056 (0.244)	0.064 (0.236)	0.023 (0.137)	0.027 (0.141)	0.025 (0.139)
Moderate Physical dating victimization	0.075 (0.289)	0.068 (0.288)	$T(1372) = -0.391$; $p = 0.696$; $d = 0.02$	0.097 (0.353)	0.125 (0.383)	0.107 (0.363)	0.085 (0.306)	0.072 (0.294)	0.080 (0.303)	0.029 (0.141)	0.051 (0.257)	0.038 (0.198)
Severe Physical dating aggression	0.043 (0.195)	0.047 (0.207)	$T(1364) = 0.389$; $p = 0.697$; $d = 0.02$	0.052 (0.186)	0.110 (0.327)	0.073 (0.246)	0.051 (0.221)	0.046 (0.227)	0.049 (0.223)	0.013 (0.076)	0.028 (0.130)	0.019 (0.103)
Severe Physical dating victimization	0.044 (0.185)	0.050 (0.237)	$T(1371) = 0.577$; $p = 0.564$; $d = 0.03$	0.050 (0.164)	0.073 (0.213)	0.058 (0.183)	0.053 (0.242)	0.054 (0.254)	0.053 (0.247)	0.017 (0.080)	0.045 (0.195)	0.029 (0.141)
Sexual dating aggression	0.044 (0.251)	0.034 (0.156)	$T(1359) = -0.908$; $p = 0.364$; $d = -0.05$	0.037 (0.162)	0.028 (0.112)	0.034 (0.147)	0.045 (0.208)	0.052 (0.333)	0.048 (0.264)	0.028 (0.131)	0.034 (0.148)	0.030 (0.139)
Sexual dating victimization	0.065 (0.293)	0.077 (0.275)	$T(1368) = 0.790$; $p = 0.430$; $d = 0.04$	0.072 (0.338)	0.045 (0.130)	0.062 (0.282)	0.089 (0.329)	0.066 (0.269)	0.075 (0.307)	0.054 (0.205)	0.081 (0.290)	0.065 (0.245)
Bullying aggression	0.439 (0.608)	0.392 (0.492)	$T(1394) = -10.563$; $p = 0.118$; $d = -0.08$	0.426 (0.539)	0.466 (0.559)	0.440 (0.546)	0.439 (0.626)	0.477 (0.624)	0.454 (0.625)	0.369 (0.451)	0.314 (0.399)	0.346 (0.431)
Bullying victimization	0.681 (0.750)	0.687 (0.749)	$T(1400) = -0.135$; $p = 0.893$; $d = -0.01$	0.578 (0.726)	0.573 (0.631)	0.576 (0.693)	0.709 (0.768)	0.782 (0.797)	0.737 (0.779)	0.618 (0.649)	0.701 (0.805)	0.652 (0.719)
Gender Boys	407 (500.7%)	327 (530.2%)	$X^2(1) = 0.862$; $p = 0.362$; $CC = 0.03$	68 (440.7%)	54 (620.8%)	122 (510.3%)	229 (490.9%)	146 (490.8%)	375 (490.9%)	138 (55%)	99 (550.9%)	237 (550.4%)
Gender Girls	396 (490.3%)	288 (460.8%)		84 (550.3%)	32 (370.2%)	116 (480.7%)	230 (500.1%)	147 (500.2%)	377 (500.1%)	113 (45%)	78 (440.1%)	191 (440.6%)
Age	140.985 (10.426)	140.977 (10.353)	$T(1413) = -0.103$; $p = 0.918$; $d = -0.00$	150.362 (10.715)	150.128 (10.423)	150.278 (10.621)	150.112 (10.433)	140.929 (10.311)	150.041 (10.389)	140.724 (10.227)	140.695 (10.202)	140.712 (10.216)

Note: CG = control group; EG = experimental group; Mean and (Standard Deviation) are displayed in the table except for gender; T = Student's T; p = *p*-value; d = Cohen's *d*; X^2 = Chi-squared; CC = Contingency coefficient.

Specifically, students who only participated at the pre-test were older and more involved in moderate physical aggression, moderate physical victimization, severe physical aggression, and bullying aggression compared to their three-wave counterparts. However, this trend was not observed for bullying victimization; pre-test-only participants were less involved than their three-wave peers. No differences were found in severe physical victimization, $F(2, 1373) = 2.058$; $p = 0.128$; eta$^2 = 0.003$, sexual aggression, $F(2, 1361) = 1.037$; $p = 0.355$; eta$^2 = 0.002$, or sexual victimization, $F(2, 1370) = 0.240$; $p = 0.787$; eta$^2 = 0.000$, among participants with different attrition characteristics. Finally, no differences were found in moderate physical aggression, $F (2, 1368) = 0.259$; $p = 0.772$; eta$^2 = 0.000$, moderate physical victimization, $F (2, 1374) = 0.653$; $p = 0.521$; eta$^2 = 0.001$, severe physical aggression, $F(2, 1366) = 2.005$; $p = 0.135$; eta$^2 = 0.003$, severe physical victimization, $F(2, 1373) = 0.612$; $p = 0.542$; eta$^2 = 0.001$, sexual aggression, $F(2, 1361) = 0.113$; $p = 0.893$; eta$^2 = 0.000$, sexual victimization, $F(2, 1370) = 0.876$; $p = 0.417$; eta$^2 = 0.001$, bullying aggression, $F(2, 1396) = 0.964$; $p = 0.382$; eta$^2 = 0.001$, or bullying victimization, $F(2, 1402) = 0.271$; $p = 0.763$; eta$^2 = 0.000$, for the interaction effect between treatment condition and attrition type, suggesting that attrition differences were similar for both control and experimental groups. Thus, we can conclude that the intervention efficacy results obtained are not influenced by sample attrition.

2.3. Procedure

A RCT design was used with a control group and an experimental group. Fifteen state high schools from the cities of Seville and Córdoba (Andalusia region) were randomly selected by the Educational Authority using a simple randomization procedure (a list of random numbers was generated following a computer-based program). Those numbers that coincided with the school identification numbers were picked for the study. Following approval from the Research Ethics Committee of the Autonomous Region of Andalusia (code: 0575-N-14), initial contact was made with all 15 schools in December 2015. All schools presented a medium economic, social and cultural level (ISC Index in Spain) in accordance with the ranking established by the autonomous region's education authority. Meetings were held with the schools' directors and counseling teams to inform them about the research, its objectives, its content and the procedure to be selected for the experimental or control groups. Seven out of 15 schools agreed to take part in the study. Informed consent forms were signed and the program details were forwarded to the families and school boards, the latter granting all centers permission to take part. The seven centers were randomly assigned to either an experimental or control group using a coin toss procedure. A member of the research group who was not in direct contact with the school did this work. The waiting list procedure was applied to the control schools that expressed interest in receiving intervention in future editions. Pre-test was carried out in January 2016, post-test in June 2016, and follow-up in December 2016. The intervention took place from February through May 2016 once a week during school hours. Anonymous self-report, paper-and-pencil questionnaires were administered in the three waves. In order to identify students at the three points in time, the names of the participants were linked to a code that was used in each wave. The code was created taking into account the school, the class, and the number of each student in his/her class (the class list having been sorted alphabetically). Data were collected during school hours. Students received no rewards or incentives for taking part.

2.4. Measures

2.4.1. Sociodemographic Variables

An ad hoc questionnaire was devised to ask participants about their gender, age, sexual orientation, locality, and nationality.

2.4.2. Dating Relationship Status

Two items from the *Dating Questionnaire* [52] were used to analyze relationship status. The first item, a multiple-choice question, assessed the participants' romantic experience. The response options were as follows: (a) Yes, I'm currently dating someone; (b) I'm not currently dating anyone, but I have done in the last two months; (c) I'm not dating anyone right now but I was, more than two months ago; and (d) I've never dated anyone before. The second item asked about the length of the current or past relationship expressed in weeks.

2.4.3. Physical Violence

Moderate and severe physical violence was evaluated using an adapted version of the physical violence scale [53] from the *Conflict Tactics Scale* (CTS2) [54]. Nine items, measured on a 5-point Likert scale (0 = Never; 1 = rarely; 2 = sometimes; 3 = often; 4 = Always), assessed the frequency with which the adolescents, in a current or past relationship, had perpetrated or received physically violent behaviors in last six months (e.g., "to shove or throw against a wall"). According to the Spanish validation of the scale for adolescents [55], the first four items represent moderate physical acts and the last five items represent more severe physical acts. CFA for two correlated factors showed a good fit for aggression, $X^2(26) = 44.191$; RMSEA = 0.023; CFI = 0.902, and for victimization, $X^2(24) = 51.182$; RMSEA = 0.029; CFI = 0.907.

2.4.4. Sexual Violence

Sexual violence was assessed using an adapted version of the sexual dating violence measure proposed by Foshee et al. [56]. Four items, measured on a 5-point Likert scale (0 = Never; 1 = rarely; 2 = sometimes; 3 = often; 4 = Always), assessed the frequency with which the adolescents, in a current or past relationship, had perpetrated or received sexually violent behaviors in last six months ("to pressure or force the other to have sex"; "to pressure or force the other to engage in a sexual act when they did not want to"; "to touch the other when they did not want to be touched"; "to make humiliating comments about sexual behavior"). CFA showed a good fit for aggression, $X^2(2) = 1.611$; RMSEA = 0.000; CFI = 1.000, and for victimization, $X^2(2) = 0.725$; RMSEA = 0.000; CFI = 1.000.

2.4.5. Bullying

Bullying perpetration and victimization was assessed using the Spanish version of the European Bullying Intervention Project Questionnaire (EBIP-Q) [57]. Fourteen items, measured on a 5-point Likert scale (0 = Never; 1 = once or twice; 2 = once or twice a month; 3 = once a week; 4 = More than once a week), assessed the frequency with which adolescents perpetrated and received direct physical abuse, indirect abuse, verbal abuse, psychological abuse, and social exclusion in the last two months (e.g., "someone has spread rumors about me"). CFA showed a good fit for aggression, $X^2(12) = 77.772$; RMSEA = 0.063; CFI = 0.934, and for victimization, $X^2(13) = 92.807$; RMSEA = 0.066; CFI = 0.949.

2.5. Analysis Plan

All analyses were performed using MPLUS 7 (Muthen & Muthen, Los Angeles, CA, USA) and SPSS 24 (SPSS Inc., Chicago, IL, USA). In order to test the comparability of the control and experimental groups, we analyzed the pre-test differences [58]. Considering the size of the sample, we included eta^2 to estimate the effect size.

Following Cheong et al.'s [59] guidelines, multiple-group latent growth models were performed to analyze the effect of intervention on dating violence and bullying. According to the authors, when a prevention program is effective, the treatment and control groups are expected to show different outcome growth. To test this hypothesis, we first analyzed (Step 1) whether the linear trajectory shape fits the data and examined whether growth rates differed by condition. To this end, the trajectory of the outcome was examined separately using a two-group model [59]. The factor loadings of the latent factors were specified to be equal across both groups. The factor loadings on the latent intercepts factor were fixed to 1.0 to define the initial starting point. The factor loadings for the slope were set to 0, 1, and 2 given the equal timing across waves. The residual variances of each wave measure were also equated across groups. The covariance between intercept and slope factor was freely estimated and allowed for differences across both groups. Next (Step 2), the common intercept was estimated and the control group's slope factor mean was set to 0. In consequence, the slope mean of the treatment group captured the mean difference in the slope factor mean between both groups. The model fit was assessed to analyze the appropriateness of using current specification for both groups and to justify the use of program group membership as a causal variable for the different trajectory shapes. Additionally, the chi-square difference test was used to choose the best model. The maximum likelihood robust (MLR) estimation method was used to estimate the models, given that the variables presented normality problems. To avoid bias due to sample attrition, all models were estimated using the full information maximum likelihood (FIML) method. Effect size was computed adhering to Raudenbush and Liu's [60] formula for GMA analyses, where between-group differences in mean growth rates is the numerator and the slope SD is the denominator of the coefficient [61]. The following indices were used to evaluate the model fit: the chi-square (X^2) statistic; the root mean square error of approximation (RMSEA); and the comparative fit index (CFI), with cut-off points of 0.08 for RMSEA and 0.90 for CFI. SPSS 24 statistics software was used for the descriptive analyses and for attrition analysis.

3. Results

In order to test the comparability of the experimental and control groups, we analyzed the pretest differences [58] (see Table 2).

Table 2. Descriptive statistics in the three waves for primary and secondary outcomes.

Outcomes	Group	Pre-Intervention			Post-Intervention			Follow-Up		
		M	SD	n	M	SD	n	M	SD	n
Moderate physical aggression	Control group	0.061	0.227	833	0.066	0.317	623	0.024	0.111	220
	Experimental group	0.053	0.224	535	0.036	0.189	421	0.021	0.094	154
Moderate physical victimization	Control group	0.071	0.280	835	0.075	0.322	629	0.039	0.161	220
	Experimental group	0.073	0.300	539	0.050	0.275	420	0.027	0.116	155
Severe physical aggression	Control group	0.040	0.184	831	0.037	0.222	623	0.023	0.094	220
	Experimental group	0.050	0.222	535	0.027	0.168	421	0.005	0.039	154
Severe physical victimization	Control group	0.041	0.194	835	0.044	0.229	629	0.027	0.119	230
	Experimental group	0.054	0.230	538	0.039	0.256	420	0.015	0.100	155
Sexual aggression	Control group	0.039	0.181	829	0.039	0.201	623	0.033	0.167	220
	Experimental group	0.042	0.259	532	0.035	0.181	420	0.015	0.082	154
Sexual victimization	Control group	0.071	0.299	833	0.060	0.259	629	0.058	0.239	220
	Experimental group	0.067	0.260	537	0.082	0.339	419	0.047	0.191	155
Bullying aggression	Control group	0.417	0.566	854	0.392	0.535	666	0.366	0.470	243
	Experimental group	0.423	0.555	542	0.408	0.588	450	0.319	0.425	173
Bullying victimization	Control group	0.659	0.729	857	0.649	0.737	667	0.626	0.674	243
	Experimental group	0.724	0.779	545	0.668	0.736	449	0.600	0.726	173

No differences were found in moderate physical dating aggression, $F(1, 1368) = 0.030$; $p = 0.863$; $\text{eta}^2 = 0.000$, moderate physical dating victimization, $F(1, 1374) = 0.462$; $p = 0.497$; $\text{eta}^2 = 0.000$, severe physical dating aggression, $F(1, 1366) = 3.455$; $p = 0.063$; $\text{eta}^2 = 0.003$, severe physical dating victimization, $F(1, 1373) = 1.880$; $p = 0.171$; $\text{eta}^2 = 0.001$, sexual dating aggression, $F(1, 1361) = 0.009$; $p = 0.923$; $\text{eta}^2 = 0.000$, sexual dating victimization, $F(1, 1370) = 0.076$; $p= 0.783$; $\text{eta}^2 = 0.000$, bullying aggression, $F(1, 1396) = 0.046$; $p = 0.830$; $\text{eta}^2 = 0.000$, and bullying victimization, $F(1, 1402) = 1.207$; $p = 0.272$; $\text{eta}^2 = 0.001$, between the control and experimental groups at pre-test. The correlations among outcome variables are shown in Table 3. Dating violence and bullying were positively correlated. For each form of violence, measures of aggression and victimization showed a strong correlation. The effect size was large for the relationship between moderate physical dating aggression and victimization, for severe physical dating aggression and victimization, and for sexual dating aggression and victimization. The effect size was medium for the relationship between bullying aggression and victimization.

3.1. Effect of the Dat-e Adolescence Program on Moderate Physical Dating Violence

For moderate physical dating aggression, the overall fit of the two-group model was unacceptable in terms of the CFI value, $X^2(7) = 12.980$; RMSEA = 0.035; CFI = 0.652. Modification indices were analyzed, suggesting that the residual variance of the post-test measure was different across groups (MI = 8.790). When freely estimating the residual variance at post-test across groups, the model showed a good fit, $X^2(6) = 4.499$; RMSEA = 0.000; CFI = 1.000. In Step 1, the growth rate factor mean for both groups was found to be negative and significant (See Table 4). This suggests that growth was not due to intervention (i.e., normative growth).

For moderate physical dating victimization, the overall fit of the two-group model was acceptable, $X^2(7) = 3.487$; RMSEA = 0.000; CFI = 1.000. In Step 1, we observed a significant decrease over time for the experimental group and a declining trend for the control group (See Table 4). This suggests that growth was not due to intervention (i.e., normative growth).

3.2. Effect of the Dat-e Adolescence Program on Severe Physical Dating Violence

For severe physical dating aggression, the overall fit of the two-groups model was acceptable, $X^2(7) = 3.870$; RMSEA = 0.000; CFI = 1.000. In Step 1, the mean and variance of the growth rate factors for the control group were not significant, whereas the slope mean for the experimental group was negative and significant (see Table 4). In light of this, the means and variances of the growth factors were constrained to be 0 for the control group (Step 2). This model showed a good fit, $X^2(10) = 5.120$; RMSEA = 0.000; CFI = 1.000, and the chi-square difference test was not significant, Trd = 0.063; df = 3; $p = 0.996$, suggesting that the best model was the constrained model. In this model, the growth rate factor mean estimated for the treatment group was the estimated program effect. When comparing the average growth rates between both groups, the average growth rate for the treatment group was negative and statistically significant. The effect size was between small to medium ($d = 0.25$). These results indicate that the treatment group's growth trajectory of severe physical aggression decreased significantly compared to the control group's growth trajectory. For severe physical dating victimization, the overall fit of the two-groups model was acceptable, $X^2(8) = 7.900$; RMSEA = 0.000; CFI = 1.000, with the residual variance of the follow-up measure fixed to 0 for both groups. In Step 1, the mean and variance of the growth rate factors for the control group were not significant, whereas the slope mean for the experimental group was negative and significant (see Table 4). In light of this, the means and variances of the growth factors were constrained to be 0 for the control group (Step 2). This model showed a good fit, $X^2(11) = 7.092$; RMSEA = 0.000; CFI = 1.000, and the chi-square difference test was not significant, Trd = 0.815; df = 3; $p = 0.846$, suggesting that the best model was the constrained model. In this model, the growth rate factor mean estimated for the treatment group was the estimated program effect. When comparing the average growth rates between both groups, the average growth rate for the treatment group was negative and statistically significant. The effect size was between small to medium ($d = 0.21$). These results indicate that the treatment group's growth trajectory of severe physical aggression decreased significantly compared to the control group's growth trajectory.

Table 3. Correlations among outcome variables.

Outcomes	Moderate Dating Physical Victimization	Severe Dating Physical Aggression	Severe Dating Physical Victimization	Sexual Dating Aggression	Sexual Dating Victimization	Bullying Aggression	Bullying Victimization
Moderate physical dating aggression	0.73 ***	0.48 ***	0.41 ***	0.30 ***	0.21 ***	0.20 ***	0.05
Moderate physical victimization	1	0.48 ***	0.53 ***	0.23 ***	0.29 ***	0.18 ***	0.14 ***
Severe physical aggression		1	0.70 ***	0.45 ***	0.27 ***	0.22 ***	0.10 ***
Severe physical victimization			1	0.37 ***	0.38 ***	0.16 ***	0.14 ***
Sexual aggression				1	0.49 ***	0.13 ***	0.05
Sexual victimization					1	0.06 *	0.18 ***
Bullying aggression						1	0.46 ***
Bullying victimization							1

Note: * $p < 0.05$; *** $p < 0.001$.

Table 4. Multiple-group estimated components of growth curves.

Outcome	Group	Step 1: Model Free				Step 2: Model Constrained			
		Intercept		Slope		Intercept		Slope	
		Mean	Variance	Mean	Variance	Mean	Variance	Mean	Variance
Moderate physical dating aggression	Control group	0.059 (0.006) ***	0.020 (0.009) **	−0.014 (0.006) *	0.004 (0.005)				
	Experimental group	0.059 (0.006) ***	0.020 (0.009) **	−0.019 (0.005) ***	0.007 (0.004)				
Moderate physical victimization	Control group	0.073 (0.008) ***	0.059 (0.034) †	−0.015 (0.008) †	0.020 (0.017)				
	Experimental group	0.073 (0.008) ***	0.059 (0.034) †	−0.023 (0.006) ***	0.026 (0.009) †				
Severe physical aggression	Control group	0.045 (0.005) ***	0.014 (0.008) †	−0.005 (0.005)	0.000 (0.002)	0.042 (0.005) ***	0.015 (0.006) **	0	0
	Experimental group	0.045 (0.005) ***	0.014 (0.008) †	−0.020 (0.003) ***	0.004 (0.002) †	0.042 (0.005) ***	0.015 (0.006) **	−0.018 (0.003) ***	0.005 (0.002) *
Severe physical victimization	Control group	0.046 (0.007) ***	0.040 (0.038)	−0.012 (0.016)	0.019 (0.034)	0.046 (0.005) ***	0.020 (0.006) **	0	0
	Experimental group	0.046 (0.007) ***	0.040 (0.038)	−0.015 (0.005) **	0.009 (0.009)	0.046 (0.005) ***	0.020 (0.006) **	−0.015 (0.004) **	0.005 (0.003) †
Sexual aggression	Control group	0.041 (0.006) ***	0.014 (0.008)	−0.001 (0.006)	0.001 (0.007)	0.041 (0.005) ***	0.015 (0.006) *	0	0
	Experimental group	0.041 (0.006) ***	0.014 (0.008)	−0.012 (0.004) **	0.001 (0.003)	0.041 (0.005) ***	0.015 (0.006) *	−0.012 (0.004) **	0.001 (0.003)
Sexual victimization	Control group	0.070 (0.007) ***	0.032 (0.022)	−0.005 (0.007)	0.002 (0.010)	0.068 (0.007) ***	0.034 (0.015) *	0	0
	Experimental group	0.070 (0.007) ***	0.032 (0.022)	−0.014 (0.006) *	0.003 (0.005)	0.068 (0.007) ***	0.034 (0.015) *	−0.013 (0.005) *	0.003 (0.004)
Bullying aggression	Control group	0.421 (0.015) ***	0.201 (0.033) ***	−0.022 (0.013) †	0.025 (0.017)				
	Experimental group	0.421 (0.015) ***	0.201 (0.033) ***	−0.024 (0.017)	0.022 (0.018)				
Bullying victimization	Control group	0.684 (0.020) ***	0.320 (0.043) ***	−0.020 (0.018)	0.008 (0.026)	0.676 (0.018) ***	0.301 (0.030) ***	0	0
	Experimental group	0.684 (0.020) ***	0.320 (0.043) ***	−0.047 (0.020) *	0.009 (0.027)	0.676 (0.018) ***	0.301 (0.030) ***	−0.044 (0.020) *	0.002 (0.019)

Note: In parenthesis SE is reported. † $p < 0.10$; * $p < 0.05$; ** $p < 0.01$; *** $p < 0.001$; In Step 1 the means of the growth rate were freely estimated in both groups; In Step 2, the mean of the growth rate was constrained to 0 for the control group and freely estimated in the experimental group.

3.3. Effect of the Dat-e Adolescence Program on Sexual Dating Violence

For sexual dating aggression, the overall fit of the two-groups model was acceptable, $X^2(7) = 8.095$; RMSEA = 0.015; CFI = 0.918, with the residual variance of the follow-up measure fixed to 0. In Step 1, the mean and variance of the growth rate factors for the control group were not significant, whereas the slope mean for the experimental group was negative and significant (see Table 4). In light of this, the means and variances of the growth factors were constrained to be 0 for the control group (Step 2). This model showed a good fit, $X^2(10) = 9.890$; RMSEA = 0.000; CFI = 1.000, and the chi-square difference test was not significant, Trd = 0.268; df = 3; $p = 0.966$, suggesting that the best model was the constrained model. In this model, the growth rate factor mean estimated for the treatment group was the estimated program effect. When comparing the average growth rates between both groups, the average growth rate for the treatment group was negative and statistically significant. The effect size was between small to medium ($d = 0.38$). These results indicate that the treatment group's growth trajectory of severe physical aggression decreased significantly compared to the control group's growth trajectory.

For sexual dating victimization, the overall fit of the two-groups model was not acceptable in terms of the CFI value, $X^2(7) = 15.290$; RMSEA = 0.041; CFI = 0.808. Modification indices were analyzed, suggesting that the residual variance of the post-test measure was different across groups (MI = 11.383). When freely estimating the residual variance at post-test across groups, the model showed a good fit, $X^2(6) = 7.740$; RMSEA = 0.020; CFI = 0.960. In Step 1, the mean and variance of the growth rate factors for the control group were not significant, whereas the slope mean for the experimental group was negative and significant (see Table 4). In light of this, the means and variances of the growth factors were constrained to be 0 for the control group (Step 2). This model showed a good fit, $X^2(9) = 8.317$; RMSEA = 0.000; CFI = 1.000, and the chi-square difference test was not significant, Trd = 0.351; df = 3; $p = 0.950$, suggesting that the best model was the constrained model. In this model, the growth rate factor mean estimated for the treatment group was the estimated program effect. When comparing the average growth rates between both groups, the average growth rate for the treatment group was negative and statistically significant. The effect size was between small to medium ($d = 0.24$). These results indicate that the treatment group's growth trajectory of sexual victimization decreased significantly compared to the control group's growth trajectory.

3.4. Effect of the Dat-e Adolescence Program on Bullying

For bullying aggression, the overall fit of the two-groups model was acceptable, $X^2(7) = 4.757$; RMSEA = 0.000; CFI = 1.000. In Step 1, we observed a declining trend over time for the control group and non-significant changes for the experimental group (See Table 4). This result suggests that intervention did not modify bullying aggression.

For bullying victimization, the overall fit of the two-groups model was acceptable, $X^2(7) = 8.321$; RMSEA = 0.016; CFI = 0.997. In Step 1, the mean and variance of the growth rate factors for the control group were not significant, whereas the slope mean for the experimental group was negative and significant (see Table 4). In light of this, the means and variances of the growth factors were constrained to be 0 for the control group (Step 2). This model showed a good fit, $X^2(10) = 9.520$; RMSEA = 0.000; CFI = 1.000, and the chi-square difference test was not significant, Trd = 1.478; df = 3; $p = 0.687$, suggesting that the best model was the constrained model. In this model, the growth rate factor mean estimated for the treatment group was the estimated program effect. When comparing the average growth rates between both groups, the average growth rate for the treatment group was negative and statistically significant. The effect size was large ($d = 0.98$). These results indicate that the treatment group's growth trajectory of bullying victimization decreased significantly compared to the control group's growth trajectory.

4. Discussion

The present study is the first efficacy evaluation of the Dat-e Adolescence program to include a follow-up measurement. On the whole, the results lend clear support to the program's effectiveness. In particular, students participating in the Dat-e Adolescence program, exhibited lower levels of severe physical dating violence (aggression and victimization); sexual dating violence (aggression and victimization); and bullying victimization six months after the intervention.

Considering the magnitude of the intervention effects, we calculated Cohen's *d* for the multiple-group latent growth models. The results revealed significant (small to medium) victimization and perpetration effects for this program at follow-up. Specifically, 0.21 for severe physical dating victimization; 0.25 for severe physical dating aggression; 0.24 for sexual dating victimization; 0.38 for sexual dating aggression; and 0.98 for bullying victimization. The results of this study are highly relevant in light of the fact that systematic reviews and meta-analyses [14–17] have emphasized how programs fail significantly to affect dating violence outcomes. Importantly, these effects at follow-up were not observed at the program's post-test evaluation stage [37]. This difference between post-test and follow-up intervention efficacy warrants deeper discussion and hypotheses. In general terms, behaviors are resistant to change because they are consolidated in relational dynamics [62]. De la Rue et al. [14] suggest that behavior modification requires time and the development of socio-emotional skills that helps students to face with conflicts and problems within the couple in a healthy way. Applied to our program, because of the post-test evaluations took place immediately after program completion, it was difficult to observe any behavioral change. In this respect we can consider some mediating variables responsible for the delayed effects observed in this study. According to De la Rue et al. [48], programs need to include skill-building components to promote students' behavioral changes when facing conflicts and problem within their romantic relationships. These socio-emotional skills would lead to healthier and more positive relationships that could prevent the expression of aggressive behaviors in dating couples. In the first efficacy assessment of the Dat-e Adolescence program, we found that students of the treatment conditions not only modified their beliefs about love and couple violence, but they also improved their socio-emotional skills. Specifically, after the intervention students showed a better control of anger, reduced the duration of anger episodes and the frequency with which they engaged in fights and arguments. Moreover, participants also reduced their negative feelings toward themselves, improving their self-esteem. We could hypothesize that the change observed in dating aggressive behavior at follow-up can be explained by means of the improved emotion regulations skills at post-test and the change of normative beliefs about love and violence shared by the peer group. Future mediation analysis could test this hypothesis confirming if the change in the behavior is produced as a result of these socio-emotional skills and the change in personal and peers' attitudes towards violence.

At follow-up, intervention and control-group students no longer showed significant differences in moderate physical dating aggression and victimization. Mean growth rates were negative in both groups, which potentially points to normative growth. To our knowledge, only one program has assessed its efficacy by differentiating between moderate and severe forms of physical dating violence [11,20]. It was Safe Dates, which successfully reduced moderate and severe physical aggression as well as moderate victimization, suggesting that moderate forms are more susceptible to change post-intervention. Unlike Safe Dates, our study reported clearer and stronger changes in more severe forms of dating violence (severe physical violence and sexual violence) than in moderate physical forms. It should be noted that decreased levels of aggression and victimization of moderate physical forms were observed in the experimental group. However, moderate physical victimization and aggression also decreased in the control group. This precludes obtaining conclusive results regarding program efficacy in relation to moderate physical violence. Given few programs have analyzed their effectiveness by comparing its impact on moderate and severe forms of physical violence, and taking into account that our results are inconclusive, future studies deepening this aspect are needed.

Considering the intervention's significant effect on bullying victimization, we can confirm that the results are also very meaningful. We hypothesized that the Dat-e Adolescence program would lead to a reduction in different problem behaviors because bullying and dating violence share protective and risk factors over which the program intervenes [9,25,63] such as emotional competence. From a developmental perspective, bullying has been described as a stepping-stone of dating violence given that relational dynamics are transferred from one context to another [9]. As such, it is possible to see adolescents modifying their behavior not only with their partner but also with their peers after receiving the program. However, the program did not modify bullying aggression. This may in part be due to the program content itself. In fact, the general skills and strategies trained in the program, such as communication, emotion regulation and coping strategies, provide victims of bullying with the necessary resources. However, we could hypothesize that this more general content, geared toward positive development, is not enough to modify aggressive behavior among peers. Dat-e Adolescence was designed originally to be a dating violence prevention program, and therefore some of the contents, including beliefs and attitudes toward violence, are specific to couples and not to peer violence. Taken together, and considering the promising effects on peer victimization, future programs should contextualize dating violence programs on a more general framework of interpersonal violence in adolescence, including new contents more closely related to peer aggression, in order to maximize the impact of these programs on different aggressive behaviors [13].

In general, the findings are considerably significant both for dating violence prevention policies in Spain and for interpersonal violence in adolescent research. The Dat-e Adolescence program was born out of a context in which most programs evaluated and analyzed under the umbrella of systematic reviews and meta-analyses come from the United States and Canada [14,15]. However, in Europe, the efficacy of already implemented programs remains an unknown [2]. To date, no previous Spanish prevention programs have been assessed using a RCT design and a large sample. Furthermore, none have delivered promising results in dating violence prevention, and to our knowledge, there is no evidence of a single program that prevents different behavioral problems in adolescents in Spain. Yet in our study, an experimental design, a large sample, and psychometrically sound measures were used. Data were also analyzed using rigorous statistical methods, which yielded promising results.

Despite the positive results of the Dat-e Adolescence program's effectiveness, future studies should focus on some key questions. A second independent trial is needed to confirm the positive results described in this study and in the program's post-test evaluation [37], adhering to standards of evidence [57,64]. In addition, research should look into whether these positive results can be replicated by changing an important program component, namely the trainers. In this first edition, the first five sessions were led by researchers; however, we believe that teachers and/or psychologists can be equally good trainers. Teacher-led training offers the opportunity to test the program's efficacy under more real and natural conditions. The Dat-e Adolescence program comes with a detailed manual, containing easy-to-follow and specific descriptions about the aims of each session, standardized instructions, and materials that can be used for this purpose. Furthermore, much more needs to be done to address several key issues concerning the effectiveness of this type of intervention; for example, the mechanism of change. In this line, the design of the Dat-e Adolescence program was based mainly on two models; DDS model [44] and a peer-led training. A systematic review of the efficacy of dating violence prevention [17] has emphasized the difficulty of preventing this complex problem where multiple risk factors intersect. For this reason, O'Leary and Slep [17] proposed to consider the DDS model [44] in the formulation of prevention programs and to include their ecological approach in the intervention design. In this line, it is necessary to analyze the impact that protective and risk factors may have on the problem using mediational models. This can help us to understand the mechanisms and processes that lead to change [2] and to test the conceptual models developed to better explain interpersonal violence in adolescence [44,64]. Moreover, the Dat-e Adolescence program included peer-led training in line with previous dating violence and bullying prevention programs [24,31]. To determine the benefits of a peer-led model component requires testing the efficacy of the program with this component and without it, and then to compare the results. In sum, it is necessary to improve our knowledge about what ingredients are responsible for the positive results, in terms of a cost-benefit approach [65].

Despite its strengths, the study has several limitations. Self-report measures were used which can be affected by social desirability bias. Our results are only generalizable to schools with similar characteristics. This study involved schools with a medium socioeconomic level, meaning it was not representative of very low-risk or very high-risk schools. In addition, a sizeable proportion of incomplete data was observed at follow-up, as four schools decided not to participate at this wave. Attrition rates were higher in older students, so future studies could benefits by including age as covariate. It is true that Attrition analysis revealed that the results were not influenced by attrition but the inclusion of this covariate could help us to conclude about the effect of age more accurately.

Closely related to this already mentioned limitation is the fact that that we did not include the differential effect of the program on boys and girls. In this respect, as reported in previous systematic reviews, an important number of dating violence prevention programs have shown to be more effective to reduce dating aggression in boys than in girls [48], which could be understood as an indicator that the programs contribute to stop the circle of violence of boys towards girls. Future studies should consider the effect of gender in the results in order to confirm the effect of this program in the reduction of gender violence.

5. Conclusions

Romantic relationships are a veritable challenge for adolescents. When faced with this scenario; some adolescents will acquire the strategies and skills enabling them to establish healthy relationships with their partners. According to the Center for Disease Control and Prevention [66], romantic relationships are healthy when the following criteria are met; both partners share the conviction that conflicts can be resolved in a non-violent way; they have the ability to adapt to and negotiate stressful situations, making decisions together; communication skills and/or assertive communication are present; couples accept that their respective partners have the right to practice their autonomy; and mutual trust lies at the heart of the relationship. Dating violence prevention programs can be a valuable resource to help young people face this difficult task and encourage them to build respectful relationships, thus encouraging positive development for both members of the dyad. In the present study, the results corresponding to the program's efficacy suggest that Dat-e Adolescence can mitigate severe forms of physical dating violence and sexual dating violence as well as bullying victimization. This last finding is critical given that cross-cutting interventions are deemed more efficient in terms of time and resources.

Author Contributions: Conceptualization, V.S.-J., J.O.-R., N.M.-F., E.M., and A.N.; Methodology, V.S.-J., J.O.-R., and N.M.-F.; Validation, N.M.-F.; Formal analysis, N.M.-F., V.S.-J. and A.N.; Investigation, V.S.-J., J.O.-R., and N.M.-F.; Resources, V.S.-J. and J.O.-R.; Data Curation, V.S.-J. and N.M.-F.; Writing—original draft preparation, N.M.-F.; Writing—Review & Editing, V.S.-J., J.O.-R., N.M.-F., E.M., and A.N.; Supervision, V.S.-J. and J.O.-R.; Project administration, V.S.-J. and J.O.-R.; Funding acquisition, V.S.-J.

Funding: The authors state that this research was funded by the Spanish Ministry of Economy, Industry and Competitiveness (PSI2013-45118-R and PSI2017-86723-R were awarded to V.S.-J.). Spanish Ministry of Education, Culture and Sport financed the fellowship of N.M.-F. (FPU2013/00830).

Acknowledgments: The authors would also like to acknowledge the anonymous reviewers of this manuscript, whose observations and suggestions improved this paper.

References

1. Centers for Disease Control and Prevention. *Preventing Intimate Partner Violence across the Lifespan: A Technical Package of Programs, Policies, and Practices*; Centers for Disease Control and Prevention: Atlanta, GA, USA, 2017.
2. Leen, E.; Sorbring, E.; Mawer, M.; Holdsworth, E.; Helsing, B.; Bowen, E. Prevalence, dynamic risk factors and the efficacy of primary interventions for adolescent dating violence: An international review. *Aggress. Violent Behav.* **2013**, *18*, 159–174. [CrossRef]
3. Rubio-Garay, F.; López-González, M.A.; Carrasco, M.Á.; Javier Amor, P. Prevalencia de la Violencia en el Noviazgo: Una Revisión Sistemática. *Papeles del Psicólogo* **2017**, *37*, 135–147. [CrossRef]
4. Wincentak, K.; Connolly, J.; Card, N. Teen Dating Violence: A Meta-Analytic Review of Prevalence Rates. *Psychol. Violence* **2017**, *7*, 224–241. [CrossRef]
5. Stonard, K.E.; Bowen, E.; Lawrence, T.R.; Price, S.A. The relevance of technology to the nature, prevalence and impact of Adolescent Dating Violence and Abuse: A research synthesis. *Aggress. Violent Behav.* **2014**, *19*, 390–417. [CrossRef]
6. Exner-Cortens, D.; Eckenrode, J.; Rothman, E. Longitudinal associations between teen dating violence victimization and adverse health outcomes. *Pediatrics* **2013**, *131*, 71–78. [CrossRef]
7. Cutbush, S.; Williams, J.; Miller, S. Teen Dating Violence, Sexual Harassment, and Bullying Among Middle School Students: Examining Mediation and Moderated Mediation by Gender. *Prev. Sci.* **2016**, *17*, 1024–1033. [CrossRef]
8. Espelage, D.L.; Hong, J.S.; Valido, A. Associations Among Family Violence, Bullying, Sexual Harassment, and Teen Dating Violence. In *Adolescent Dating Violence. Theory, Research and Prevention*; Wolfe, D.A., Temple, J.R., Eds.; Academic Press: London, UK, 2019; pp. 85–102. [CrossRef]
9. Josephson, W.L.; Pepler, D. Bullying: A stepping stone to dating aggression. *Int. J. Adolesc. Med. Health* **2012**, *24*, 37–47. [CrossRef]
10. Pepler, D.J.; Craig, W.M.; Connolly, J.A.; Yuile, A.; McMaster, L.; Jiang, D. A developmental perspective on bullying. *Aggress. Behav.* **2006**, *32*, 376–384. [CrossRef]
11. Foshee, V.A.; Bauman, K.E.; Ennett, S.T.; Linder, G.F.; Benefield, T.; Suchindran, C. Assessing the long-term effects of the Safe Dates program and a booster in preventing and reducing adolescent dating violence victimization and perpetration. *Am. J. Public Health* **2004**, *94*, 619–624. [CrossRef]
12. Wolfe, D.A.; Crooks, C.; Jaffe, P.; Chiodo, D.; Hughes, R.; Ellis, W.; Stitt, L.; Donner, A. A school-based program to prevent adolescent dating violence: A cluster randomized trial. *Arch. Pediatr. Adolesc. Med.* **2009**, *163*, 692–699. [CrossRef]
13. Taylor, B.G.; Stein, N.D.; Mumford, E.A. Shifting Boundaries: An Experimental Evaluation of a Dating Violence Prevention Program in Middle Schools. *Prev. Sci.* **2013**, *14*, 64–76. [CrossRef]
14. De La Rue, L.; Joshua, P.; Dorothy, E.; Pigott, T. School-based interventions to reduce dating and sexual violence: A systematic review. *Campbell Syst. Rev.* **2014**, *7*, 1–110. [CrossRef]
15. Fellmeth, G.L.T.; Heffernan, C.; Nurse, J.; Habidula, S.; Sethi, D. Educational and skills-based interventions for preventing relationship and dating violence in adolescents and young adults: A systematic review. *Campbell Syst. Rev.* **2014**, *31*, 441–443. [CrossRef]
16. Martínez Gómez, J.A.; Rey-Anacona, C.A. Prevention of Dating Violence: A Review of Programs Published Between 1990 and 2012. *Pensam Psicológico* **2014**, *12*, 117–132. [CrossRef]
17. O'Leary, K.D.; Slep, A.M.S. Prevention of Partner Violence by Focusing on Behaviors of Both Young Males and Females. *Prev. Sci.* **2012**, *13*, 329–339. [CrossRef]
18. Foshee, V.A.; Reyes, H.L.M.; Ennett, S.T.; Cance, J.D.; Bauman, K.E.; Bowling, M. Assessing the Effects of Families for Safe Dates, a Family-Based Teen Dating Abuse Prevention Program. *J. Adolesc. Health* **2012**, *51*, 349–356. [CrossRef]
19. Wolfe, D.A.; Wekerle, C.; Scott, K.; Straatman, A.L.; Grasley, C.; Reitzel-Jaffe, D. Dating violence prevention with at-risk youth: A controlled outcome evaluation. *J. Consult. Clin. Psychol.* **2003**, *71*, 279–291. [CrossRef]
20. Foshee, V.A.; Bauman, K.E.; Ennett, S.T.; Suchindra, C.; Benefield, T.; Linder, G.F. Assessing the effects of the dating violence prevention program "safe dates" using random coefficient regression modeling. *Prev. Sci.* **2005**, *6*, 245–258. [CrossRef]

21. Coker, A.L.; Bush, H.M.; Cook-Craig, P.G.; DeGue, S.A.; Clear, E.R.; Bancato, C.J.; Fisher, B.S.; Recktenwald, E.A. RCT Testing Bystander Effectiveness to Reduce Violence. *Am. J. Prev. Med.* **2017**, *52*, 566–578. [CrossRef]

22. Levesque, D.A.; Johnson, J.L.; Welch, C.A.; Prochaska, J.M.; Paiva, A.L. Teen Dating Violence Prevention: Cluster-Randomized Trial of Teen Choices, an Online, Stage-Based Program for Healthy, Nonviolent Relationships. *Psychol. Violence* **2016**, *6*, 421–432. [CrossRef]

23. Miller, E.; Tancredi, D.J.; Mccauley, H.L.; Decker, M.R.; Virata, M.C.D.; Anderson, H.A.; O'Connor, B.; Silverman, J.G. One-Year Follow-Up of a Coach-Delivered Dating Violence Prevention Program. *Am. J. Prev. Med.* **2013**, *45*, 108–112. [CrossRef]

24. Connolly, J.; Josephson, W.; Schnoll, J.; Simkins-Strong, E.; Pepler, D.; MacPherson, A.; Wieser, J.; Moran, M.; Jiang, D. Evaluation of a youth-led program for preventing bullying, sexual harassment, and dating aggression in middle schools. *J. Early Adolesc.* **2015**, *35*, 403–434. [CrossRef]

25. Foshee, V.A.; Reyes, H.L.M.; Chen, M.S.; Ennett, S.T.; Basile, K.C.; DeGue, S.; Vivolo-Kantor, A.M.; Moracco, K.E.; Bowling, J.M. Shared Risk Factors for the Perpetration of Physical Dating Violence, Bullying, and Sexual Harassment Among Adolescents Exposed to Domestic Violence. *J. Youth Adolesc.* **2016**, *45*, 672–686. [CrossRef]

26. Foshee, V.A.; Reyes, H.L.M. Primary prevention of adolescent dating abuse perpetration: When to begin, whom to target, and how to do it. In *Preventing Partner Violence: Research and Evidence-Based Intervention Strategies*; Whitaker, D.J., Lutzker, J.R., Eds.; American Psychological Association: Washington, DC, USA, 2009; pp. 141–168. [CrossRef]

27. Whitaker, D.J.; Murphy, C.M.; Eckhardt, C.I.; Hodges, A.E.; Cowart, M. Effectiveness of Primary Prevention Efforts for Intimate Partner Violence. *Partner Abuse* **2013**, *4*, 175–196. [CrossRef]

28. De Koker, P.B.; Mathews, C.C.; Zuch, M.D.; Bastien, S.; Mason-Jones, A.J. systematic review of interventions for preventing adolescent intimate partner violence. *J. Adolesc. Heath* **2014**, *54*, 3–13. [CrossRef]

29. Storer, H.L.; Casey, E.; Herrenkohl, T. Efficacy of Bystander Programs to Prevent Dating Abuse Among Youth and Young Adults: A Review of the Literature. *Trauma Violence Abuse* **2016**, *17*, 256–269. [CrossRef]

30. Williford, A.; Elledge, L.C.; Boulton, A.J.; DePaolis, K.J.; Little, T.D.; Salmivalli, C. Effects of the Kiva Antibullying Program on Cyberbullying and Cybervictimization Frequency Among Finnish Youth. *J. Clin. Child Adolesc. Psychol.* **2013**. [CrossRef]

31. Palladino, B.E.; Nocentini, A.; Menesini, E. Evidence-Based Intervention against Bullying and Cyberbullying: Evaluation of the NoTrap! Program in Two Independent Trials. *Aggress. Behav.* **2016**, *42*, 194–206. [CrossRef]

32. Del Rey, R.; Casas, J.A.; Ortega-Ruiz, R. El programa ConRed: Una práctica basada en la evidencia. *Comunicar* **2012**, *39*, 129–138. [CrossRef]

33. Hernando, Á. La prevención de la violencia de género en adolescentes. Una experiencia en el ámbito educativo. *Apunt Psicol.* **2007**, *25*, 325–340.

34. Garrido, V.; Casas, M. La prevención de la violencia en la relación amorosa entre adolescentes a través del taller « La Máscara del Amor ». *Rev. Educ.* **2009**, *349*, 335–360.

35. Fernández-González, L.; Muñoz-Rivas, M.J. Evaluación De Un Programa De Prevención De La Violencia En Las Relaciones De Noviazgo: Indicaciones Tras Un Estudio Piloto. *Behav. Psychol.* **2013**, *21*, 229–247. [CrossRef]

36. Muñoz, B.; Ortega-Rivera, F.; Sánchez-Jiménez, V. El DaViPoP: Un programa de prevención de violencia en el cortejo y las parejas adolescentes. *Apunt Psicol.* **2013**, *31*, 215–224.

37. Sánchez-Jiménez, V.; Muñoz-Fernández, N.; Ortega-Rivera, J. Efficacy evaluation of "Dat-e Adolescence": A dating violence prevention program in Spain. *PLoS ONE* **2018**, *13*, e0205802. [CrossRef]

38. Chiodo, D.; Crooks, C.V.; Wolfe, D.A.; McIsaac, C.; Hughes, R.; Jaffe, P.G. Longitudinal Prediction and Concurrent Functioning of Adolescent Girls Demonstrating Various Profiles of Dating Violence and Victimization. *Prev. Sci.* **2012**, *13*, 350–359. [CrossRef]

39. Fernández-González, L.; Calvete, E.; Orue, I. Adolescent Dating Violence Stability and Mutuality: A 4-Year Longitudinal Study. *J. Interpers. Violence* **2017**. [CrossRef]

40. Collins, W.A.; van Dulmen, M. "The course of the true love(s) . . . ": Origins and pathways in the development of romantic relationships. In *Romance and Sex in Adolescence and Emerging Adulthood: Risks and Opportunities*; Crouter, A.C., Booth, A., Snyder, A., Eds.; Routledge: New York, NY, USA, 2016; pp. 63–86.

41. Espelage, D.L.; Holt, M.K. Dating violence & sexual harassment across the bully-Victim Continuum among middle and high school students. *J. Youth Adolesc.* **2007**, *36*, 799–811. [CrossRef]

42. Sánchez-Jiménez, V.; Viejo, C.; Ortega-Ruíz, R. El contexto de los iguales y de la pareja como factores predictores de la agresión física y sexual en las parejas adolescentes. *Prolepsis* **2012**, 123–130. Available online: https://idus.us.es/xmlui/handle/11441/32782 (accessed on 31 January 2019).

43. Reyes, H.L.M.; Foshee, V.A.; Bauer, D.J.; Ennett, S.T. Heavy Alcohol Use and Dating Violence Perpetration During Adolescence: Family, Peer and Neighborhood Violence as Moderators. *Prev. Sci.* **2012**, *13*, 340–349. [CrossRef]

44. Capaldi, D.M.; Shortt, J.W.; Kim, H.K. A Life Span Developmental Systems Perspective on Aggression toward a Partner. In *Oxford Series in Clinical Psychology. Family Psychology: The Art of the Science*; Pinsof, W.M., Lebow, J.L., Eds.; Oxford University Press: New York, NY, USA, 2005; pp. 160–187.

45. Capaldi, D.M.; Knoble, N.B.; Shortt, J.W.; Kim, H.K. A Systematic Review of Risk Factors for Intimate Partner Violence. *Partner Abuse* **2012**, *3*, 231–280. [CrossRef]

46. Vagi, K.J.; Rothman, E.; Latzman, N.E.; Tharp, A.T.; Hall, D.M.; Breiding, M. Beyond Correlates: A Review of Risk and Protective Factors for Adolescent Dating Violence Perpetration. *J. Youth Adolesc.* **2014**, *42*, 633–649. [CrossRef]

47. Shortt, J.W.; Capaldi, D.M.; Kim, H.K.; Kerr, D.C.R.; Owen, L.D.; Feingold, A. Stability of Intimate Partner Violence by Men across 12 Years in Young Adulthood: Effects of Relationship Transitions. *Prev. Sci.* **2012**, *13*, 360–369. [CrossRef]

48. De La Rue, L.; Polanin, J.R.; Espelage, D.L.; Pigott, T.D. A Meta-Analysis of School-Based Interventions Aimed to Prevent or Reduce Violence in Teen Dating Relationships. *Rev. Educ. Res.* **2017**, *87*, 7–34. [CrossRef]

49. Fanti, K.A.; Henrich, C. Effects of Self-Esteem and Narcissism on Bullying and Victimization during Early Adolescence. *J. Early Adolesc.* **2014**. [CrossRef]

50. O'Moore, M.; Kirkham, C. Self-Esteem and Its Relationship to Bullying Behaviour. *Aggress. Behav.* **2001**, *27*, 269–283. [CrossRef]

51. Patchin, J.W.; Hinduja, S. Cyberbullying and self-esteem. *J. Sch. Health* **2016**, *8*, 614–621.

52. Connolly, J.; Craig, W.; Goldberg, A.; Pepler, D. Mixed-Gender Groups, Dating, and Romantic Relationships in Early Adolescence. *J. Res. Adolesc.* **2004**, *14*, 185–207. [CrossRef]

53. Nocentini, A.; Menesini, E.; Pastorelli, C.; Connolly, J.; Pepler, D.; Craig, W. Physical Dating Aggression in Adolescence. Cultural and Gender invariance. *Eur. Psychol.* **2011**, *16*, 278–287. [CrossRef]

54. Straus, M. Measuring Intrafamily Conflict and Violence: The Conflict Tactics (CT) Scales. *J. Marriage Fam.* **1979**, *41*, 75–88. [CrossRef]

55. Viejo, C.; Sánchez-Jiménez, V.; Ortega-Ruiz, R. Physical dating violence: The potential understating value of a bi-factorial model. *Anales de Psicologia* **2014**, *30*, 171–179. [CrossRef]

56. Foshee, V.A.; Benefield, T.S.; Ennett, S.T.; Bauman, K.E.; Suchindran, C. Longitudinal predictors of serious physical and sexual dating violence victimization during adolescence. *Prev. Med.* **2004**, *39*, 1007–1016. [CrossRef]

57. Ortega-Ruiz, R.; Del Rey, R.; Casas, J.A. Evaluar el bullying y el cyberbullying validación española del EBIP-Q y del ECIP-Q. *Psicol. Educ.* **2016**, *22*, 71–79. [CrossRef]

58. Flay, B.; Biglan, A.; Boruch, R.; González, F.; Gottfredson, D.; Kellam, S.; Mościcki, E.K.; Schinke, S.; Valentine, J.C.; Ji, P. Standards of Evidence Criteria for Efficacy, Effectiveness and Dissemination. *Prev. Sci.* **2005**, *6*, 151–175. [CrossRef]

59. Cheong, J.; MacKinnon, D.P.; Khoo, S.L. Investigation of Mediational Processes Using Parallel Process Latent Growth Curve Modeling. *Struct. Equ. Model.* **2003**, *10*, 238–262. [CrossRef]

60. Raudenbush, S.W.; Xiao-Feng, L. Effects of Study Duration, Frequency of Observation, and Sample Size on Power in Studies of Group Differences in Polynomial Change. *Psychol. Methods* **2001**, *6*, 387–401. [CrossRef]

61. Feingold, A. Trials in the Same Metric as for Classical Analysis. *Psychol. Methods* **2009**, *14*, 43–53. [CrossRef]

62. Cornelius, T.L.; Resseguie, N. Primary and secondary prevention programs for dating violence: A review of the literature. *Aggress. Violent Behav.* **2007**, *12*, 364–375. [CrossRef]

63. Espelage, D.L.; Low, S.K.; Anderson, C.; Ru, L.D. *Bullying, Sexual, and Dating Violence Trajectories from Early to Late Adolescence*; The United States Department of Justice: Washington, DC, USA, 2014.

64. Gottfredson, D.C.; Cook, T.D.; Gardner, F.E.M.; Gorman-Smith, D.; Howe, G.W.; Sandler, I.N.; Zafft, K.M. Standards of Evidence for Efficacy, Effectiveness, and Scale-up Research in Prevention Science: Next Generation. *Prev. Sci.* **2015**, *16*, 893–926. [CrossRef]

65. Menesini, E.; Salmivalli, C. Bullying in schools: The state of knowledge and effective interventions. *Psychol. Health Med.* **2017**, *22*, 240–253. [CrossRef]

66. Centers for Disease Control and Prevention. *Strategic Direction for Intimate Partner Violence Prevention: Promoting Respectful, Nonviolent Intimate Partner Relationships through Individual, Community, and Societal Change*; Centers for Disease Control and Prevention: Atlanta, GA, USA, 2008.

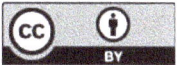

International Journal of
Environmental Research and Public Health

MDPI

Article

For Whom Is Anti-Bullying Intervention Most Effective? The Role of Temperament

Annalaura Nocentini *, Benedetta Emanuela Palladino and **Ersilia Menesini**

Department of Educational Science and Psychology, University of Florence, Ital Via di San Salvi, 12, Complesso di San Salvi Padiglione 26, 50135 Florence, Italy; benedettaemanuela.palladino@unifi.it (B.E.P.); menesini@psico.unifi.it (E.M.)

* Correspondence: annalaura.nocentini@unifi.it; Tel.: +0039-055-6237870

Received: 28 December 2018; Accepted: 24 January 2019; Published: 30 January 2019

Abstract: Studying moderators of the effects of anti-bullying universal interventions is essential to elucidate what works for whom and to tailor more intensive, selective, and indicated programs which meet the needs of non-responders. The present study investigated whether early adolescents' temperament—effortful control (EC), negative emotionality (NE), and positive emotionality (PE)—moderates the effects of the KiVa anti-bullying program. The sample consisted of 13 schools, with 1051 sixth-grade early adolescents (mean age = 10.93; SD = 0.501), randomly assigned to the KiVa intervention (seven schools; n = 536) or to the control condition (six schools; n = 516). Adolescents reported bullying and victimization before the intervention (pre-test) and after (post-test). Temperament was assessed by a self-report pre-test. Findings showed that EC and NE moderated intervention effects on bullying, indicating that subgroups with high levels of EC, and with low and medium levels of NE were those who benefited most from the intervention. The low-EC subgroup showed a lower increase compared to the control condition, with a considerable effect size. Conversely, the high-NE subgroup did not show any positive effects compared to the control group. Regarding victimization, findings showed that early adolescents with high and medium levels of PE were the subgroups who benefited the most from the intervention, whereas the low-PE subgroup was the most resistant. The present study confirms the relevance of considering temperament as a moderator of intervention effects, since interventions tailored to early adolescents with specific traits might yield larger effects.

Keywords: effectiveness; moderators; temperament; anti-bullying; subgroup analyses

1. Introduction

Evidence-based research about anti-bullying interventions needs to move beyond basic questions related to anti-bullying intervention efficacy. The mechanisms through which ameliorative effects may be exerted, the factors that alter the efficiency of the intervention within different subsamples, and the identification of those who are most likely to benefit from a given intervention are relevant research questions that need to be addressed. The modest effect size of reduction estimates found in studies on the efficacy of anti-bullying interventions, as well as the existing variability between studies and programs, suggests the need to pay more attention to potential moderators of the response to these interventions. Identifying children and adolescents who do not respond to interventions is, therefore, an important objective for tailoring more intensive selective and indicated programs which meet the needs of non-responders. The present study aimed to evaluate whether specific subgroups of early adolescents defined by their temperamental traits can be differently affected by a universal school-based anti-bullying program.

School bullying increasingly became a topic of both public concern and research efforts. The literature on the effectiveness of anti-bullying programs showed that they are effective in reducing bullying by 20% to 23%, and victimization by 17% to 20% [1]. These findings were substantially confirmed by the recent update by Gaffney and colleagues [2]. Overall, although these percentages correspond to a substantial amount of bullying prevention, the effect sizes are considered as small (standardized mean difference (d) values ranging from 0.14 to 0.17). There is still much to understand about why programs vary in effectiveness, and much to learn about improving prevention strategies to optimize the effect size of prevention programs.

Prevention science also recommends the testing of moderation models to better understand what works and for whom [3]. The importance of examining the consistency of intervention effects across subgroups was incorporated into the standards of evidence for identifying effective prevention programs adopted by the Society for Prevention Research [4,5]. In the literature on the effectiveness of anti-bullying interventions, only a few studies focused on uncovering these individual moderating factors, investigating the role of demographic characteristics (age and gender) [1,6,7], initial severity of behaviors and symptoms [7,8], type of involvement in either bullying or victimization or both (i.e., pure bullies, pure victims, or bully/victims) [9], and a general personality child trait called environmental sensitivity [10].

In relation to gender moderation, studies showed mixed results, with some suggesting that gender does not have a moderating effect on bullying and victimization decrease [7,11], and others reporting boys obtaining higher results for bullying reduction compared to girls [6,10]. The stronger positive effects on boys may be a consequence of boys' initially higher scores on bullying and pro-bullying behavior that make them suitable targets for the intervention to reduce bullying, assisting, and reinforcing. Age is another variable showing contrasting moderating effects; greater reductions in bullying were documented for younger children compared to their older counterparts [12–15]. Other studies reported no differences between age groups [7], and others [1] asserted that greater intervention success can be attained when working with slightly older youths (age 11 or older). The initial severity of the behaviors was found to be a significant moderator of the effectiveness of anti-bullying programs. In agreement with the literature on other outcomes [8,16–19], those most involved in problematic behaviors at the baseline level were those benefiting the most from the intervention. The KiVa program was particularly effective in facilitating the perception of a caring school environment for the students who were most victimized before the intervention, and intervention effects on depression and self-esteem were strong only among the most victimized sixth graders [8]. In the study on the ViSC Social Competence Program [7], youths with initially high levels of aggressive behavior (including bullying) or victimization changed more in the respective variable compared with initially not-so-involved youths. Another interesting individual moderator included the involvement of children in both bullying and victimization roles. Specific subgroups of children (e.g., bullies, victims, bully/victims) followed a different trend after the KiVa intervention. Yang and Salmivalli [9] suggested that KiVa is effective in reducing the prevalence of bully/victims, and these effects are comparable or even larger than the effects on pure bullies and pure victims. Finally, an individual variable able to predict interindividual variability in the effectiveness estimates is a general personality trait called environmental sensitivity, which is defined as the inherent ability to perceive and process environmental stimuli [10]. A recent study showed that low-sensitivity children seem to be relatively resistant to the program's effects in relation to reducing victimization, and low-sensitivity boys in relation to reducing internalizing behaviors. On the other side, highly sensitive children were more responsive to the anti-bullying program in relation to a decrease in victimization and on internalizing behaviors [10].

Environmental sensitivity may constitute a non-specific personality predictor for victimization. In relation to bullying, more specific personality or temperamental traits could play a key role in identifying children and adolescents who respond better or worse to the intervention.

However, studies are yet to investigate the moderating role of personality or temperament in relation to anti-bullying prevention programs, and very few investigated this role in the more general literature of externalizing behaviors. In particular, two studies conducted in the Netherlands showed that highly conscientious and highly agreeable juvenile delinquents [20], and highly conscientious and low extroverted children [21] benefited most from interventions targeted at reducing externalizing problems. These two studies showed that youth with a lower-risk personality profile for the development of delinquency benefited most from the intervention.

The association between personality traits and bullying and victimization was analyzed in a few studies [22–29]. Using the Eysenck Personality Inventory Junior, a study conducted in Ireland reported heightened levels of psychoticism and modest increases in extroversion and neuroticism among bullies [24]. Using the five-factor model, studies conducted in the United States (US) and in Italy confirmed that victimization is associated with higher levels of neuroticism, and lower levels of agreeableness and conscientiousness [22,26,28], and that bullying is associated with low agreeableness and low conscientiousness [22,23,26,28]. In the Italian studies, bullying was also associated with high levels of neuroticism [26,28]. Using the HEXACO Personality Inventory, Book et al. [23] found that bullying was significantly negatively correlated with traits of honesty–humility, emotionality, agreeableness, and conscientiousness. Finally, using the EATQ (Early Adolescent Temperament Questionnaire), Terranova and colleagues [29] showed the role played by fear reactivity and effortful control in bullying. Starting from these associations, we might expect differential effectiveness as a function of effortful control and negative emotionality in reducing bullying and victimization.

Given the considerable variability in anti-bullying intervention effects, additional research is required to identify the characteristics of the most responsive early adolescents. The issue of variation in effectiveness based on subgroup membership is particularly relevant for the development of the tiered framework in anti-bullying interventions. This model, including a universal, a selective, and an indicated tier [16], is essential for tailoring interventions according to the risk profile of subgroups of students.

Starting from these considerations, the current study evaluates whether the impact of the KiVa anti-bullying program varied as a function of early adolescents' temperament defined using the three superordinate dimensions: effortful control (EC), negative emotionality (NE), and positive emotionality (PE).

General recommendations for testing the moderation of the impact of an intervention proposed by Supplee et al. [30] and Wang et al. [31] were followed. Results were based first on the test of the heterogeneity of treatment effects, and secondly on subgroup analyses presented along with effect estimates within each level of each baseline moderator. Subgroups were specified using an empirical distribution: top 30%, medium 40%, and bottom 30%.

2. Methods

2.1. Participants

Participants of this study were part of a randomized controlled trial (RCT), which was not associated to an ethical code because an ethical committee was not established in our University until 2016. At that time, we were requested to strictly adhere to the ethical code of the Italian Association of Psychology. This RCT aimed at testing the effectiveness of the KiVa anti-bullying program in Italy, involving 13 comprehensive schools located in three cities in Tuscany. A detailed description of the trial design, and the recruitment and retention of participants in the RCT is reported in Nocentini and Menesini [12]. Data were collected in two waves: September–October 2013 (T1: pre-treatment) and May–June 2014 (T2: post-treatment). The sample included in this study is limited to secondary schools because the EATQ questionnaire is not adequate for primary school and was used only with the secondary subsample. In order to recruit children, parents were sent information letters together with a consent form. In total, 94% of the target sample provided active consent for study participation. Overall, 1052 early adolescents from grade 6 filled out the questionnaires at T1 and 984 at T2. The attrition is mainly explained by absences of some students at T2, randomly distributed in the sample.

2.2. Procedure

Data were collected in classrooms with paper/pencil questionnaires during school hours in two waves, conducted by trained psychologists, researchers, and master students. The intervention took place at schools after baseline data collection.

2.3. KiVa Intervention

KiVa is an intensive and systematic universal school-based anti-bullying program focused on actions targeting individual children, classrooms, and schools. It was developed in the University of Turku, Finland, and it was adapted to the Italian schools in 2013–2014. It is based on the participant role model, where bullying is seen as a group process [32]. The intervention focuses on the bystanders' reactions to a bullying situation; it aims to change their attitudes and behaviors, which assist and reinforce the bully. KiVa aims to prevent bullying and victimization and to intervene in existing bullying cases [32]. The prevention involves universal actions targeted at all students, which are delivered through 10 student lessons taught by the teachers throughout the school year. Methods used in the KiVa lessons are discussion, group work, role-play exercises, and short films about bullying, and they aim to raise awareness of the role bystanders play in the bullying process, to increase empathy toward the victim, and to provide students with safe strategies to support and defend their victimized peers. Other universal components include school posters and information for parents. Furthermore, more specific actions are targeted at students who were identified as targets or perpetrators of bullying. Both universal and indicated actions are conducted by teachers and school personnel trained in the KiVa program in two full-day face-to-face trainings and supervised in four to five meetings during school. More information about the program and the Italian adaptation can be found in Nocentini and Menesini [12].

2.4. Measures

The Florence Bullying–Victimization Scales (FBVS) [11] each consist of 14 items asking how often respondents experience particular behaviors either as a perpetrator or victim (e.g., "I threatened someone" for bullying, and "I was threatened" for victimization) during the past couple of months. Each item is rated on a five-point scale ranging from 1 = "never" to 5 = "several times a week". The scales were presented after a definition of the constructs was presented. The FBVS scale showed consistent psychometric properties [11,12]. Internal reliability for both scales at T1 and T2 ranged from $\alpha = 0.82$ to 0.86.

The Early Adolescent Temperament Questionnaire, Revised Short Form (EATQ-RSF) [33] was administered at T1. EATQ-RSF contains 65 questions in a self-report form asking adolescents how true each statement is for them. Response options for both forms used a five-point Likert-type scale ranging from 1 = "almost always untrue: to 5 = "almost always true". The questionnaire measures 10 aspects of temperament (activation control, affiliation, attention, fear, frustration, high-intensity pleasure, inhibitory control, perceptual sensitivity, pleasure sensitivity, and shyness). According to the authors [34], for the present study, we used the classification based on the three superordinate dimensions of temperament: (a) effortful control (EC; based on attention, activation control, and inhibitory control), (b) negative emotionality (NE; based on fear, frustration, and shyness), and (c) positive emotionality (PE; based on surgency, pleasure sensitivity, perceptual sensitivity, and affiliation). All the subscales showed acceptable reliability coefficients: 0.71 for EC, 0.81 for NE, and 0.75 for PE.

2.5. Statistical Analysis

Hypotheses were tested in SPSS (SPSS Inc., Chicago, IL, USA) with linear mixed-effects models (MIXED) with full-information maximum-likelihood (ML) estimation [35]. The analysis featured a three-level (measurement occasion within individuals within schools) random-intercept model, to account for within-subject and within-school correlations. Analyses were conducted in two steps. Firstly, we tested whether EATQ temperament subscales moderated the efficacy of the KiVa program through the interaction time by group by temperament. The model tested the main effect of time, group, the three temperamental traits, and all the two- and three-level interactions. Secondly, significant moderation interactions (time by group by temperament) were followed up by creating three subgroups: top 30%, medium 40%, and bottom 30%. Subgroup analyses included the following: (a) using the same linear mixed-effect models, we tested the significance of the interaction treatment condition by time separately for subgroups of high, medium, and lower levels of temperament trait. These analyses yielded intervention effects indicating the improvement in the KiVa group relative to the control group for each subgroup defined by a different level of the temperamental traits (moderator); (b) a comparison of the effect sizes in the three subgroups separately. Effect size estimates from pre-test, post-test, and control group designs were calculated following suggestions from Morris [36]. In particular, the results from the Morris study [36] favored an effect size based on the mean pre–post change in the treatment group minus the mean pre–post change in the control group, divided by the pooled pre-test standard deviation, according to the definition of Carlson and Schmidt [37].

3. Results

3.1. Preliminary Results

Table 1 shows descriptive statistics for the outcome variables across time in both experimental and control groups. As preliminary analyses, we confirmed the finding of the previous study conducted with grade 4 and grade 6. A significant group-by-time interaction emerged for bullying ($B = -0.014$; standard error (SE) = 0.004; $p = 0.000$) and victimization ($B = -0.024$; $SE = 0.006$; $p = 0.000$), with children in the KiVa group displaying a decrease in bullying and victimization between T1 and T2, whereas children in the control group displayed a significant increase in both variables. Effect sizes estimated using all the information available from pre-test/post-test/control group designs were calculated. The estimation of effect sizes was different as compared to the previous study [12]. In the first effectiveness study, we used Cohen's d comparing the intervention effects with the control schools at T2. Specifically, Cohen's d was calculated as the adjusted group mean difference divided by unadjusted pooled within-group standard deviation. Results showed that, for victimization, the d pre-test/post-test/control was 0.27, and for bullying the d pre-test/post-test/control was 0.25.

Table 1. Descriptive statistics for the behavioral outcomes: means (M) and standard deviations (SD).

Outcomes	Data Collection	Middle School	
		Experimental M (SD)	Control M (SD)
Victimization	T1 ($n = 1049$)	$n = 533$; 0.062 (0.096)	$n = 516$; 0.056 (0.080)
	T2 ($n = 987$)	$n = 494$; 0.057 (0.073)	$n = 493$; 0.075 (0.086)
Bullying	T1 ($n = 1045$)	$n = 529$; 0.032 (0.059)	$n = 516$; 0.030 (0.050)
	T2 ($n = 986$)	$n = 493$; 0.029 (0.053)	$n = 493$; 0.041 (0.063)

Notes: Differences in the number of subjects within the same time are due to missing data in the specific variable. Means and standard deviations are based on subjects with full information available used in the analysis.

3.2. Temperamental Moderation of Treatment Effects

Significant findings of the linear mixed models aimed at evaluating the moderation effect of temperament subscales are presented in Table 2 for both bullying and victimization outcomes. Findings showed that the trend of bullying across time is dependent on the experimental condition (KiVa vs. control) interacting with the level of effortful control and negative affectivity. Furthermore, the trend of victimization across time is dependent on the experimental condition (KiVa vs. control) interacting with the level of positive emotion.

Table 2. Mixed model predicting the moderating role of effortful control (EC), negative emotionality (NE), and positive emotionality (PE) on bullying and victimization outcomes.

Predictor	Outcome: Bullying		Outcome: Victimization	
	B (SE)	*p*	*B* (SE)	*p*
Intercept	**0.093 (0.022)**	**0.000**	**0.065 (0.032)**	**0.040**
Time	−0.018 (0.025)	0.445	0.029 (0.037)	0.424
Group	**0.087 (0.032)**	**0.006**	−0.034 (0.045)	0.449
EC	**−0.007 (0.002)**	**0.000**	**−0.005 (0.002)**	**0.028**
NE	0.001 (0.001)	0.202	**0.005 (0.002)**	**0.002**
PE	0.000 (0.001)	0.772	−0.001 (0.002)	0.466
Time × group	−0.062 (0.035)	0.073	−0.014 (0.053)	0.791
EC × time	0.000 (0.002)	0.741	−0.002 (0.003)	0.460
NE × time	**−0.003 (0.001)**	**0.010**	−0.002 (0.002)	0.233
PE × time	**0.003(0.001)**	**0.006**	0.001 (0.002)	0.516
EC × group	**−0.006(0.002)**	**0.004**	−0.001(0.003)	0.712
NE × group	**−0.003 (0.001)**	**0.010**	0.000 (0.003)	0.830
PE × group	0.002(0.002)	0.218	**0.005(0.002)**	**0.050**
Time × EC × group	**0.005 (0.002)**	**0.039**	0.006 (0.004)	0.080
Time × NE × group	**0.004 (0.002)**	**0.046**	−0.002 (0.003)	0.611
Time × PE × group	−0.003 (0.002)	0.127	**−0.005 (0.002)**	**0.049**
Residual variance	**0.002 (0.000)**	**0.000**	**0.004 (0.000)**	**0.000**
Subjects: random intercept	**0.001 (0.000)**	**0.000**	**0.002 (0.000)**	**0.000**
Schools: random intercept	0.000 (0.000)	0.126	0.000 (0.000)	0.188

Note: Boldface type indicates statistically significant results ($p < 0.05$) from the deviance tests for fixed effects and from the Wald tests for random effects.

3.3. Bullying Outcome: Follow-Up Analyses of High, Medium, and Low Effortful Control Levels

A significant interaction (group by time) was found in the high-EC ($B = −0.0121$; $SE = 0.005$; $p = 0.020$) and medium-EC ($B = −0.0120$; $SE = 0.005$; $p = 0.026$) subgroups, while a trend was found in the low-EC subgroup ($B = −0.018$; $SE = 0.009$; $p = 0.060$). As we can see from Table 3 and from Figure 1, the highest effect size was found in the high-EC group, where the KiVa group showed a decreasing trend over time, and the control group showed an increase over time. The same trend was found for the medium group, although with a lower effect size. The result of the low-EC subgroup was interesting; the KiVa group showed an increase over time, but this was very small as compared to the large increase in bullying over time in the low-EC participants in the control group. Thus, comparing the trend over time of KiVa and the control group within this subgroup, the effect size showed a considerable estimate, although the KiVa group did not show a significant decrease over time.

Table 3. Effect sizes (Cohen's *d*) estimates from pre-test/post-test/control group designs in each temperamental subgroup.

Subgroup	*d* **Pre-Test/Post-Test/Control**
High effortful control	0.30
Medium effortful control	0.22
Low effortful control	0.24
High negative emotionality	0.09
Medium negative emotionality	0.28
Low negative emotionality	0.30
High positive emotionality	0.35
Medium positive emotionality	0.48
Low positive emotionality	0.01

Notes: The effect size is based on the mean pre–post change in the treatment group minus the mean pre–post change in the control group, divided by the pooled pre-test standard deviation (see Morris, 2008).

EFFORTFUL CONTROL SUBGROUPS

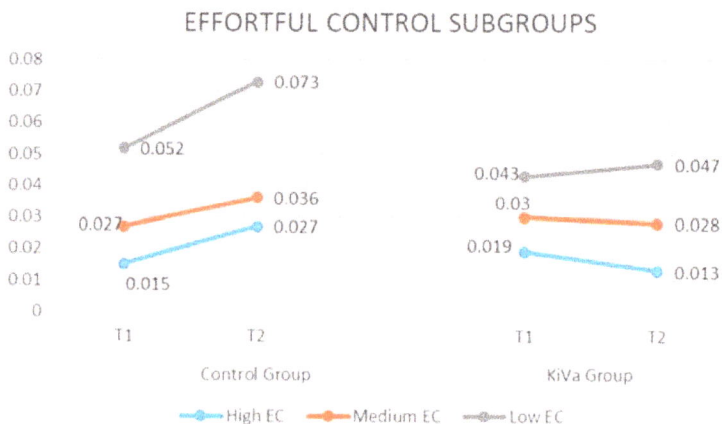

Figure 1. Bullying across time distinguishing between control and KiVa groups, and high, medium, and low levels of effortful control.

3.4. Bullying Outcome: Follow-Up Analyses for High, Medium, and Low Negative Emotionality

Significant interactions (group by time) were found in the low-NE ($B = -0.016$; $SE = 0.007$; $p = 0.030$) and medium-NE ($B = -0.016$; $SE = 0.006$; $p = 0.010$) subgroups, but not in the high-NE subgroup ($B = 0.006$; $SE = 0.006$; $p = 0.379$). This means that the treatment had an effect, compared to the control group, only in the low- and medium-NE subgroups. As we can see from Table 3 and Figure 2, the highest effect size was found for the low-NE subgroup, where the KiVa group showed a decreasing trend over time and the control group showed an increase over time. The same trend was found in the medium group, although with a smaller effect. Within the high-NE subgroup, the effect size comparing the trend across time of the experimental and control groups was very small, because, in both groups, these early adolescents considerably increased their level of bullying.

Negative Emotionality Subgroups

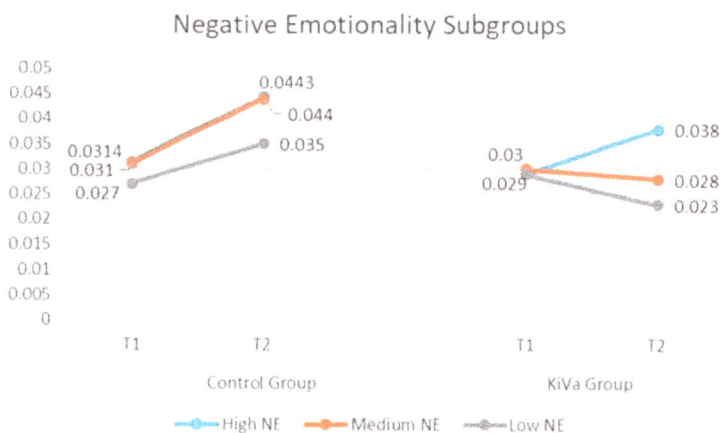

Figure 2. Bullying across time distinguishing between control and KiVa groups, and high, medium, and low levels of negative emotionality.

3.5. Victimization Outcome: Follow-Up Analyses for High, Medium, and Low Positive Emotionality

Significant interactions (group by time) were found in the high-PE ($B = -0.032$; $SE = 0.011$; $p = 0.007$) and medium-PE ($B = -0.042$; $SE = 0.009$; $p = 0.000$) subgroups, but not in the low-PE subgroup ($B = -0.000$; $SE = 0.012$; $p = 0.977$). This means that the treatment had an effect, compared to the control group, only in the high- and medium-PE subgroups. As we can see from Table 3 and Figure 3, the highest effect was found for the medium-PE and the high-PE subgroups, where the KiVa group showed a decreasing trend over time and the control group showed an increase over time. The effect size within the low-PE subgroup was close to 0, because, in both experimental and control groups, these young adolescents increased their level of victimization.

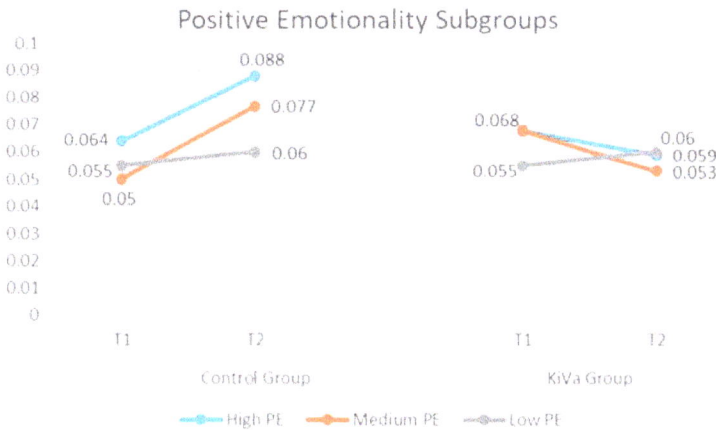

Figure 3. Victimization across time distinguishing between control and KiVa groups, and high, medium, and low levels of positive emotionality.

4. Discussion

The present study suggests that specific subgroups of early adolescents defined by their temperament are able to benefit most from the KiVa anti-bullying intervention, while others are more resistant to the beneficial effect of this experience. In particular, young adolescents with high levels of effortful control, and with low and medium levels of negative emotionality are the subgroups who benefit the most from the intervention in the reduction of bullying, whereas the high-NE subgroup is the most resistant. In the low-EC subgroup (a subgroup at high risk for bullying), although bullying did not decrease over time, the KiVa intervention altered the normative strong increase in bullying over time found in the control condition, with a considerable effect size. In relation to victimization, findings showed that early adolescents with high and medium levels of positive emotionality are the subgroups who benefit most from the intervention in the reduction of victimization, whereas the low-PE subgroup is the most resistant.

Findings related to the bullying outcome highlighted that the most responsive early adolescents to a universal anti-bullying intervention are those high in EC; they are able to regulate negative emotions and behaviors in the context of stressful interpersonal interactions, to employ flexible and effective coping strategies to modulate high levels of emotional reactivity, and/or to activate appropriate responses in light of changing task demands. On the other hand, the most resistant adolescents high in NE present dysregulated expression of negative affect, a high level of affective reactivity, an increased sensitivity to threat and vigilance for negative cues, and attentional bias to threatening emotional information, fear, anxiety, and threat-based reactive aggressions.

We had interesting findings in relation to the low-EC and high-NE subgroups, both potentially more at risk of bullying perpetration. The subgroup with high NE was not able to benefit from the universal anti-bullying program. On the other hand, the subgroup with low EC was affected by the program, even more than the medium-EC subgroup (see the comparison with the control group), but intervention dosage was not sufficient to decrease their level of bullying. These findings give relevant suggestions for planning selected or indicated actions. Firstly, anti-bullying programs such as KiVa are able to reduce bullying based on emotion regulation difficulties, but this is not enough for individuals with a low level of EC; for those individuals, a more intensive module on emotion regulation seems necessary. Moreover, anti-bullying programs such as KiVa are not able to reduce bullying when high levels of NE are present. The study confirmed that the NE trait is the most severe personality risk factor, because the subgroup with high NE did not respond to the intervention. This is in line with previous literature where high NE was found to be correlated with mental and physical health problems to a greater extent in comparison to other personality traits [38]. Perhaps, for these adolescents, a more intensive module which attempts to reduce high levels of NE in order to indirectly reduce risk for bullying would be more appropriate. Adaptations of cognitive and behavioral interventions, such as those developed for stress management, or to prevent anxiety disorders and depression, might be more effective in improving this dimension (e.g., for a review, see Lahey) [38]. Decreasing levels of depression and anxiety may be favorable to reduce factors triggering situations in which aggressive confrontations and bullying are likely to arise. Self-regulatory abilities may moderate the impact of NE, providing children with the capability to modulate and cope with emotionality. Increasing self-regulation may enhance children's ability to be more flexible or competent in dealing with stressors that provoke negative emotions.

Findings related to the victimization outcome supported a previous study where boys scoring high in environmental sensitivity benefited the most from the effects of the KiVa intervention in terms of reduced victimization scores and internalizing symptoms, but not bullying. In contrast, boys with low sensitivity did not respond to treatment at all [10]. Positive emotionality is a broad construct also involving a general sensitivity trait, and it overlaps with constructs such as extraversion and behavioral activation [39]. Thus, the findings of the present study, where the subgroup of low PE did not respond to the universal anti-bullying program, support previous findings where a specific measure of sensory-processing sensitivity was used [10].

To summarize, the subgroups most resistant to the KiVa universal anti-bullying intervention are high NE for bullying—but not low EC—and low PE for victimization. One possible explanation is the fact that the KiVa program addressed the vulnerability of the low-EC adolescents' profile through specific activities, but not the vulnerability of the high-NE and low-PE subgroups. More specific components covering these aspects are needed if we want anti-bullying interventions to be able to address bullying and victimization in these high-risk subgroups of early adolescents as well.

Limitations and Future Studies

The current study presents some limitations. Firstly, we relied on self-report data for the evaluation of bullying and victimization and of temperament, which raises the probability of reporter bias. Secondly, the effect sizes in the current study ranged from 0.09 to 0.30, representing a small effect size. However, we need to specify that these are the effects of a universal program on subgroups. The effect sizes are typically smaller in universal prevention studies than in more indicated interventions, and the effect sizes in effectiveness studies are also typically smaller than in efficacy studies [4]. Thirdly, other relevant moderators should be considered in a more articulated design assessing the moderation effect of different types of variables, such as socio-demographic, temperamental, individual, and contextual variables. Fourthly, the findings of the current study could be specific for Italian culture and cannot be generalized to other countries. Further research should also be focused on interesting research questions such as whether temperament interacts with the "pure condition" (bully or victim) or the double role (bully/victim). Moreover, this study evaluated the moderation of temperament on the effectiveness of a universal anti-bullying program. Finally, future studies could evaluate whether temperament is also able to moderate the effectiveness of selective and indicated actions devoted to the decrease of bullying and victimization, contributing to Tier 2 and Tier 3 as well.

5. Conclusions

Despite these limitations, the present study moved beyond merely examining the average treatment effect by identifying which part of the distribution is most affected by the intervention, and by giving suggestions for future targeting and program roll-out. The analyses used in this study were able to account for the nested design, using a subject and school random effect. Furthermore, the test of moderation effects in a single model without conducting multiple moderation tests, as well as the subgroups analyses conducted following the most recent literature [17,30], represents a strength of the current study.

The identification of non-responders to the universal anti-bullying interventions has relevant implications because of their impact on Tier 2 and Tier 3 interventions. Overall, the current study showed that high-NE and low-PE early adolescents are more resistant to the intervention. Maybe these subgroups need a longer intervention or an intervention with a more intense dosage or with a different component (Tier 2 and Tier 3). The higher the number of students responding to the universal (Tier 1) preventive interventions is, the lower the number of students to be involved in advanced tier supports (Tier 2 and Tier 3) will be. Given that students involved in Tier 2 and Tier 3 for bullying prevention are at increased risk for future psychological, social, and school consequences, providing better universal prevention that meets the needs of high-risk early adolescents is crucial.

Author Contributions: Conceptualization, A.N. and E.M.; methodology, A.N.; software, A.N.; validation, E.M. and B.E.P.; formal analysis, A.N.; investigation, A.N. and B.E.P.; resources, A.N. and B.E.P.; data curation, A.N. and B.E.P.; writing—original draft preparation, A.N.; writing—review and editing, E.M.; supervision, E.M.; project administration, E.M.

Funding: This research received no external funding.

Conflicts of Interest: The authors declare no conflicts of interest.

References

1. Tofi, M.M.; Farrington, D.P. Effectiveness of school-based programs to reduce bullying: A systematic and meta-analytic review. *J. Exp. Criminol.* **2011**, *7*, 27–56. [CrossRef]
2. Gaffney, H.; Tofi, M.M.; Farrington, D.P. Evaluating the effectiveness of school-bullying prevention programs: An updated meta-analytical review. *Aggress. Violent Behav.* **2018**. [CrossRef]
3. Rothman, A.J. Exploring connections between moderators and mediators: Commentary on sub-group analysis for intervention research. Subgroup analysis in prevention and intervention research. *Prev. Sci.* **2013**, *14*, 189–192. [CrossRef] [PubMed]
4. Flay, B.R.; Biglan, A.; Boruch, R.F.; González Castro, F.; Gottfredson, D.; Kellam, S.; Ji, P. Standards of evidence: Criteria for efficacy, effectiveness and dissemination. *Prev. Sci.* **2005**, *6*, 151–175. [CrossRef] [PubMed]
5. Gottfredson, D.C.; Cook, T.D.; Gardner, F.E.M.; Gorman-Smith, D.; Howe, G.W.; Sandler, I.N.; Zafft, C.M. Standards of evidence for efficacy, effectiveness, and scale up research in prevention science: Next generation. *Prev. Sci.* **2015**, *16*, 893–926. [CrossRef] [PubMed]
6. Kärnä, A.; Voeten, M.; Little, T.D.; Alanen, E.; Poskiparta, E.; Salmivalli, C. Effectiveness of the KiVa anti-bullying program: Grades 1–3 and 7–9. *J. Educ. Psychol.* **2013**, *105*, 535–551. [CrossRef]
7. Yanagida, T.; Strohmerier, D.; Spiel, C. Dynamic change of aggressive behavior and victimization among adolescents: effectiveness of the ViSC program. *J. Clin. Child Adolescent Psychol.* **2016**, *45*, 1–15. [CrossRef]
8. Juvonen, J.; Schacter, H.L.; Sainio, M.; Salmivalli, C. Can a school-wide bullying prevention program improve the plight of victims? Evidence for risk × intervention effects. *J. Consult Clin. Psychol.* **2016**, *84*, 334–344. [CrossRef]

9. Yang, A.; Salmivalli, C. Effectiveness of the KiVa antibullying programme on bully-victims, bullies and victims. *Educ. Res.* **2013**, *57*, 80–90. [CrossRef]
10. Nocentini, A.; Menesini, E.; Pluess, M. The Personality trait of environmental sensitivity predicts children's positive response to school-based antibullying intervention. *Clin. Psychol. Sci.* **2018**, *6*, 848–859. [CrossRef]
11. Palladino, B.E.; Nocentini, A.; Menesini, E. Evidence-based intervention against bullying and cyberbullying: Evaluation of the Noncadiamointrappola! program in two independent trials. *Aggress. Behav.* **2016**, *42*, 194–206. [CrossRef] [PubMed]
12. Nocentini, A.; Menesini, E. KiVa Anti-bullying program in Italy: Evidence of effectiveness in a randomized control trial. *Prev. Sci.* **2016**, *17*, 1012–1023. [CrossRef] [PubMed]
13. Pepler, D.J.; Craig, W.M.; O'Connell, P.; Atlas, R.; Charach, A. Making a difference in bullying: Evaluation of a systemic school-based program in Canada. In *Bullying in Schools: How Successful Can Interventions Be?* Smith, P.K., Pepler, D., Rigby, K., Eds.; Cambridge University Press: Cambridge, UK, 2004; pp. 125–140.
14. Smith, P.K. Bullying in primary and secondary schools: Psychological and organizational comparisons. In *Handbook of Bullying in Schools: An International Perspective*; Jimerson, S.R., Swearer, S.M., Espelag, D.L., Eds.; Routledge: New York, NY, USA, 2010; pp. 137–150.
15. Yeager, D.S.; Fong, C.J.; Lee, H.Y.; Espelage, D. Declines in efficacy of anti-bullying programs among older adolescents: Theory and meta-analysis. *J. Appl. Dev. Psychol.* **2015**, *37*, 36–51. [CrossRef]
16. Bradshaw, C.P.; Waasdorp, T.E.; Leaf, P.J. Examining variation in the impact of school-wide positive behavioral interventions and supports: Findings from a randomized controlled effectiveness trial. *J. Educ. Psychol.* **2015**, *107*, 546–557. [CrossRef]
17. Farrell, A.D.; Henry, D.B.; Bettencourt, A. Methodological challenges examining subgroup differences: Examples from universal school-based youth violence prevention trials. *Prev. Sci.* **2013**, *14*, 121–133. [CrossRef] [PubMed]
18. Muthén, B.O.; Brown, C.H.; Masyn, K.; Jo, B.; Khoo, S.T.; Yang, C.C.; Liao, J. General growth mixture modeling for randomized preventive interventions. *Biostatistics* **2002**, *3*, 459–475. [CrossRef]
19. Van Lier, P.A.C.; Vuijk, P.; Crijnen, A.A.M. Understanding mechanisms of change in the development of antisocial behavior: The impact of a universal intervention. *J. Abnormal Child Psychol.* **2005**, *33*, 521–535. [CrossRef]
20. Ascher, J.; Dekovic, M.; van den Akker, A.L.; Manders, W.A.; Prins, P.J.M.; van der Laan, P.H.; Prinzie, P. Do personality traits affect responsiveness of juvenile delinquents to treatment? *J. Res. Pers.* **2016**, *63*, 44–50. [CrossRef]
21. Stoltz, S.; Dekovic, M.; de Catro, B.O.; Prinzie, P. What works for whom, how, and under what circumstances? Testing moderated mediation of intervention effects on externalzing behavior in children. *Soc. Dev.* **2013**, *22*, 406–425. [CrossRef]
22. Bollmer, J.M.; Harris, M.J.; Milich, R. Reactions to bullying and peer victimization: Narratives, physiological arousal, and personality. *J. Res. Pers.* **2006**, *40*, 803–828. [CrossRef]
23. Book, A.S.; Volk, A.A.; Hosker, A. Adolescent bullying and personality: An adaptive approach. *Pers. Individ. Differ.* **2012**, *52*, 218–223. [CrossRef]
24. Connolly, I.; Moore, M.O. Personality and family relations of children who bully. *Pers. Individ. Differ.* **2003**, *35*, 559–567. [CrossRef]
25. Jensen-Campbell, L.A.; Rosseli, M.; Workman, K.A.; Santisi, M.; Rios, J.D.; Bojan, D. Agreeableness, conscientiousness and effortful control processes. *J. Res. Pers.* **2002**, *36*, 476–489. [CrossRef]
26. Menesini, E.; Camodeca, M.; Nocentini, A. Bullying among siblings: The role of personality and relational variables. *Br. J. Dev. Psychol.* **2010**, *28*, 921–939. [CrossRef]
27. Pronk, J.; Olthof, T.; Goossens, F.A. Differential personality correlates of early adolescents' bullying-related outsider and defender behavior. *J. Early Adolesc.* **2015**, *35*, 1069–1091. [CrossRef]
28. Tani, F.; Greenman, P.S.; Schneider, B.H.; Fregoso, M. Bullying and the big five. *Sch. Psychol. Int.* **2003**, *24*, 131–146. [CrossRef]
29. Terranova, A.M.; Morris, A.S.; Boxer, P. Fear reactivity and effortful control in overt relational bullying: A six-month longitudinal study. *Aggress. Behav.* **2008**, *34*, 104–115. [CrossRef]
30. Supplee, L.H.; Kelly, B.C.; MacKinnon, D.M.; Barofsky, M.Y. Introduction to the special issue: Subgroup analysis in prevention and intervention research. *Prev. Sci.* **2013**, *14*, 107–110. [CrossRef]

31. Wang, R.; Lagakos, S.W.; Ware, J.H.; Hunter, D.J.; Drazen, J.M. Statistics in medicine—Reporting of subgroup analyses in clinical trials. *New Engl. J. Med.* **2007**, *357*, 2189–2194. [CrossRef]

32. Salmivalli, C.; Kärnä, A.; Poskiparta, E. Development, evaluation, and diffusion of a national anti-bullying program, KiVa. In *Handbook of Youth Prevention Science*; Doll, B., Pfohl, W., Yoon, J., Eds.; Routledge: New York, NY, USA, 2010; pp. 238–252.

33. Ellis, L.K.; Rothbart, M.K. Revision of the early adolescent temperament questionnaire. In Proceedings of the Poster presented at The Biennial Meeting of the Society for Research in Child Development, Minneapolis, MN, USA, April 2001.

34. Putnam, S.P.; Ellis, L.K.; Rothbart, M.K. The structure of temperament. In *Advances in Research on Temperament*; Eliasz, A., Angleitner, A., Eds.; Pabst Scientific Publishers: Lengerich, Germany, 2001; pp. 165–182.

35. West, B.T. Analyzing longitudinal data with the linear mixed models procedure in SPSS. *Eval. Heal. Prof.* **2009**, *32*, 207–228. [CrossRef]

36. Morris, S.B. Estimating effect sizes from pretest-posttest-control group designs. *Organ. Res. Methods* **2008**, *11*, 364–386. [CrossRef]

37. Carlson, K.D.; Schmidt, F.L. Impact of experimental design on effect size: Findings from the research literature on training. *J. Appl. Psychol.* **1999**, *84*, 851–862. [CrossRef]

38. Lahey, B.B. Public health significance of neuroticism. *Am. Psychol.* **2009**, *64*, 241–256. [CrossRef] [PubMed]

39. Snyder, H.R.; Gulley, L.D.; Bijttebier, P.; Hatman, C.A.; Oldehinkel, A.J.; Mezulis, A.; Young, J.F.; Hankin, B.L. Adolescent emotionality and effortful control: Core latent constructs and links to psychopathology and functioning. *J. Pers. Soc. Psychol.* **2015**, *109*, 1132–1149. [CrossRef] [PubMed]

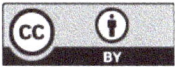

International Journal of
*Environmental Research
and Public Health*

MDPI

Article

Developing Wellbeing Through a Randomised Controlled Trial of a Martial Arts Based Intervention: An Alternative to the Anti-Bullying Approach

Brian Moore *, Stuart Woodcock and Dean Dudley

Department of Educational Studies, Faculty of Human Sciences, Macquarie University, North Ryde, NSW 2109, Australia; stuart.woodcock@mq.edu.au (S.W.); dean.dudley@mq.edu.au (D.D.)
* Correspondence: brian.william.moore@det.nsw.edu.au

Received: 17 December 2018; Accepted: 27 December 2018; Published: 29 December 2018

Abstract: Anti-bullying policies and interventions are the main approach addressing bullying behaviours in Australian schools. However, the evidence supporting these approaches is inconsistent and its theoretical underpinning may be problematic. The current study examined the effects of a martial arts based psycho-social intervention on participants' ratings of resilience and self-efficacy, delivered as a randomised controlled trial to 283 secondary school students. Results found a consistent pattern for strengths-based wellbeing outcomes. All measures relating to resilience and self-efficacy improved for the intervention group, whereas results declined for the control group. These findings suggest that a martial arts based psycho-social intervention may be an efficacious method of improving wellbeing outcomes including resilience and self-efficacy. The study proposes utilising alternatives to the anti-bullying approach and that interventions should be aimed towards helping individuals develop strengths and cope more effectively, which has specific relevance to bullying and more generalised importance to positive mental health.

Keywords: bullying; martial arts; mental health; resilience; self-efficacy; wellbeing

1. Introduction

Bullying is a complex and controversial subject that receives frequent media and academic attention. However, there is no standard definition of bullying [1–3], and definitions inclusive of all bullying behaviours are difficult to establish [4]. Bullying behaviours can occur directly and indirectly; and include verbal, physical, and/or relational characteristics. Research suggests bullying can be defined as: (a) a type of aggression [5], (b) systematic and repeated [6], and (c) based upon an imbalance of power [7,8].

Anti-bullying policies and interventions are the main approach addressing bullying behaviours in Australian schools [9]. However, the evidence supporting these approaches is indeterminate (for example: [1,10,11]) and their theoretical underpinnings are problematic [4,5].

Examining Australian state and territory educational policies and related documents suggests there is a relatively consistent approach to bullying policy across Australia. While education is primarily a state and territory responsibility in Australia, there has been a collaborative approach to addressing bullying across Australian education jurisdictions. For example, the Bullying. No way! website [9] is a collaborative product of the Australian Government's (AG) Department of Education, the state and territory government education departments, the National Catholic Education Commission, and the Independent Schools Council of Australia. This consistency is also due to school-based anti-bullying interventions being the main strategy addressing bullying behaviours [12]. Table 1 lists key policies across Australia, and Table 2 provides details of the characteristics of anti-bullying programs across Australian education jurisdictions.

Table 1. Australian educational bullying policy and associated documents.

Education Jurisdiction	Bullying Policy Accessible Online	Policy Document Title
ACT (Territory)	Yes	Safe and supportive schools policy [13]
AG (Federal)	No [a]	Disability Discrimination Act 1992 [14] Human Rights and Equal Opportunity Commission (HREOC) Act 1986 [15] Racial Discrimination Act 1975 [16] Racial Hatred Act 1995 [17] Sex Discrimination Act 1984 [18]
NSW (State)	Yes	Bullying of students—Prevention and response policy [19]
NT (Territory)	Limited	Health and wellbeing of students: Bullying, cyberbullying and cybersafety [20]
QLD (State)	Yes	Preventing bullying and violence [21]
SA (State)	Limited	Keeping children safe from bullying [22]
TAS (State)	No	n/a
VIC (State)	Yes	School Policy—Bullying [23]
WA (State)	Yes	Guidelines for preventing and managing bullying in schools [24]

Note. ACT: Australian Capital Territory, AG: Australian Government, NSW: New South Wales, NT: Northern Territory, QLD: Queensland, SA: South Australia, TAS: Tasmania, VIC: Victoria, WA: Western Australia. [a] While there is no specific Federal policy regarding school bullying the listed Federal legislation is relevant to this area.

As indicated by Table 2, Australian anti-bullying policies have relatively consistent characteristics. Policies typically define bullying as: (a) involving the misuse of power in a relationship, (b) ongoing and repeated behaviour, and (c) involving behaviours intended to cause harm [9]. It is important to consider differences between the former (research oriented) and latter (policy oriented) definitions of bullying. First, the latter definition omits the notion that bullying is a form of aggression [5]. Second, while the issue of power is noted in the latter definition, the meaning of this is moderated by including the term misuse. Third, the latter definition includes a focus on intent and harm causation. While this issue is not excluded from the former definition, its use in the latter frames the way bullying is conceptualised in terms of victims and perpetrators of bullying.

In response to these definitions, anti-bullying interventions typically fall into several categories. These include behavioural rule-based, non-punitive, social-emotional learning, and student intervention approaches. Policies typically mandate schools have official bullying or anti-bullying plans but suggest a flexible approach to implementation. Consequently, while policy and associated documents suggest a variety of strategies, it is difficult to know what anti-bullying actions are enacted at the school level.

Table 2. Characteristics of Australian anti-bullying programs based on policy and associated documents.

Education Jurisdiction	Defines Bullying	Mandates Bullying Plan	Whole School	Preventative Strategies	Awareness Raising	Staff Training	Engage Carers	Behaviour Sanctions	Non-Punitive	Social-Emotional	Bystander Intervention
ACT (Territory)	√	√	√	√	√	√	√	√	√	√	×
AG (Federal)	√	n/a	√	√	√	√	√	√	√	√	√
NSW (State)	√	√	√	√	√	√	√	√	√	√	√
NT (Territory)	√	×	×	×	×	×	×	×	×	×	×
QLD (State)	√	√	√	√	√	√	√	×	√	√	√
SA (State)	√	√	√	√	×	√	√	×	×	×	×
TAS (State)	n/a	n/a	n/a	n/a	n/a	n/a	n/a	n/a	n/a	n/a	n/a
VIC (State)	√	√	√	√	√	√	√	×	√	√	√
WA (State)	√	√	√	√	√	√	√	×	√	√	×

Note. ACT: Australian Capital Territory, AG: Australian Government, NSW: New South Wales, NT: Northern Territory, QLD: Queensland, SA: South Australia, TAS: Tasmania, VIC: Victoria, WA: Western Australia, √ = yes, x = not stated, n/a = not applicable.

1.1. The Failure of Anti-Bullying Policy

Anti-bullying literature frequently claims substantial empirical support to address bullying [1,25]. However, these claims should be viewed with caution. Case in point, a meta-analysis published by the Australian Government's Attorney General's Department reported that "with several exceptions . . . the outcomes from the evaluations reviewed were . . . positive in reducing overall bullying behaviour" [1] (p. 2). Despite Rigby's [1] assertion that research shows bullying behaviours among school children can be "significantly reduced" (p. 1), this is not wholly supported by the evidence presented in the meta-analysis. Notably, of the 13 studies reviewed by the meta-analysis three studies reported no change and six studies cited increased bullying behaviour post-intervention.

Evidence provided by other meta-analyses vary considerably in the level of support they provide for the efficacy of anti-bullying approaches. Ttofi and Farrington [11], reported that anti-bullying programs reduced bullying behaviours by an average of 20–23 per cent; and Jiménez-Barbero, Ruiz-Hernández, Llor-Zaragoza, Pérez-García, and Llor-Esteban [26] reported that anti-bullying programs resulted in significant reductions in the frequency of bullying behaviours. By contrast, Merrell, Gueldner, Ross and Isava [10] reported mixed results regarding anti-bullying programs changing rates of bullying; and Smith, Schneider, Smith and Ananiadau [27] reported that only a small number of programs produced positive outcomes regarding bullying and victimisation. Despite claims of substantial empirical support, the evidence to date is largely inconclusive.

The published meta-analyses raise another issue regarding anti-bullying policy and interventions to-date. It appears that the construct has become so broad that included studies contain almost any program that mentions bullying as a potential outcome variable. This leads to complicated methodologies and instruments being applied and it is therefore unsurprising that research to-date has not established what elements of anti-bullying strategies are crucial for reducing bullying behaviours [1]. Nonetheless, Farrington and Ttofi's [12] meta-analysis suggested that several anti-bullying strategies appear to be associated with decreased bullying. The most important of these being disciplinary methods including using explicit consequences regarding bullying, followed by parent training and meetings, and the duration and intensity of bullying programs.

1.2. An Evolutionary Perspective of Bullying

Bullying is a complex phenomenon that resists simple solutions [9]. Consequently, it is important to consider the narrative underpinning the anti-bullying approach to understand why the evidence regarding anti-bullying programs is inconclusive. As noted, anti-bullying policies typically omit the notion that bullying is a form of aggression [5] from their definitions. Aggression can be conceptualised as an exercise of power and relational power imbalances are critical to understanding bullying behaviours [28]. While anti-bullying literature proposed that bullying involves the abuse and exploitation of power [3,8], an evolutionary psychology perspective explores the use of power and rationalises why power imbalances exist.

Evolutionary psychology proposes that behaviours exist because they are adaptive [28]. Consequently, it is important to consider the adaptive nature of bullying, which appears to be a ubiquitous human behaviour [3,4]. Social dominance theory proposed that bullying can be used as a strategy to establish and maintain social dominance which facilitates access to valued resources, and can be understood in terms of the costs and benefits associated with using aggression [5]. It appears that many of the strategies used by the anti-bullying approach attempt to shift the relational balance of power without accounting for an evolutionary understanding of bullying behaviour. This occurs across behavioural, non-punitive, and student intervention anti-bullying strategies.

Bystander intervention has been identified as a "core tenant" of anti-bullying programs [29] (pp. 31–32), and involves shifting bystanders to become "active defenders of bullied students" [25] (p. 8). This approach can be interpreted as attempting to change the relational balance of power and may be a conceptually optimistic strategy. Research regarding the bystander effect was developed due to the observation that bystanders are unlikely to help others [30]. Latane and Darley [30] suggested that there are many factors that inhibit helping and make bystander intervention less likely including bystanders noticing that something is happening, interpreting the event and deciding something is wrong, assuming personal responsibility for helping, and deciding how to help.

1.3. Resilience and Bullying

Resilience is a complex construct [31] that is often defined as the attainment of positive outcomes despite significant adversity, risk, or stress [32,33]. This is evident in the varying operational definitions of resilience which include hardiness, optimism, competence, self-esteem, social-skills, achievement, and absence of pathology in the face of adversity [34]. Resilience can be conceptualised as a multi-level construct that includes: (a) protective processes, (b) the interaction of protection and risks, and (c) conceptual tools used in predictive models [35]. Examining resilience in terms of protective factors offers a viable means of measuring the construct [36] and recent research has suggested specific resilience factors may have greater efficacy in developing resilience based approaches to bullying [37].

Generally, the research examining the relationship between resilience and bullying is limited. Positively, students who reported higher levels of resilience were found to be less likely to engage in bullying behaviours or be victims of bullying [38]. Resilience towards bullying behaviours appeared to improve when individuals could disclose their experiences to a peer or family member [39] which is supported by research finding family factors, such as warm relationships and positive home environments were associated with greater resilience to bullying [40]. Resilience programs that improved social skills also appeared to decrease bullying behaviours [41]. Greater resilience and self-efficacy to bullying was reported as correlating with students completing an adventure based anti-bullying initiative [42], however the study reported weak correlations (ranging from $r = 0.25$ to $r = 0.26$) to support its claims.

A recent study by Moore and Woodcock [28] examining the mental health impacts of bullying considered resilience from a factorial perspective and conceptualised resilience as incorporating a sense of mastery, relatedness to others, and emotional reactivity. The study found higher levels of mastery and relatedness were a protective factor regarding depression, lower levels of emotional reactivity were a protective factor regarding depression and anxiety, and that higher levels of emotional reactivity were associated with an increased likelihood of bullying and being a victim of bullying behaviours. In a follow-up study, Moore and Woodcock [37] examined the resilience sub-scales underpinning these factors and found a pattern of effect sizes that suggested the sub-scale factors optimism, trust, tolerance, sensitivity and impairment may be more important for developing efficacious interventions that promote resilience to the effects of bullying.

1.4. Martial Arts Based Therapeutic Intervention and Developing Wellbeing

Martial arts are an ancient human behaviour which are often associated with promoting psychological benefits such as increased well-being, self-esteem and confidence [43]. The term martial arts are often used to describe many of the combat arts that developed in Eastern cultures [44] and martial arts participation exhibited substantial growth during the 20th century [45]. Perceptions of the martial arts are mixed [46]. The views range from martial arts promoting psychological benefits [43] to the assumption that martial arts training results in negative socialization processes such as increased aggression and hostility [46]. The focus of existing research has examined the physical aspects of martial arts training, such as health benefits and injuries resulting from martial arts practice [44]. Few studies have examined whether martial arts training can address mental health problems or promote mental health and wellbeing.

In a recent meta-analysis Moore, Dudley and Woodcock [47] reported that martial arts training had a positive effect on mental health outcomes. The analysis found that martial arts training had a small effect size regarding increasing wellbeing, and medium effect size regarding reducing internalising mental health issues, such as anxiety and depression. Several studies have reported martial arts training promoted characteristics associated with wellbeing. For example, a study examining a six-month taekwondo program reported increased self-esteem following the intervention [48]; while another found that participants reported higher self-concept compared to a comparison group after studying taekwondo for eight weeks [49]. Similarly, several studies reported that martial arts training reduced the symptoms associated with anxiety and depression. For example, karate students have been reported as being less prone to depression compared to reported norms for male college students [50]; and training in tai-chi reduced anxiety and depression compared to a non-treatment condition [51]. However, studies examining the psychological effects of martial arts training exhibit significant methodological problems that limit the generalisability of findings [46,52]. These include theoretical problems such as conceptual and definitional issues; and research design problems including a reliance on cross-sectional designs, small sample sizes, self-selection effects, limited use of follow-up measures, and not accounting for gender differences.

1.5. Bullying and a Martial Arts Based Psycho-Social Intervention

This study proposes an evolutionary perspective of bullying and considers the term bullying as a synonym for power imbalances in relationships. If it is assumed that bullying behaviours have an adaptive function, it may be optimistic to believe that bullying behaviours can be systemically modified.

An alternative approach could involve more generalised interventions promoting mental health through developing strengths, wellbeing and the ability to cope. Martial arts training can be conceptualised as a sports-based mental health intervention, where sport provides "the hook" [53] (p. 124) with which to deliver psycho-social interventions. Given its emphasis on respect, self-regulation and health promotion, martial arts training may be efficacious alternative to the anti-bullying approach. However, the efficacy of martial arts based interventions has received little research attention [54]. This study examined a martial arts based intervention using a randomised controlled trial design, and considered whether this type of sports-based psycho-social approach has the potential to improve participants' ratings of resilience and self-efficacy.

1.6. Theoretical Framework

The theoretical framework of this study is based on the bipartite martial arts model. Research examining the effects of martial arts training on mental health outcomes has typically used a bipartite model [55] which distinguishes between traditional and modern martial arts practice. This model assumes that the martial arts can be classified according to various criteria. The distinction between traditional and modern martial arts is based upon whether mediation, patterns practice and ethical and philosophical teachings are included (traditional martial arts) or excluded (modern martial arts) [56]. Traditional martial arts emphasize the non-aggressive aspects of martial arts, whereas modern martial arts typically emphasize competition and aggression [57]. The study is based on a traditional martial arts perspective.

1.7. Research Questions

Based on the literature review including identified gaps, methodological issues, and theoretical orientation; the following questions are proposed for investigation:

1. How does participation in a 10-week martial arts based intervention affect mental health factors, including resilience and self-efficacy?; and,
2. What is the relationship of mental health factors, including resilience and self-efficacy:

   a) before a 10-week martial based intervention (pre-intervention)?
   b) immediately after a 10-week martial based intervention (post-intervention)? and,
   c) three months after a 10-week martial based intervention (follow-up)?

2. Materials and Methods

2.1. Research Design

The study was a 10-week secondary school-based intervention that has been evaluated using a randomised controlled trial. Ethics approval for the study was obtained from an Australian University Human Research Ethics Committee. The study was registered with the Australian and New Zealand Clinical Trials Registry (ACTRN12618001405202). Additionally, the study protocol was also reviewed externally by school psychologists employed by the NSW Department of Education.

The researchers conducted pre-intervention (baseline) assessments at participating schools after the initial recruitment process. Following pre-intervention assessments and randomisation, the intervention group received the intervention program after which post-intervention assessment was conducted. At the time of writing this article results from the planned 12-week post-intervention (follow-up) assessment were not available. The control group received the same intervention program after the first post-intervention assessment. The design, conduct and reporting of this study adhered to the Consolidation Standards of Reporting Trials (CONSORT) guidelines for a randomised controlled trial [58]. Participants and caregivers provided written informed consent.

2.2. Participants

Two hundred and eighty-three (*N* = 283) students from five secondary schools in NSW, Australia were recruited to participate in the study. Participants had an age range of 12 to 14 years (*M* = 12.76, *SD* = 0.68) and were recruited from grade 7 (*n* = 192) and grade 8 (*n* = 91) at participating schools. One hundred and forty-three females and 136 males participated in the program. Four participants did not identify their biological sex. The socio-economic status of participants was reported as high (*n* = 70), high average (*n* = 85), low average (*n* = 49), and low (*n* = 78). The cultural background of the sample was predominantly reported as Australian (*n* = 251). Other reported cultural backgrounds included Aboriginal (*n* = 2), African (*n* = 1), Arabic (*n* = 1), Asian (*n* = 14), European (*n* = 3), and Pacific (*n* = 8). Two hundred and forty-one (*N* = 241) participants completed the post-intervention assessment. Of the 42 drop-outs from the study 20 participants chose to discontinue participation, 13 participants changed schools, and nine participants did not complete the assessment for unknown reasons.

Power calculations were conducted to determine the sample size required to detect changes in resilience and self-efficacy outcomes resulting from martial arts training. Statistical power calculations assumed baseline-post-test expected effect size gains of *d* = 0.3, and were based on 90% power with alpha levels set at *p* < 0.05. The minimum completion sample size was calculated as *N* = 234. As participant drop-out rates of 20% are common in randomised controlled trials [59] the maximum proposed sample size was *N* = 293.

2.3. Intervention Program

The intervention was delivered in a face-to-face group format onsite at participating schools. The intervention dose was 10 × 50 min sessions, once per week for 10 weeks. Each intervention session included:

(a) Psycho-education—based on facilitator guided group discussion. Topics included respect, goal-setting, self-concept and self-esteem, courage, resilience, bullying and peer pressure, self-care and caring for others, values, and, optimism and hope;
(b) Warm up activities—basic exercises including jogging, star jumps, push ups, and sit ups;
(c) Stretching activities—a variety of stretching activities were used during the program including hamstring stretch, triceps stretch, figure four stretch, butterfly stretch, lunging hip flexor stretch, knee to chest stretch, and standing quad stretch; and,
(d) Technical martial arts practice—including stances, blocks, punching, and kicking.

Additionally, the following activities were alternated during the program:

(e)   Patterns practice—a pattern is a choreographed sequence of movements consisting of combinations of blocks, punches and kicks, performed as though defending against imaginary opponents;

(f)   Sparring—an activity based on the tai-chi sticking hands exercise was included as an alternative to traditional martial arts sparring; and,

(g)   Meditation—based on breath focusing exercise.

It should be noted that aggressive physical contact was not part of the intervention program. The intervention was delivered by a (1) registered psychologist with minimum 6 years of experience, and (2) 2nd Dan/level black-belt taekwondo instructor with minimum 5 years of experience.

2.4. Instruments

Evaluation of the intervention program involved a variety of standardised psychometric instruments to report on mental health related outcomes. Instruments included the Strengths and Difficulties Questionnaire (SDQ) [60], Child and Youth Resilience Measure (CYRM-28) [61], and the Self-Efficacy Questionnaire for Children (SEQ-C) [62].

The SDQ is a 25-item instrument that measures various aspects of children's and adolescents' behaviour. The scale provided a total problems scale and five subscales including an emotional scale, conduct scale, hyperactivity-inattention scale, peer problems scale, and a prosocial behaviour scale. The English language self-report version of the scale was used which has a good internal consistency (0.76) [63] and good convergent validity. Items are scored on a 3-point Likert scale with 0 = not true, 1 = somewhat true, and 2 = certainly true. An example of SDQ items include: (1) I have one good friend or more, and (2) I am kind to younger children.

The CYRM-28 is a 28-item instrument that measures various aspects of children's and adolescents' resilience. The scale provided a total resilience scale and three subscales including an individual capacities and resources scale, relationship with primary caregiver scale, and contextual factors scale. The self-report version of the scale was used which has good internal consistency (.66 to .81) [64] and good construct validity. Items are scored on a 5-point Likert scale with 0 = not at all, 1 = a little, 2 = somewhat, 3 = quite a bit, and 4 = a lot. An example of CYRM-28 items include: (1) I have people I look up to, and (2) I feel supported by my friends.

The SEQ-C is a 24-item instrument that measures various aspects of children's and adolescents' self-efficacy. The scale provided a total self-efficacy scale and three subscales including an academic self-efficacy scale, a social self-efficacy scale, and an emotional self-efficacy scale. The SEQ-C scales have good internal consistency (>0.70) [65]. Items are scored on a 5-point Likert scale with 0 = not at all, 1 = a little, 2 = somewhat, 3 = quite a bit, and 4 = very well. An example of SEQ-C items include: (1) How well can you become friends with other children? and (2) How well can you control your feeling?.

2.5. Data Collection

The sampling plan utilised a randomised controlled sample to generate data for the study. All eligible government or catholic secondary schools in an urban area of New South Wales, Australia (n = 140) were sent an initial email with an invitation to participate in the study. Schools that responded to the initial email were pooled and received a follow up call in random order from the project researchers to discuss their participation. The first five schools that demonstrated interest were then recruited into the study.

All students enrolled in grades 7 and 8 (target age range 12–14 years) at participating schools were invited to participate in the study. Participant and caregiver information and consent forms were provided to students. Two follow-up letters were subsequently sent at two week intervals. Students who responded to the invitation were pooled and randomly allocated into the study, or not included in the study. Concurrent martial arts training were exclusion criteria for participation in the study, however previous experience of martial arts training was not an exclusion criterion.

Data was collected at pre-intervention (baseline), post-intervention, and 12-week post-intervention (follow-up). Randomisation into intervention and control group occurred after pre-intervention assessments. A simple computer algorithm was used to randomly allocate participants into intervention or control groups. The researchers were blinded to this randomisation of intervention and control group allocations.

During data collection participants were withdrawn from regular classes in small groups (pre-intervention), or the groups in which they completed the program (post-intervention). This enabled the researchers to explain, monitor and provide assistance while participants completed the survey. Participants were reminded that the survey was confidential and that they could discontinue the survey at any point. Instructions given to participants included: (a) an explanation of rating scales, and (b) how to make corrections if necessary. Surveys were then given to participants. Upon completion participants placed the survey into a locked box to ensure confidentiality.

2.6. Data Analysis

Statistical analysis of the psychometric test data was conducted using Statistical Package for the Social Sciences version 25 (IBM SPSS Statistics, Chicago, IL, USA) and alpha levels were set at $p < 0.05$.

The collected psychometric test data was consolidated into subscale variables using factor analysis and the internal consistency of each variable was examined to determine reliability. This was completed for pre-intervention and post-intervention measures. Table 3 reports pre-intervention and post-intervention internal consistency for the SDQ, CYRM-28 and SEQ-C. During factor analysis the SDQ converged in four factors (the conduct subscale and attention subscale converged in one factor which was renamed behaviour problems). For the emotional problems subscale item 6 did not converge across pre-intervention and post-intervention factor analysis and was discarded from the study. Internal consistency for the emotional problems scale was good. For the behaviour problems subscale items 12 and 22 did not converge across pre-intervention and post-intervention factor analysis and were discarded from the study. Internal consistency for the behaviour problems scale was good. For the peer problems subscale items 12, 14 and 19 did not converge across pre-intervention and post-intervention factor analysis and were discarded from the study. Internal consistency for the peer problems scale was poor and the subscale was discarded from the study. All items converged for the prosocial behaviour subscale across pre-intervention and post-intervention factor analysis, however internal consistency for the prosocial behaviour scale was poor and the scale was discarded from the study. The internal consistency for the SDQ total problems scale was good across pre-intervention and post-intervention factor analysis.

Table 3. Internal consistency for SDQ, CYRM-28 and SEQ-C across pre-intervention and post-intervention measures.

Measure	Scale	Pre-Intervention α	Post-Intervention α
SDQ	Emotional problems	0.72	0.73
	Behaviour problems	0.81	0.81
	Peer problems	0.18	0.12
	Prosocial behaviour	0.50	0.45
	Total problems	0.72	0.76
CYRM-28	Individual capacities and resources	0.85	0.89
	Relationship with primary carer	0.80	0.81
	Contextual factors	0.73	0.74
	Total resilience	0.89	0.91
SEQ-C	Academic self-efficacy	0.83	0.84
	Social self-efficacy	0.78	0.82
	Emotional self-efficacy	0.81	0.85
	Total self-efficacy	0.89	0.91

During factor analysis the CYRM-28 converged in three factors. For the individual capacities and resources subscale all factors converged across pre-intervention and post-intervention factor analysis, and internal consistency for the scale was good. For the relationship with primary caregiver subscale all factors converged across pre-intervention and post-intervention factor analysis, and internal consistency for the scale was good. For the contextual factors subscale all factors converged across pre-intervention and post-intervention factor analysis, and internal consistency for the scale was good. The internal consistency for the CYRM-28 total resilience scale was good across pre-intervention and post-intervention factor analysis.

During factor analysis the SEQ-C converged in three factors. For the academic self-efficacy subscale all factors converged across pre-intervention and post-intervention factor analysis, and internal consistency for the scale was good. For the social self-efficacy subscale all factors converged across pre-intervention and post-intervention factor analysis, and internal consistency for the scale was good. For the emotional self-efficacy subscale item 8 did not converge across pre-intervention and post-intervention factor analysis and was discarded from the study. Internal consistency for the emotional self-efficacy scale was good. The internal consistency for the SEQ-C total self-efficacy scale was good across pre-intervention and post-intervention factor analysis.

Items to be included in the scale variables were added and computed to create composite scores for pre-intervention and post-intervention data. Multivariate analysis of variance (MANOVA), analysis of variance (ANOVA) and Chi-square analyses were used to examine test data. Interpretation of effect sizes reflected Cohen's suggested small, medium, and large effect sizes, where η_p^2 sizes are equal to 0.10, 0.25, and 0.40 respectively [66].

3. Results

3.1. Behaviour and Emotion Problems

The hypothesis that martial arts training would decrease total problems and related sub-factors was not supported. Using Pillai's trace, martial arts training had no significant effect on participants' emotional problems, $V = 0.004$, $F(2, 238) = 0.52$, $p = 0.59$, $\eta_p^2 = 0.004$; behavioural problems, $V = 0.014$, $F(2, 237) = 1.65$, $p = 0.19$, $\eta_p^2 = 0.014$; or total problems, $V = 0.006$, $F(2, 237) = 0.75$, $p = 0.47$, $\eta_p^2 = 0.006$. Means and standard deviations are summarized in Table 4.

Table 4. Means and standard deviations for SDQ strengths and difficulties scales by experimental condition.

Scale	Condition	Baseline		Post-Test	
		Mean	SD	Mean	SD
Emotional difficulties	Intervention	0.69	0.51	0.66	0.47
	Control	0.74	0.51	0.73	0.51
Behavioural difficulties	Intervention	0.77	0.42	0.77	0.45
	Control	0.78	0.48	0.68	0.43
Total difficulties	Intervention	0.82	0.23	0.81	0.24
	Control	0.81	0.24	0.78	0.25

3.2. Resilience

The intervention improved levels of the overall resilience and resilience sub-factors. Means and standard deviations are summarized in Table 5.

Individual capacities and resources: Using Pillai's trace, there was a significant effect of the experimental condition on participants' individual capacities and resources, $V = 0.10$, $F(2, 238) = 13.35$, $p < 0.001$, $\eta_p^2 = 0.10$. Separate univariate ANOVAs revealed no significant difference between the intervention and control condition pre-intervention, $F(1, 239) = 1.64$, $p = 0.20$, $\eta_p^2 = 0.007$; however there was a significant difference between the intervention and control condition post-intervention, $F(1, 239) = 18.87$, $p < 0.001$, $\eta_p^2 = 0.07$.

Relationship with primary caregiver: There was a significant effect of the experimental condition on participants' relationship with primary caregiver, $V = 0.09$, $F(2, 238) = 11.59$, $p < 0.001$, $\eta_p^2 = 0.09$. Separate univariate ANOVAs revealed no significant difference between the intervention and control condition pre-intervention, $F(1, 239) = 1.06$, $p = 0.30$, $\eta_p^2 = 0.004$; however there was a significant difference between the intervention and control condition post-intervention, $F(1, 239) = 23.04$, $p < 0.001$, $\eta_p^2 = 0.09$.

Contextual factors: There was a significant effect of the experimental condition on participants' contextual factors, $V = 0.09$, $F(2, 238) = 11.94$, $p < 0.001$, $\eta_p^2 = 0.09$. Separate univariate ANOVAs revealed no significant difference between the intervention and control condition pre-intervention, $F(1, 239) = 1.54$, $p = 0.22$, $\eta_p^2 = 0.006$; however there was a significant difference between the intervention and control condition post-intervention, $F(1, 239) = 22.10$, $p < 0.001$, $\eta_p^2 = 0.09$.

Total resilience: There was a significant effect of the experimental condition on participants' total resilience score, $V = 0.14$, $F(2, 238) = 18.58$, $p < 0.001$, $\eta_p^2 = 0.14$. Separate univariate ANOVAs revealed no significant difference between the intervention and control condition pre-intervention, $F(1, 239) = 0.00$, $p = 0.98$, $\eta_p^2 = 0.000$; however there was a significant difference between the intervention and control condition post-intervention $F(1, 239) = 32.80$, $p < 0.001$, $\eta_p^2 = 0.12$.

Table 5. Means and standard deviations for CYRM-28 resilience scales by experimental condition.

Scale	Condition	Baseline		Post-Test	
		Mean	SD	Mean	SD
Individual capacities and resources	Intervention	2.96	0.60	3.10	0.53
	Control	3.06	0.59	2.75	0.69
Relationship with primary carer	Intervention	3.14	0.68	3.17	0.65
	Control	3.05	0.74	2.73	0.79
Contextual factors	Intervention	2.51	0.76	2.62	0.72
	Control	2.38	0.77	2.18	0.71
Total resilience	Intervention	2.90	0.51	3.01	0.45
	Control	2.90	0.56	2.62	0.61

3.3. Self-Efficacy

In terms of self-efficacy, the intervention improved levels of the overall self-efficacy and self-efficacy sub-factors. Means and standard deviations are summarized in Table 6.

Table 6. Means and standard deviations for SEQ-C self-efficacy scales by experimental condition.

Scale	Condition	Baseline		Post-Test	
		Mean	SD	Mean	SD
Academic self-efficacy	Intervention	2.56	0.71	2.77	0.64
	Control	2.48	0.73	2.41	0.69
Social self-efficacy	Intervention	2.57	0.74	2.84	0.62
	Control	2.78	0.57	2.60	0.67
Emotional self-efficacy	Intervention	2.23	0.80	2.63	0.70
	Control	2.34	0.73	2.25	0.79
Total self-efficacy	Intervention	2.45	0.60	2.75	0.52
	Control	2.54	0.52	2.42	0.59

Academic self-efficacy: Using Pillai's trace, there was a significant effect of the experimental condition on participants' academic self-efficacy, $V = 0.07$, $F(2, 238) = 9.19$, $p < 0.001$, $\eta_p^2 = 0.07$.

Separate univariate ANOVAs revealed no significant difference between the intervention and control condition pre-intervention, $F(1, 239) = 0.67$, $p = 0.41$, $\eta_p^2 = 0.003$; however there was a significant difference between the intervention and control condition post-intervention $F(1, 239) = 17.98$, $p < 0.001$, $\eta_p^2 = 0.07$.

Social self-efficacy: There was a significant effect of the experimental condition on participants' social self-efficacy, $V = 0.09$, $F(2, 238) = 12.14$, $p < 0.001$, $\eta_p^2 = 0.09$. Separate univariate ANOVAs revealed a significant difference between the intervention and control condition pre-intervention, $F(1, 239) = 6.24$, $p < 0.05$, $\eta_p^2 = 0.03$; and there was a significant difference between the intervention and control condition post-intervention, $F(1, 239) = 8.58$, $p < 0.01$, $\eta_p^2 = 0.04$.

Emotional self-efficacy: There was a significant effect of the experimental condition on participants' emotional self-efficacy, $V = 0.09$, $F(2, 238) = 11.64$, $p < 0.001$, $\eta_p^2 = 0.09$. Separate univariate ANOVAs revealed no significant difference between the intervention and control condition pre-intervention, $F(1, 239) = 1.24$, $p = 0.27$, $\eta_p^2 = 0.005$; however there was a significant difference between the intervention and control condition post-intervention, $F(1, 239) = 15.95$, $p < 0.001$, $\eta_p^2 = 0.06$.

Total self-efficacy: There was a significant effect of the experimental condition on participants' total self-efficacy, $V = 0.11$, $F(2, 238) = 14.94$, $p < 0.001$, $\eta_p^2 = 0.11$. Separate univariate ANOVAs revealed no significant difference between the intervention and control condition pre-intervention, $F(1, 239) = 1.48$, $p = 0.23$, $\eta_p^2 = 0.006$; however there was a significant difference between the intervention and control condition post-intervention, $F(1, 239) = 21.16$, $p < 0.001$, $\eta_p^2 = 0.08$.

3.4. Post-Program Martial Arts Participation

The intervention condition was asked whether they would like to continue practising martial arts after completing the program. Of the 125 participants who completed the intervention condition, 94 (75.2%) reported they would like to continue the program or participate in another martial art based program after the intervention. Chi square analysis of covariates found no significant differences for age, $\chi^2 = 2.86$, $p > 0.05$; grade, $\chi^2 = 0.14$, $p > 0.05$; biological sex, $\chi^2 = 5.25$, $p > 0.05$; cultural background $\chi^2 = 4.85$, $p > 0.05$; or socio-economic status $\chi^2 = 7.83$, $p > 0.05$.

4. Discussion

The results of the current study found a consistent pattern for wellbeing outcomes. All primary and secondary measures relating to resilience and self-efficacy improved for the intervention group and declined for the control group at statistically significant levels, which supports previous research [48,49]. The results provide valid and reliable evidence that psycho-social interventions based on a traditional martial arts model can be considered as an efficacious method of improving strengths and wellbeing outcomes. Interventions using this approach should promote an individual's ability to cope with the effects of bullying.

For resilience, the intervention had the greatest effect on total resilience which observed the largest effect size in the study. This is an important result given that students who report higher levels of resilience are less likely to become victims of bullying [38]. The resilience sub-factors relationship with primary caregivers and contextual factors exhibited the same effect size which was slightly smaller than for total resilience; and the resilience sub-factor individual capacities and resources exhibited the smallest resilience effect size resulting from the intervention program. The result regarding improved relationships with primary caregivers is particularly important given previous resilience research found that family factors including warm relationships and positive home environments are associated with greater resilience to bullying [40], and that resilience to bullying behaviours was improved when individuals could disclose their experiences to a family member [39]. The result that participants' resilience improved for the intervention group and declined for the control group suggests the intervention may improve participants' resilience to bullying.

A similar pattern was evident for self-efficacy insofar as the intervention had the greatest effect for total self-efficacy when compared to the self-efficacy sub-scales. Academic and emotional self-efficacy exhibited a similar effect size, which was slightly smaller than for total self-efficacy; while social self-efficacy exhibited the smallest self-efficacy effect size resulting from the intervention program. As the victims of bullying report lower self-efficacy compared to non-victims [37] the result that all self-efficacy scales improved for the intervention group and declined for the control group suggests the intervention may improve participants' ability to cope with bullying.

While the study exhibited increased resilience and self-efficacy for the intervention group and decreases for the control group, comparison of effect sizes suggests that the intervention had a greater effect on resilience outcomes. To this end, it is notable that the intervention program had a greater effect regarding total resilience and two of the resilience subscales (relationship with primary caregivers and contextual factors); than for total self-efficacy. It is also interesting that the relationship with primary caregivers resilience sub-scale exhibited a larger effect size compared to the social self-efficacy sub-scale, as they are intuitively related scales. Further, it is important to note that while the specific wellbeing scales considered in the current study differ from previous research, the current results support previous findings which reported martial arts training improved wellbeing factors such as self-esteem [48] and self-concept [49].

Although the effect sizes for resilience and self-efficacy were in the small range, this is nonetheless an important result. First, the meta-analyses conducted by Moore, Dudley and Woodcock [47] found that martial arts training resulted in improvements to factors associated with wellbeing, but that observed effect sizes were small. Results from the current study are consistent with this. Second, as noted there is a clear pattern regarding all resilience and self-efficacy scales increasing for the intervention group and decreasing for the control group. Third, the study recruited a randomised sample from a normal population and the intervention program was a 10-week group program. Consequently, the intervention's resilience and self-efficacy results should be viewed as promising.

However, results from the current study do not support previous research findings [50,51] and a meta-analysis [47] suggesting that martial arts training had a significant impact on internalising mental health issues. The current study found no significant internalising mental health differences between the intervention and control groups post-intervention, which is intriguing in view of previous research and positive finding from the current study regarding wellbeing outcomes.

It is encouraging that a large majority of the intervention group reported they would elect to continue martial arts participation post-program. Co-variate analysis was similarly encouraging, finding no differences for age, grade, biological sex, cultural background or socio-economic status regarding participants choosing to continue practicing martial arts. While the issue of self-selection effects cannot be entirely discounted, the result suggests the intervention program successfully engaged participants and may be applicable for a variety of different groups.

4.1. Explanation of Intervention Effects

The positive wellbeing outcomes found by the study are important, however explaining the casual factors associated with these effects is difficult. Resilience is a complex construct, and there are many elements in the intervention program incorporated from resilience literature that could result in improving resilience outcomes. These include empathic modelling, changing negative scripts, accepting participants for who they are and establishing realistic goals, encouraging participants to learn from mistakes, developing a social conscience, and encouraging problem solving and self-discipline [67]. Additionally, other social psychological constructs may have utility in explaining the intervention effects. For example, participants in the intervention program may have benefited from the development of an in-group identity [68] and the development of group superordinate goals [69]. From the current results the authors do not propose to isolate which factors may have been more important for developing greater resilience, however the above may be a useful conceptualisation towards this. These factors may also have utility in explaining participants' improved self-efficacy resulting from the intervention program.

The lack of observed effect post-intervention regarding internalising mental health issues may be explained by a variety of factors including scale issues, sample issues, as well as consideration of the null hypothesis. Scale issues may have impacted the study's capacity to measure participants' reports of internalising mental health issues. The SDQ exhibited problems regarding factor analysis and poor internal reliability, which resulted in several elements of the scale being discarded from the study. Consequently, it would be interesting to examine the effects of martial arts training regarding internalising mental health using an alternate measure. Sample bias may also have contributed to the study not detecting changes regarding internalising mental health. Given that the sample was randomly recruited from a normal population, the current study may not have had the same capacity to detect changes to participants' internalising mental health issues compared to previous research that recruited from targeted pathological samples. For example, Trulson's [48] study recruited from a sample of males diagnosed with behaviour disorders. Finally, it is important to consider the null hypothesis. It is possible that martial arts based training does not have a significant effect on internalising mental health outcomes. However, the authors propose that the noted scale and sample issues require further investigation before making conclusions regarding the null hypothesis.

4.2. Limitations

Several issues may limit the results of the current study. First, while the study has addressed many of limitations evident in prior research, the current study did not obtain third party corroboration of self-report measures. Inclusion of third party report measures should be considered in future research. Longer term effects of martial art training on mental health outcomes are unclear, given that follow-up data was not available at the time of writing this article. Finally, the issue of psycho-education versus martial arts training may be a confound in the current study. Psycho-education and martial arts training were presented as part of a single intervention program, hence it is not possible to separate their effects. However, it is arguable that combined psycho-education and martial arts training is consistent with the practice of many traditional martial arts, hence this issue may only have superficial significance.

4.3. Implications Regarding Interventions to Reduce Bullying

The current study's results have multiple implications to policy, practice and future research regarding bullying. Bullying behaviours are difficult to address, and the results attributed to the anti-bullying approach are inconsistent. Despite this, the anti-bullying approach maintains a dominant position informing educational policy regarding bullying. Arguably, the theoretical underpinning informing educational policy should be modified to account for other explanations of bullying behaviour, such as evolutionary perspectives on power and bullying. This should lead to questions regarding whether the aims of the anti-bullying approach (namely: no bullying) are achievable. The current study proposes an alternate approach to educational policy and suggests that instead of focusing resources towards eliminating bullying behaviours, policy should focus on promoting mental health through developing wellbeing. Results from the current study suggest that martial arts based psycho-social interventions have the potential to improve participants' strengths, wellbeing and ability to cope; which is important to consider in terms of educational policy regarding bullying.

The study has significant implications to practice regarding bullying behaviour. The institutional failure of the anti-bullying approach is potentially damaging to individuals. It is important to consider the impact and message understood by students when they continue to experience bullying behaviours despite the explicit anti-bullying policies and strategies used by schools. Further, because schools combine a wide variety of anti-bullying strategies flexibly, it is difficult to know what anti-bullying actions occur at the school level, and concerns should exist regarding whether the specific combinations used by schools are empirically supported. Given the inconsistent results attributed to the anti-bullying approach, alternate practices regarding bullying behaviour should be considered. Specifically, the current results have implications for practice by suggesting that intervention programs that develop strengths, including resilience and self-efficacy, have the potential to improve participants' sense of wellbeing and ability to cope with bullying.

The current study employed a robust design and rigorous evaluation, and suggests a promising approach to addressing bullying behaviours through improving wellbeing and mental health. The current results have a variety of implications for future research including sample considerations, methodological variations and developing a teacher professional learning program based on the study. Future research should examine the intervention program's effects on different population samples. Consideration should be given to implementing the intervention as a universal program with primary school students (ages 10–11); targeting specific populations such as participants diagnosed with (a) mental health issues such as anxiety and depression, (b) Autism Spectrum Disorder, (c) intellectual disability, and (d) behavioural disorders such as Oppositional Defiance Disorder, and participants who have experienced violent incidents including domestic and sexual violence; and extending the study to international settings to examine the intervention's efficacy in different cultural milieus. Future research should incorporate methodological changes including utilising third party measures to corroborate self-report measures, using alternate measures of mental health pathology such as the Kessler 10 Psychological Distress Scale [70], including a qualitative approach to supplement quantitative information, and varying the longitudinal parameters of the study by extending the follow-up period and lengthening the intervention program (e.g., 3/6/12 month interventions). Finally, future research should develop a professional learning program for teachers to facilitate similar programs which could be embedded within a physical education curriculum or welfare/pastoral care curriculum. Such a program would require piloting and ongoing measurement to ensure program efficacy.

5. Conclusions

Despite inconsistent evidence, the anti-bullying approach dominates educational policy and practice regarding bullying behaviours. While bullying is a complex phenomenon, the inconsistent evidence regarding the anti-bullying approach may be explained by problems with its theoretical underpinning. The authors propose the primary aim regarding bullying behaviours should change from attempted reduction of the behaviour, to improving individual ability to cope with the effects of bullying. The current study offers a strengths-based method of achieving this which is consistent with previous research. The results suggest that psycho-social interventions based on a traditional martial arts model can successfully promote wellbeing characteristics such as resilience and self-efficacy. Interventions that promote these strengths can help individuals develop better mental health and should be a focus of efforts to address the effects of bullying.

Author Contributions: B.M. conceptualized the article. Methodology was developed by all authors. B.M. conducted the investigation. Formal analysis was conducted by B.M., and all authors provided feedback and approved the final analysis. The paper was written by B.M., and all the authors provided feedback on the draft manuscript and approved the final version.

Funding: This research received no external funding.

Conflicts of Interest: The authors declare no conflict of interest.

References

1. Rigby, K. *A Meta-Evaluation of Methods and Approaches to Reducing Bullying in Pre-Schools and Early Primary School in Australia*; Commonwealth Attorney-General's Department: Canberra, Australia, 2002.
2. Rigby, K. An overview of approaches to managing bullying and victim problems. In *Bullying Solutions: Evidence Based Approaches to Bullying in Australian Schools*; McGrath, H., Noble, T., Eds.; Pearson: Sydney, Australia, 2006; pp. 161–173.
3. Rigby, K. *Children and Bullying: How Parents and Educators Can Reduce Bullying at Schools*; Blackwell: Victoria, Australia, 2008.
4. Lines, D. *The Bullies: Understanding Bullies and Bullying*; Jessica Kingsley: London, UK, 2008.

5. Pellegrini, A. Bullying during the middle school years. In *Bullying: Implications for the Classroom*; Saunders, C., Pyne, G., Eds.; Elsevier Academic Press: New York, NY, USA, 2004.

6. Olweus, D. *Bullying at School*; Blackwell: Oxford, UK, 1993.

7. Bouman, T.; van der Meulen, M.; Goossens, F.; Olthaf, T.; Vermande, M.; Aleva, E. Peer and self-reports of victimization and bullying: Their differential association with internalizing problems and social adjustment. *J. Sch. Psychol.* **2012**, *50*, 759–774. [CrossRef]

8. Smith, P.; Sharp, S. *School Bullying: Insights and Perspectives*; Routledge: London, UK, 1994.

9. Australian Education Authorities. Bullying. No Way! Available online: https://bullyingnoway.gov.au (accessed on 15 December 2018).

10. Merrell, K.; Gueldner, B.; Ross, S.; Isava, D. How effective are school bullying intervention programs? A meta-analysis of intervention research. *Sch. Psychol. Q.* **2008**, *23*, 26–42. [CrossRef]

11. Ttofi, M.; Farrington, D. Effectiveness of school-based programs to reduce bullying: A systematic and meta-analytic review. *J. Exp. Criminol.* **2011**, *7*, 27–56. [CrossRef]

12. Farrington, P.; Ttofi, M. School-Based Programs to Reduce Bullying and Victimization. Campbell Collaboration, 2009. Available online: https://www.ncjrs.gov/pdffiles1/nij/grants/229377.pdf (accessed on 28 December 2018).

13. ACT Education Directorate. Safe and Supportive Schools Policy. Available online: https://www.education.act.gov.au/publications_and_policies/School-and-Corporate-Policies/wellbeing/safety/safe-and-supportive-schools-policy (accessed on 15 December 2018).

14. Australian Government. Disability Discrimination Act 1992. Available online: https://www.legislation.gov.au/Details/C2018C00125 (accessed on 15 December 2018).

15. Australian Government. Human Rights and Equal Opportunity Commission (HREOC) Act 1986. Available online: https://www.legislation.gov.au/Details/C2017C00143 (accessed on 15 December 2018).

16. Australian Government. Racial Discrimination Act 1975. Available online: https://www.legislation.gov.au/Details/C2014C00014 (accessed on 15 December 2018).

17. Australian Government. Racial Hatred Act 1995. Available online: https://www.legislation.gov.au/Details/C2004A04951 (accessed on 15 December 2018).

18. Australian Government. Sex Discrimination Act 1984. Available online: https://www.legislation.gov.au/Details/C2014C00002 (accessed on 15 December 2018).

19. NSW Department of Education. Bullying of Students—Prevention and Response Policy. Available online: https://education.nsw.gov.au/policy-library/policies/bullying-of-students-prevention-and-response-policy (accessed on 15 December 2018).

20. NT Department of Education. Health and Wellbeing of Students: Bullying, Cyberbullying and Cybersafety. Available online: https://nt.gov.au/learning/primary-and-secondary-students/health-and-wellbeing-of-students/bullying-cyberbullying-and-cybersafety (accessed on 15 December 2018).

21. QLD Department of Education. Preventing Bullying and Violence. Available online: http://behaviour.education.qld.gov.au/bullying-and-violence/Pages/default.aspx (accessed on 15 December 2018).

22. SA Department for Education. Keeping Children Safe from Bullying. Available online: https://www.education.sa.gov.au/supporting-students/health-e-safety-and-wellbeing/keeping-children-safe-bullying (accessed on 15 December 2018).

23. VIC Department of Education and Training. School Policy—Bullying. Available online: https://www.education.vic.gov.au/school/principals/spag/safety/Pages/bullying.aspx (accessed on 15 December 2018).

24. WA Department of Education. Guidelines for Preventing and Managing Bullying in Schools. Available online: http://det.wa.edu.au/studentsupport/behaviourandwellbeing/detcms/school-support-programs/behaviour-and-wellbeing/safe-and-supportive-schools/guidelines-for-preventing-and-managing-bullying-in-schools.en?title=Guidelines+for+preventing+and+managing+bullying (accessed on 15 December 2018).

25. Centre for Education Statistics and Evaluation. Anti-Bullying Interventions in Schools—What Works? NSW Department of Education, 2017. Available online: https://www.cese.nsw.gov.au/images/stories/PDF/anti_bullying_in_schools_what_works_AA.pdf (accessed on 28 December 2018).

26. Jiménez-Barbero, J.; Ruiz-Hernández, J.; Llor-Zaragoza, L.; Pérez-García, M.; Llor-Esteban, B. Effectiveness of anti-bullying school programs: A meta-analysis. *Child. Youth Serv. Rev.* **2016**, *61*, 165–175. [CrossRef]

27. Smith, J.; Schneider, B.; Smith, P.; Ananiadau, K. The effectiveness of whole-school antibullying programs: A synthesis of evaluation research. *Sch. Psychol. Rev.* **2004**, *33*, 547–560.

28. Moore, B.; Woodcock, S. Bullying and resilience: Towards an alternative to the anti-bullying approach. *Educ. Psychol. Pract.* **2017**, *33*, 65–80. [CrossRef]

29. Ansary, N.; Elias, M.; Greene, M.; Green, S. Guidance for schools selecting antibullying approaches: Translating evidence-based strategies to contemporary implementation realities. *Educ. Res.* **2015**, *44*, 27–36. [CrossRef]

30. Latane, B.; Darley, J. *The Unresponsive Bystander: Why Doesn't He Help?* Appleton Century Crofts: New York, NY, USA, 1970.

31. Kaplan, H. Understanding the concept of resilience. In *Handbook of Resilience in Children*; Goldstein, S., Brooks, R., Eds.; Springer: New York, NY, USA, 2006; pp. 39–48.

32. Goldstein, S.; Brooks, R. Why study resilience? In *Handbook of Resilience in Children*; Goldstein, S., Brooks, R., Eds.; Springer: New York, NY, USA, 2006; pp. 3–16.

33. Naglieri, J.; LeBuffe, P. Measuring resilience in children. In *Handbook of Resilience in Children*; Goldstein, S., Brooks, R., Eds.; Springer: New York, NY, USA, 2006; pp. 107–123.

34. Prince-Embury, S. *Resilience Scales for Children and Adolescents: A Profile of Personal Strengths*; Pearson: Minneapolis, MN, USA, 2007.

35. Elias, M.; Parker, S.; Rosenblatt, J. Building educational opportunity. In *Handbook of Resilience in Children*; Goldstein, S., Brooks, R., Eds.; Springer: New York, NY, USA, 2006; pp. 315–336.

36. Fuller, A. A resilience based approach to helping the victims of bullying and their families. In *Bullying Solutions: Evidence Based Approaches to Bullying in Australian Schools*; McGrath, H., Noble, T., Eds.; Pearson: Sydney, Australia, 2006; pp. 161–173.

37. Moore, B.; Woodcock, S. Resilience, bullying, and mental health: Factors associated with improved outcomes. *Psychol. Sch.* **2017**, *54*, 689–702. [CrossRef]

38. Donnon, T. Understanding how resiliency development influences adolescent bullying and victimization. *Can. J. Sch. Psychol.* **2010**, *25*, 101–113. [CrossRef]

39. Rivers, I.; Cowie, H. Bullying and homophobia in UK schools: A perspective on factors affecting resilience and recovery. *J. Gay Lesbian Issues Educ.* **2006**, *3*, 11–43. [CrossRef]

40. Bowes, L.; Maughan, B.; Caspi, A.; Moffitt, T.; Arseneault, L. Families promote emotional and behavioural resilience to bullying: Evidence of an environmental effect. *J. Child Psychol. Psychiatry* **2010**, *51*, 809–814. [CrossRef] [PubMed]

41. Lisboa, C.; Killer, S. Coping with peer bullying and resilience promotion: Data from Brazilian at-risk children. *Int. J. Psychol.* **2008**, *43*, 711.

42. Beightol, J.; Jevertson, J.; Gray, S.; Carter, S.; Gass, M. The effect of an experiential, adventure-based 'anti-bullying initiative' on levels of resilience: A mixed methods study. *J. Exp. Educ.* **2009**, *31*, 420–424. [CrossRef]

43. Daniels, K.; Thornton, E. An analysis of the relationship between hostility. *J. Sport Sci.* **1990**, *8*, 95–101. [CrossRef] [PubMed]

44. Burke, D.; Al-Adawi, S.; Lee, Y.; Audette, J. Martial Arts as sport and therapy and training in the martial arts. *J. Sport Med. Phys. Fit.* **2007**, *47*, 96–102.

45. Cox, J. Traditional Asian martial arts training: A review. *Quest* **1993**, *45*, 366–388. [CrossRef]

46. Vertonghen, J.; Theeboom, M. The socio-psychological outcomes of martial arts practice among youth: A review. *J. Sport Sci. Med.* **2010**, *9*, 528–537.

47. Moore, B.; Dudley, D.; Woodcock, S. The effect of martial arts training on mental health outcomes: A systematic review and meta-analysis. *BMC Public Health* **2018**, under review.

48. Trulson, M. Martial arts training: A "novel" cure for juvenile delinquency. *Hum. Relat.* **1986**, *39*, 1131–1140. [CrossRef]

49. Finkenberg, M. Effect of participation in Taekwondo on college women's self-concept. *Percept. Mot. Skill* **1990**, *71*, 891–894. [CrossRef]

50. McGowan, R.; Jordan, C. Mood states and physical activity. *Louis Assoc. Health Phys. Educ. Rec. Dan J.* **1988**, *15*, 32.

51. Li, F.; Fisher, K.; Harmer, P.; Irbe, D.; Tearse, R.; Weimer, C. Tai Chi and self rated quality of sleep and daytime sleepiness in older adults: A randomised controlled trial. *J. Am. Geriatr. Soc.* **2004**, *52*, 892–900. [CrossRef] [PubMed]

52. Tsang, T.; Kohn, M.; Chow, C.; Singh, M. Health benefits of Kung Fu: A systematic review. *J. Sport Sci.* **2008**, *26*, 1249–1267. [CrossRef] [PubMed]

53. Hartmann, D. Theorizing sport as social intervention: A view from the grassroots. *Quest* **2003**, *55*, 118–140. [CrossRef]

54. Macarie, I.; Roberts, R. Martial arts and mental health. *Contemp. Psychother.* **2010**, *2*, 1–4.

55. Donohue, J.; Taylor, K. The classification of the fighting arts. *J. Asian Martial Art* **1994**, *3*, 10–37.

56. Nosanchuk, T.; MacNeil, C. Examination of the effects of traditional and modern martial arts training on aggressiveness. *Aggress. Behav.* **1989**, *15*, 153–159. [CrossRef]

57. Twemlow, S.; Biggs, B.; Nelson, T.; Venberg, E.; Fonagy, P.; Twemlow, S. Effects of participation in a martial arts based antibullying program in elementary schools. *Psychol. Sch.* **2008**, *45*, 947–959. [CrossRef]

58. Moher, D.; Liberati, A.; Tetzlaff, J.; Altman, D. PRISMA Group Preferred reporting items for systematic reviews and meta-analyses: The PRISMA statement. *PLoS Med.* **2009**, *6*. [CrossRef]

59. Wood, A.; White, I.; Thompson, S. Are missing outcome data adequately handled? A review of published randomized controlled trials in major medical journals. *Clin. Trials* **2004**, *1*, 368–376. [CrossRef]

60. Goodman, R. Strengths and Difficulties Questionnaire. Available online: http://www.sdqinfo.com (accessed on 14 December 2018).

61. Ungar, M.; Liebenberg, L. Assessing Resilience across Cultures Using Mixed-Methods: Construction of the Child and Youth Resilience Measure-28. *J. Mixed-Methods Res.* **2011**, *5*, 126–149. [CrossRef]

62. Muris, P. A Brief Questionnaire for Measuring Self-Efficacy in Youths. *J. Psychopathol. Behav. Assess.* **2001**, *23*, 145–149. [CrossRef]

63. Muris, P.; Meesters, C.; Eijkelenboom, A.; Vincken, M. The self-report version of the Strengths and Difficulties Questionnaire: Its psychometric properties in 8- to 13-year-old non-clinical children. *Br. J. Clin. Psychol.* **2004**, *43*, 437–448. [CrossRef] [PubMed]

64. Sanders, J.; Munford, R.; Thimasarn-Anwar, T.; Liebenberg, L. Validation of the Child and Youth Resilience Measure (CYRM-28) on a Sample of At-Risk New Zealand Youth. *Res. Soc. Work Pract.* **2017**, *27*, 827–840. [CrossRef]

65. Minter, A.; Pritzker, S. Measuring Adolescent Social and Academic Self-Efficacy: Cross-Ethnic Validity of the SEQ-C. *Res. Soc. Work Pract.* **2015**, *27*, 818–826. [CrossRef]

66. Richardson, J. Eta squared and partial eta squared as measures of effect size in educational research. *Educ. Res. Rev.* **2011**, *6*, 135–147. [CrossRef]

67. Brooks, R. The power of parenting. In *Handbook of Resilience in Children*; Goldstein, S., Brooks, R., Eds.; Springer: New York, NY, USA, 2006; pp. 297–313.

68. Kurzban, R.; Leary, M. Evolutionary origin of stigmatization: The functions of social exclusion. *Psychol. Bull.* **2001**, *127*, 187–208. [CrossRef]

69. Sherif, M.; Harvey, L.; White, B.; Hood, W.; Sherif, C. *The Robbers Cave Experiment: Intergroup Conflict and Cooperation*; Wesleyan University Press: Middletown, CT, USA, 1961.

70. Kessler, R.; Barker, P.; Colpe, L.; Epstein, J.; Gfroerer, J.; Hiripi, E.; Howes, M.J.; Normand, S.L.T.; Manderscheid, R.W.; Walters, E.E.; et al. Screening for serious mental illness in the general population. *Arch. Gen. Psychiatry* **2003**, *60*, 184–189. [CrossRef]

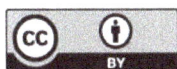

International Journal of
Environmental Research and Public Health

MDPI

Article

The Efficacy of the Tabby Improved Prevention and Intervention Program in Reducing Cyberbullying and Cybervictimization among Students

Anna Sorrentino [1], Anna Costanza Baldry [1,2,*] and David P. Farrington [2]

[1] Department of Psychology, Università degli Studi della Campania "Luigi Vanvitelli", 81100 Caserta, Italy;
     anna.sorrentino1@unicampania.it
[2] Institute of Criminology, University of Cambridge, Cambridge CB3 9DA, UK; dpf1@cam.ac.uk
*   Correspondence: annacostanza.baldry@gmail.com

Received: 24 September 2018; Accepted: 8 November 2018; Published: 13 November 2018

Abstract: *Background.* This article presents results from the evaluation of the Tabby Improved Prevention and Intervention Program (TIPIP) for cyberbullying and cybervictimization. TIPIP is theoretically designed to address cyberbullying and cybervictimization. It is the first program in this field developed combining the Ecological System Theory and the Threat Assessment Approach. *Method.* The Tabby Improved program was evaluated using an experimental design with 759 Italian students (aged 10–17 years) randomly allocated via their classes to either the Experimental or Control Group. *Results.* Repeated measures ANOVAs showed a significant decrease both in cyberbullying and cybervictimization among students who received the intervention with a follow-up period of six months. The program was more effective for boys than for girls. *Conclusions.* Because cyberbullying is a cruel problem negatively affecting those involved, validated interventions that prove their efficacy in reducing the problem using experimental designs should be widely tested and promoted, paying particular attention to implementing a program fully to increase and guarantee its effectiveness.

Keywords: cyberbullying; cybervictimization; prevention program; tabby intervention program; risk factors; threat assessment; ecological system theory

1. Introduction

In the first decade of the 21st century, parallel to the development and the dissemination of the new communication technologies especially among youngsters, a new phase in school bullying studies started [1]. Researchers began to show interest in harmful behavior involving the use of information and communication technologies (ICTs) and the possible consequences, resulting in what has been since then identified as cyberbullying [2,3].

Cyberbullying is an increasing problem, involving students of all ages from many countries [4–7]. Several studies have found that involvement in cyberbullying is associated with negative behavioral, psychological, and psychosomatic outcomes for both cyberbullies and cybervictims [5,6,8,9]. Because of such negative consequences, studies have multiplied, and several cyberbullying prevention programs have been developed, implemented and tested [4].

Compared to the four decades of research on school bullying, research on the effectiveness of cyberbullying prevention programs is relatively recent. This means that effective and successful school bullying prevention strategies are known [5,10–13], but, to date, only a limited number of studies have evaluated the effectiveness of cyberbullying and cybervictimization prevention programs [14].

Based on the meta-analyses carried out by Mishna et al. [14], Tokunaga [15] and Slonje, Smith and Frisén [16], it is clear that although several cyberbullying prevention programs have been developed and evaluated, few have been specifically conceptualized for the prevention of cyberbullying by adopting sound theoretical frameworks. As pointed out by Tokunaga [15] and Slonje, Smith and Frisén [16], most programs are not based on any theoretical framework and there is a doubt whether they are effective, or if they are, why, and which component is working. Tanrikulu [6], in his systematic review of seventeen studies, assessing the effectiveness of cyberbullying prevention and intervention programs, found that four of these programs were not theoretically based while the other thirteen had very little or no theoretical background, making it difficult to understand the underlying theoretical structure of such programs and the criteria for using one or another component.

Regarding studies that assess the effectiveness of cyberbullying and cybervictimization prevention programs, consistent with Palladino et al. [17], we can identify three main types of programs designed to: (1) prevent school bullying that have been subsequently adapted to prevent cyberbullying; (2) specifically deal with cyberbullying; and (3) prevent both school bullying and cyberbullying. The KiVa program (Kiusaamista Vastaan) and the ViSC Social Competence Program, originated respectively in Finland and Austria for preventing school bullying, were then adopted and extended to address cyberbullying and cybervictimization. The KiVa program proved to be effective in reducing both cyberbullying and cybervictimization [18,19], while the ViSC Social Competence Program [20] was effective in reducing cyberbullying but not cybervictimization.

Regarding other programs, the *MedienHelden* (Media Heroes), developed in Germany by Schultze-Krumbholz, Wölfer, Jäkel, Zagorscak and Scheithauer [21], includes as its components empathy training and peer-to-peer tutoring on Internet safety, as well as teacher and parent training. This program proved to be effective in decreasing cyberbullying incidents [22,23]. The Spanish *"ConRed"* cyberbullying prevention program [24,25] also showed a significant reduction for both cyberbullying and cybervictimization. The Australian *"Cyber Friendly School Program"* [26] was assessed longitudinally and the results indicated a significant decrease in students' likelihood of being involved in both cyberbullying and cybervictimization between the pre-test to the post-stages However, no significant differences were found between the intervention and control groups with regard to cyberbullying or cybervictimization. The *"Noncadiamointrappola!"* (*Let's not fall into the trap!*) Program [27] consists of a peer-led approach to prevent both school bullying and cyberbullying. Evaluations of its effectiveness have shown a significant decrease in both cyberbullying and cybervictimization [17,27,28].

Many of these programs are limited as they only include a few components (e.g., a curriculum and training for teachers and/or activities with students) [29], and evidence about how many and which components are most relevant in preventing and reducing cyberbullying and cybervictimization is still scarce [5].

The present study aimed to overcome some of the above-mentioned limitations, by presenting results of the effectiveness on the so-called Tabby Improved Prevention and Intervention Program (TIPIP). This program is the first prevention and intervention program developed specifically for cyberbullying and cybervictimization by combining two sound theoretical frameworks: The Ecological System Theory [30,31] and the threat assessment approach [32–35].

1.1. Theoretical Background of the Program

Adopting and combining Bronfenbrenner's Ecological System Theory (EST) and the Threat Assessment Approach seems to be a promising way to understand, explain and prevent youth involvement in cyberbullying and cybervictimization, deriving its roots from other fields of antisocial behavior and social psychology [36,37]. The EST [30,31] provides a comprehensive theoretical framework of the extent to which an individual's involvement in cyberbullying and/or cybervictimization is affected by several factors: the students' involvement, their families, peers, school, and community. The threat assessment approach [32–35] helps us to recognize and evaluate the presence of those risk factors that the international literature suggests are significant for students' involvement in cyberbullying and cybervictimization [36].

The Threat Assessment Approach (TAA) [32–35] is applied to understand how to best prevent a threat for antisocial behaviors to occur. In the field of cyberbullying and cybervictimization, based on certain risk factors and needs, how likely is that these conducts will take place or will take place again in the future? The TAA was developed to address the threats taking place before a massive disaster (e.g., a shooting) or other violent act (e.g., in the workplace) could take place, to intervene in time.

Cyberbullying is characterized by many threatening behaviors and attitudes that might or might not result in attacking a child/adolescent online. The Ecological Systems Theory [30,31], on the other hand, allows for identifying the levels (individual, interpersonal, social, community) where those risk factors are, and by influencing each other, they could increase the risk of involvement of a certain individual in these aggressive behaviors. To this aim, dimensions identified by reviewing the international literature as risk factors for cyberbullying and/or cybervictimization were classified accordingly to the ecological systems identified by Bronfenbrenner [30,31].

By adopting this classification, it is possible to look at the relationship between risk factors and involvement in cyberbullying and cybervictimization [32–35] and evaluating the presence of risk factors at one or more of the four ecological levels identified by Bronfenbrenner [30,31,36] and assess the individual likelihood of being at risk.

The Tabby Improved Prevention and Intervention Program (TIPIP) has been designed to assess not only the presence of risk factors for cyberbullying and cybervictimization, but to identify the ecological levels in which those risk factors operate and interact with each other, in the directing of assessing future risk of any threatening circumstances (risk factors) taking place.

1.2. The Tabby (Threat Assessment of Bullying Behavior among Youngsters) Improved Prevention and Intervention Program (TIPIP)

The TIPIP program was developed in two previous projects [4] and then 'improved' after evaluating the two previous projects' results and validating the instruments and by analyzing the results derived by the review of the international literature on risk factors for youngsters' involvement in cyberbullying and cybervictimization [36]. The program has four main components: (i) training activities with teachers, (ii) school conferences with parents; (iii) online materials for students, teachers and parents (available at www.tabby.eu); and (iv) in-class activities with students (see Figure 1).

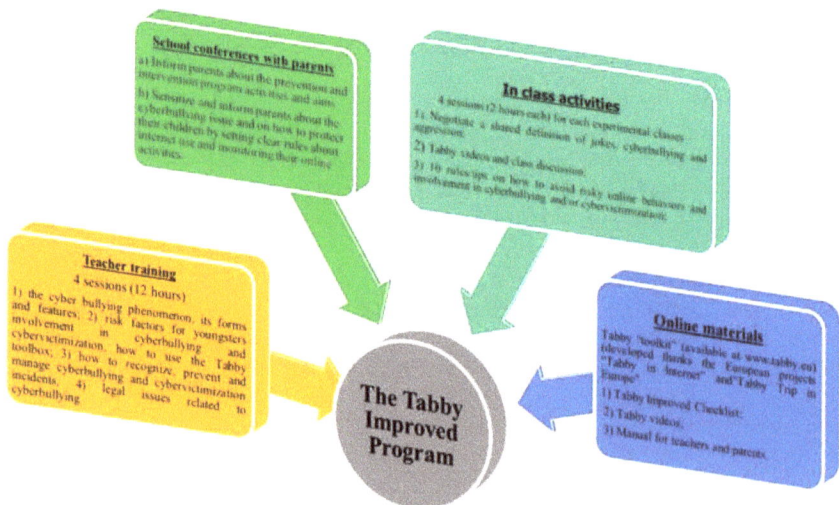

Figure 1. Components of the Tabby Improved Prevention and Intervention Program (TIPIP).

Each of them is included in the program according to the Ecological System Theory [30,31] to address relevant dimensions involved in cyberbullying and cybervictimization prevention, that is the individual, his/her family, the peer group and the school by raising and increasing their awareness about risk factors for the involvement in those behaviors [32–35].

(i) The teacher training activities lasted three days, approximately three hours per session, once a week for three weeks, plus an additional day on the possible civil, criminal and administrative legal implications of cyberbullying and on age of responsibility. The training was scheduled as follows: (a) the cyberbullying phenomenon, its forms and features, similarity to and differences from school bullying; (b) risk factors for youngsters' involvement in cyberbullying and cybervictimization, how to use the Tabby toolbox (the checklist, the booklet and the videos); (c) how to recognize, prevent and manage cyberbullying and cybervictimization incidents; (d) legal issues related to cyberbullying.

(ii) The School conferences with parents were scheduled in each of the participating schools. The main aims of these conferences were to: (a) inform parents about the prevention and intervention program activities and aims, and (b) sensitize and inform parents about the cyberbullying problem and how to protect their children by setting clear rules about internet use and how to best monitor their online activities. (iii) The third component of the program is the Tabby "toolkit" [4,38]. This is an extensive combination of three tools, including: the first consists of the updated version of the online self-report questionnaire, the Tabby Improved checklist, used to measure risk factors for students' involvement in cyberbullying and cybervictimization; the second includes) four short videos, used as stimuli to make youngsters think about the cyberbullying phenomenon and its consequences. Each video addresses one of the most common types of cyberbullying and aims to increase youngsters' awareness about the risks they face when using the Internet and the new communication technologies in a distorted or inattentive way. The central theme in each of the four videos is the idea that there is always an alternative, which helps to avoid either getting into trouble or causing trouble. For this reason, at the end of each video, after each cyber scenario, the story 'rewinds', showing what would or could have happened if the character(s) in the video had opted for another alternative (desirable) possible choice. At the end of the rewind scene, some recommendations on the safe use of the web are provided. Finally, the third tool is a manual for teachers, parents and students with useful information on cyberbullying, consisting of several short chapters with definitions and some scientific information on cyberbullying, is also a guide for trained teachers for them to organize class groups' activities to raise students' awareness about cyberbullying and cybervictimization. All are available at www.tabby.eu.

In-class activities with students were organized in each of the participating schools by scheduling four sessions (2 h each) for each of the experimental classes. The sessions with students were scheduled as follows: first, a group work aimed at negotiating a shared definition of jokes, cyberbullying and aggression. Once each group had defined these phenomena, they then had to identify differences and similarities between them. At the end of this activity, a representative from each group read to the class what emerged from their group discussion. Then all students chose the best definitions. The most highly voted work was exhibited in the classroom so that all students could share the same definitions of jokes, aggression, and cyberbullying. Then, during the second meeting, the Tabby videos described above were used. The videos were used as a stimuli from which to start a guided discussion regarding students' experiences in the cyberspace and to discuss useful strategies to protect themselves and/or to put an end to cyberbullying and/or cybervictimization incidents. Then in a third meeting, students were again divided into small working groups. Each group had to prepare at least ten rules or tips on how to avoid risky online behaviors and involvement in cyberbullying and/or cybervictimization. Students were also asked to think about *rules* that they would comply to, and that the whole class would then be able to adopt as new rules. These *rules* drawn up by the experimental classes were then presented to the school principal. At the end of the project, these rules were disseminated to the whole school, and they were included in the participating schools' policies on cyberbullying. In the fourth meeting, students had the opportunity to learn more about the legal consequences related to cyberbullying. During this last meeting a young boy who had been cyberbullying in the past met all classes to share his story and explain his point of view, answer questions and discuss what made him realize the damage caused by his actions and what he was doing to address it to change

The present study aimed to validate the effectiveness of the TIPIP by comparing pre and post and Experimental vs. Control Groups involvement in cyberbullying and cybervictimization.

2. Method

2.1. Design and Procedure

Five schools located in the Campania region, South Italy, participated in the project. Students were randomly assigned to one of two conditions (Experimental vs. Control), via their classes. Classes had to be randomly allocated to the research conditions because none of the contacted schools agreed to participate as a pure control school. To avoid possible teacher selection bias or class bias, the first author did the random assignment to the study conditions. Possible contamination effects were controlled by the first author, who was present and coordinated all the activities scheduled with students of the Experimental Group. In particular, most of the activities carried out with students were group work where students interacted with each other to understand what cyberbullying is, the dynamic and its impact and how to distinguish a credible and risky threat from a 'joke' or something that is not potentially harmful.

Before the data collection, the authors had obtained research approval from the Departmental Ethics committee for the procedure (29/2015), and consent from the custodial adults, and the participating students. All students filled in the Tabby online questionnaire before and six months after the whole intervention stages (T1 and T2). The first data collection was scheduled within the third month from the beginning of the school year, and then the procedure varied according to the condition (Experimental Group = EG, Control Group = CG); only students, teachers and parents of the EG received the intervention. The second data collection (follow-up T2), took place after six months, a few weeks before the end of the same school year.

To collect data, regardless of the research condition, the first author approached students in their classes, and, class by class, they all went with the teachers to the Computer Technology Room (CTR) that all participating school had to fill in the online questionnaire. Here, each student sat in front of a PC connected to the website questionnaire page and received instructions on how to proceed. Students were told that they should fill in an online, anonymous self-report questionnaire regarding their experiences on the use of new communication technologies and their online experiences, referring to a time period of six months.

Before filling in the questionnaire, the first author briefly explained the meaning of term cyberbullying so to make sure they had a common understanding of the main topic of the questionnaire and understood how their answers would not be available to anyone but collected and analyzed in an aggregated way. The following definition was provided:

"Cyberbullying as an aggressive and intentional act, carried out by a group or an individual, using electronic forms of contact, repeatedly over time against a victim who cannot easily defend himself/herself" [39].

Students were then instructed on how to generate an individualized ID code following a procedure to allow them to anonymously match their answers provided on that day (T1) with those on the following data collection (T2). The rule provided students was as follows: "Insert your personal code (two numbers of your date of birth- for example 03if you were born on the 3rd the, last two letters of your surname, and the last 3 numbers of your mobile or home phone number/if you don't have it, e.g., 03BA362, for Barba born on the 3rd, with mobile nr: ++362). After completing the questionnaire, all students returned to their classes.

Only classes in the EG participated in the next stages of the study, which included the teacher training on cyberbullying (trained teachers did not teach in any of the classes assigned to the control condition); the in-school conferences with parents, and the class activities with students. Six months after the end of all stages of the intervention, students were again brought in the CTR fill in the same online questionnaire, this time referring to what had happened in the last six months. Students, at the beginning of the T2 questionnaire had to fill inn their ID following the same rule. Only matched students ended up in the final sample. Data for the Control Group were collected during the same period as for the EG.

2.2. Participants

The initial sample consisted of 759 students randomly recruited from five schools (49 classes). Classes were randomly divided into two groups corresponding to the conditions: 20 classes (40.8%) were in the Experimental Group (students who received the intervention), and 29 classes (59.2%) were in the Control Group (students who did not receive any intervention, but filled in the Tabby Improved Checklist).

Overall, 622 students were included in the analyses as they had taken part and completed phases T1 and T2 (82% of the initial sample) and their questionnaire could be correctly matched. Attrition rates were checked, and analyses did not show any significant differences in any of the variables investigated. The dropping out of just over one hundred students was namely due to mistakes in filling in the matching ID code that students themselves had to create to guarantee their anonymity or absence on the day of data collection. Of all students, 45.9% were males, (54.1% females), with an age range between 10 to 17 years old (M = 12.14, SD = 1.44).

With regard to the use of cyber communication, 29.4% of all students reported at least one profile on a social network. Of those who had a profile, 7.2% personally knew only half of their online contacts and 35.7% of students on average spent 2–4 h a day online (see Table 1 for details). With regard to students' experiences of cyberbullying and cybervictimization, 15.0% reported cyberbullying others least once in the past six months, and 43.9% being cybervictimized at least once in the past six months. Boys were more likely to be cyberbullies but not cybervictims (see Table 1).

More boys were also reported having parents who did not talk with them about Internet security more than girls, control more their online activities, r spending more time per day on the Internet, being involved in both school bullying and victimization, and having poorer academic achievement.

Table 1. Descriptive statistics for the sample.

Age	Answer Criteria	Overall (622) M = 12.14 (SD = 1.44)	Boys (286) M = 12.11 (SD = 1.44)	Girls (336) M = 12.18 (SD =1.44)	OR (C.I.)
Presence of social network profile(s)	At Least One	29.4%	31.7%	27.0%	0.71 * (0.54–0.94)
Personally know friends on social network	Only half	7.2%	6.8%	7.5%	1.01 (0.87–1.16)
Parents talk with students about Internet Safety	Never	18.6%	11.0%	4.8%	1.37 *** (1.16–1.62)
Parents control students' online activities	Never	33.2%	29.7%	19.9%	1.48 *** (1.24–1.75)
Teachers talk with students about Internet Safety	Never	34.3%	18.7%	15.0%	1.01 (0.87–1.16)
Hours per day online	2–4 h	35.7%	41.9%	30.2%	0.83 * (0.70–0.97)
School achievement	Below average	7.6%	9.5%	6.0%	1.19 * (1.01–1.41)
School bully	At least sometimes	20.6%	28.2%	14.1%	2.45 *** (1.64–3.65)
School victim	At least sometimes	47.7%	53.2%	43.0%	1.49 * (1.08–2.04
Cyberbully	At least once	15.0%	21.5%	9.6%	2.59 *** (1.63–4.11)
Cybervictim	At least once	43.9%	43.0%	45.1%	0.92 (0.67–1.26)

Notes: * $p < 0.05$, *** $p < 0.001$, OR = Odds Ratio, C.I. = Confidence Interval.

2.3. Measures

The online Tabby Improved checklist was developed by analyzing the results of a review of the international literature on risk factors for youngsters' involvement in cyberbullying and cybervictimization and how these risk factors operate and interact at different levels according to the ecological theoretical framework, and the short-term predictive ability of the risk the previous instrument [4,38].

The Tabby Improved checklist consists of 12 scales and a total of 130 items; for the purposes of the current study only certain dimension were used. All dimensions were selected to measure ontogenetic, microsystem, and community level risk factors. For the purpose of the present paper, two different scales were analyzed: Involvement in cyberbullying and cybervictimization (in the past six months). For both cyberbullying and cybervictimization, participants' previous involvement in these behaviors was measured adopting the taxonomy by Willard [40]: flaming (A *'flame'* is a deliberately hostile and provocative message sent from one user to the community or an individual. Flaming is done by sending violent or vulgar electronic messages, in order to arouse verbal conflicts within the network between two or more users), denigration, impersonation, outing, and exclusion (5 items for cyberbullying and 5 items for cybervictimization for each scale). Students rated their experiences of cyberbullying and cybervictimization on 5-point Likert scales ranging from 0 = "it has never happened in this period" to 4 = "it happened several times a week". Example items: 'I pretended to be someone else, created a fake profile in order to send or post damaging messages about another person', 'I disclosed online private information or images without the person consent', and 'I was actively engaged in excluding someone from an online group'.

At the end of the cyberbullying and cybervictimization items, students were asked about their involvement as cyberbullies and cybervictims in the past six months, using a final global question only used as a check item ('In the last six months, have you ever been involved in cyberbullying?').

To measure cyberbullying and cybervictimization, scores on the 5-items measuring different types of cyberbullying and cybervictimization were added, total scores ranged from 0 to 20. Reliability coefficients at T1 and T2 were respectively $\alpha = 0.64$ and $\alpha = 0.75$ for cyberbullying and $\alpha = 0.72$ and $\alpha = 0.71$ for cybervictimization. Even if the reliability coefficient of the cyberbullying measure at T1 was just sufficient values <0.60 are considered acceptable given the short scale dimension [41–43].

2.4. Analysis

Data analyses were carried out using the SPSS statistical package (version 21.0, IBM Milano, Milan, Italy). First, the possible differences between the Experimental and the Control Groups with regard to cyberbullying and cybervictimization pre-intervention measures were analyzed. Next, the Intraclass Correlation coefficients for the outcome measures (ICC) [44] were calculated. Because of the clustered randomization design of the study, the presence of any clustering effects could lead to an inaccurate test for statistical significance [45]. This analysis takes into account the possible similarity of the responses of individuals within each cluster (classes). Finally, to evaluate the impact of the program, we used repeated-measures ANOVAs. We analyzed the longitudinal differences (pre- and post-intervention) in cyberbullying and cybervictimization between the Control and Experimental Groups.

3. Results

The main scores revealed non-significant differences between the Experimental and the Control Group with regard to cyberbullying ($F_{(6)} = 0.56$, $p > 0.05$) and cybervictimization ($F_{(15)} = 1.67$, $p > 0.05$) measured at baseline (T1). Because of the clustered randomization design of the study, the Intraclass Correlation coefficients for the dependent measures were calculated, obtaining $\varrho = -0.002$ for the cyberbullying pre-test score and $\varrho = -0.001$ for the cybervictimization pre-test score. These results indicated that clustering effects were very small and negligible compared with the 0.05 value that has sometimes been used in clustering designs [46]. Therefore, the clustering would not affect the outcomes of the intervention.

Table 2 shows descriptive analyses for both groups in the outcome variables (pre- and post-intervention). Repeated measures-ANOVA tests were carried out to evaluate whether any change in the Experimental Group was significantly different to the change in the Control Group.

Table 2. Pre–post differences in outcome variables.

Cyberbullying	Group	Pre M (SD)	Post M (SD)	Cyberbullying	Gender	Group	Pre M (SD)	Post M (SD)
	EG	0.29 (0.79)	0.21 (0.61) [a]		Boys	EG	0.35 (0.79)	0.24 (0.65) [c]
	CG	0.28 (0.84)	0.50 (1.78)				0.47 (1.08)	0.93 (2.55)
					Girls	CG	0.23 (0.79)	0.19 (0.58) [d]
							0.15 (0.57)	0.17 (0.58)
Cybervictimization	EG	1.10 (2.11)	0.74 (1.27) [b]	Cybervictimization	Boys	EG	1.18 (2.17)	0.63 (1.12) [e]
	CG	1.12 (1.73)	1.31 (2.34)			CG	1.08 (1.75)	1.52 (2.92)
					Girls	EG	1.03 (2.07)	0.83 (1.40) [f]
						CG	1.16 (1.72)	1.16 (1.77)

Notes: EG = Experimental Group; CG = Control Group. [a] $F_{(1,620)} = 6.46$; $p < 0.05$; [b] $F_{(1,620)} = 10.77$; $p < 0.001$; [c] $F_{(1,1000)} = 6.20$; $p < 0.05$; [d] $F_{(1,1000)} = 0.61$; $p > 0.05$; [e] $F_{(1,1000)} = 10.68$; $p < 0.001$; [f] $F_{(1,1000)} = 1.28$; $p > 0.05$.

For cyberbullying (see Figure 2), the results showed a significant effect of the condition (Experimental vs. Control) ($F_{(1,620)} = 4.10$; $p = 0.043$) and a significant interaction time * condition ($F_{(1,620)} = 6.46$; $p = 0.011$). Bonferroni post hoc analyses indicated an increase of cyberbullying at T2 in the Control Group ($F_{(1,620)} = 6.83$; $p = 0.009$). Also, for cybervictimization (see Figure 3), the results showed a significant effect of condition (Experimental vs. Control) ($F_{(1,620)} = 5.23$; $p = 0.022$) and a significant interaction time * condition ($F_{(1,620)} = 10.77$; $p = 0.001$). Post hoc analyses indicated a decrease of cybervictimization at T2 in the Experimental Group compared with the Control Group ($F_{(1,620)} = 13.71$; $p = 0.000$).

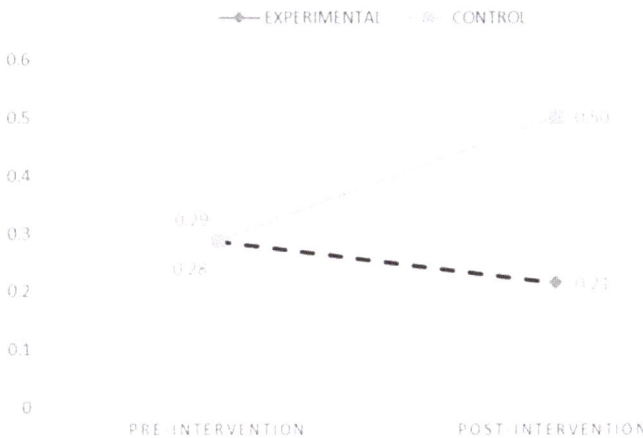

Figure 2. Changes in cyberbullying over time.

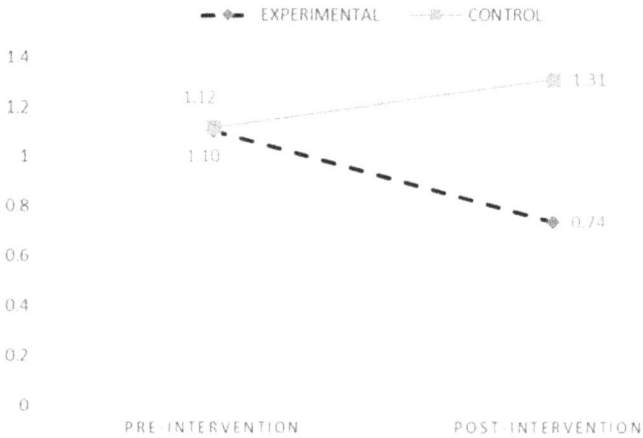

Figure 3. Changes in cybervictimization over time.

We tested the effectiveness of the intervention for boys and girls. For this purpose, repeated measures ANOVAs were carried out separately for boys and girls. For cyberbullying (see Figure 4), the results showed a significant interaction time * condition ($F_{(1,1000)}$ = 6.20; p = 0.013) among boys, but a non-significant interaction time * condition among girls ($F_{(1,1000)}$ = 0.61; p = 0.44). Bonferroni post hoc analyses indicated an increase of cyberbullying at T2 among boys of the Control Group ($F_{(1,282)}$ = 9.66; p = 0.002). For cybervictimization (see Figure 5), the results showed a significant interaction time * condition ($F_{(1,1000)}$ = 10.68; p = 0.001) among boys, but not for girls ($F_{(1,1000)}$ = 1.28; p = 0.26). The results revealed that both cyberbullying and cybervictimization varied across groups and gender, indicating a significant decrease of both cyberbullying and cybervictimization over time among boys in the EG (but not girls). Post hoc analyses underlined a decrease in cybervictimization at T2 among boys for the Experimental Group ($F_{(1,282)}$ = 11.14; p = 0.001).

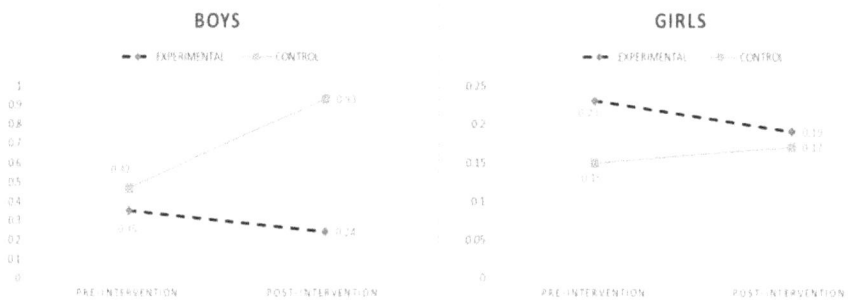

Figure 4. Changes in cyberbullying over time by gender.

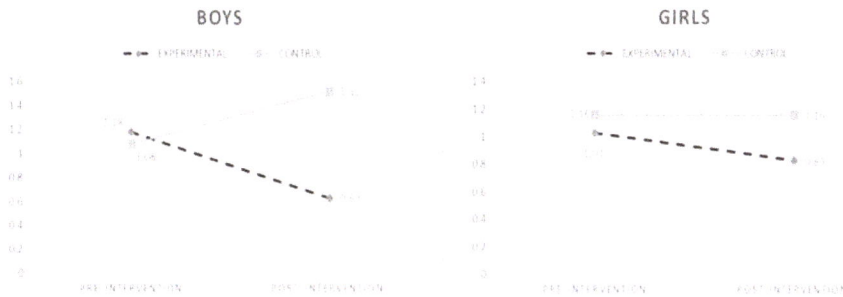

Figure 5. Changes in cybervictimization over time by gender.

4. Discussion

The present study aimed to present results of the effectiveness of the Tabby Improved Prevention Program (TIPIP), a multi-component program developed by combining the Ecological System Theory [30,31] and the Threat Assessment Approach [32–35]. We evaluated the short-term impact of the TIPIP on reducing cyberbullying and cybervictimization, by also looking at gender differences.

The results clearly show the efficacy of the TIPIP after six months of its extensive and thorough application, with reductions of cyberbullying and cybervictimization reported by students. The decreases in cyberbullying and cybervictimization in the Experimental Group has proved to be significant independently of student characteristics [20]. In particular, it is possible to assume that the inclusion of components of the program such as dedicated videos and cooperative work addressing cyberbullying and cybervictimization were those increasing its effectiveness [12].

With regard to the program's impact on boys and girls, the results showed that the program is effective in reducing both cyberbullying and cybervictimization among boys. In particular, cyberbullying significantly decreased both among boys of the Experimental Group, while boys' cyberbullying overall increased in the Control Group; for girls reported the same trend, the reduction was not significant. Similar to cyberbullying, the results showed a significant decrease in cybervictimization only among boys of the Experimental Group, while no significant differences were found among girls. However, it should be noticed that, even if not significant, a decrease in both cyberbullying and cybervictimization was observed among girls of the Experimental Group.

It is clear that the Tabby Improved Prevention and Intervention Program (TIPIP) works better for boys. These results are similar to those reported by Menesini and colleagues [28], who found a significant reduction of cyberbullying only among boys, and by Del Rey and colleagues [25], who found that the ConRed program was successful in reducing both cyberbullying and cybervictimization among boys. However, further studies are needed to understand whether this difference has to do with the components of the program, or on the role of other dimensions here not analyzed that might mediate such an effect such as empathy or moral disengagement [25,47].

We believe that one of the main strengths of this intervention program lies in the comprehensive cyberbullying and cybervictimization multicomponent theoretically driven approach. Furthermore, the activities undertaken with students were all planned to include curricula on classroom rules and cooperative group work, all elements that have been proven to be effective in preventing school bullying [10–13,29,48–52]. Also, all steps of the program were delivered, monitored and controlled one by one by the researchers, in cooperation with teachers and students. This reduces a risk of those programs where just a few days presence of an expert is provided as part of the program and material is distributed without any supervision or implementation check.

5. Conclusions

The current study has certain limitations. As in the majority of educational research, straightforward randomization is not always possible, and students were allocated to the conditions via their class [46]. Classes were randomly allocated to the research conditions by the researcher (to avoid possible teacher selection bias) and the Intraclass Correlation Coefficient was calculated. Possible contamination effects due to students of Experimental and Control Groups talk to each other were handled by the first author, which carried out all the activities with students of the Experimental Group. We cannot exclude, however, that some students from different groups talked to each other, although we did include this question at the end of the questionnaire and no contamination appeared from the analyses of the responses. However, we believe that due to the nature of the activities undertaken, that are most related to group work, negotiating and sharing common definitions and knowledge, the possible and simple word of mouth would not have affected the effectiveness of the program in its final results. A second possible limitation of the present study is related to the sole use of self-reported measures. In fact, despite their advantages [53], students could under-report their involvement in cyberbullying and/or cybervictimization or they could answer in a socially desirable manner [54]. As suggested by Topcu and Erdur-Backer [55], to overcome this limitation, multiple sources of information (for example peer, teacher and parent reports) could be used to investigate cyberbullying and cybervictimization. A third limitation concerns the short time of the follow-up measure (six months) and the lack of a long-term follow-up. According to the standards of evidence of prevention science [56], to claim that a program is effective, it would be necessary to report program efficacy in at least one long-term follow-up. Finally, repeated Anovas measures to test the program efficacy in reducing cyberbullying and cybervictimization for boys and girls as these are somehow skewed. However, even if our data were not normally distributed, we believe, consistent with Norman [57], that due to our sample size *'the means would be approximately normally distributed regardless of the original distribution'*.

Despite the aforementioned limitations, to the best of our knowledge, the present study is the first one aimed at investigating the effectiveness of a holistic, theoretically based cyberbullying and cybervictimization prevention program developed by combining the Ecological System Theory and the Threat Assessment Approach, and the use of an actuarial self-reported instrument which has vast potential of use. We can conclude and show that this program and its components and its procedure is worth extending and promoting as a promising solution to address cyberbullying and cybervictimization as a vicious public health concern.

Author Contributions: A.C.B. and A.S. conducted the research project; A.S. delivered the program, A.S., A.C.B., and D.P.F. analyzed the data; A.S., A.C.B., and D.P.F. wrote the paper.

Funding: This intervention program and its components have been developed and assessed and delivered thanks to the European funded "Tabby Trip in Europe" (European Project N° JUST/2011-2012/DAP/AG/3259) granted to the second author.

Acknowledgments: Authors wish to thank all participants that took part to this project and the anonymous reviewers and the special guest editors for all their precious comments.

Conflicts of Interest: The authors declare no conflict of interest.

References

1. Sánchez, V.; Ortega, R. El estudio científico del fenómeno bullying. In *Agresividad Injustificada, Bullying y Violencia Escolar*; Ortega, R., Ed.; Alianza Editorial: Madrid, Spain, 2010; pp. 55–80, ISBN 978-84-206-5461-4.
2. Ortega, R.; Elipe, P.; Monks, C.P. The emotional responses of victims of cyberbullying: Worry and indifference. *Br. J. Educ. Psychol. Monogr. Ser. II Psychol. Behav. Antisoc. Sch.* **2012**, *9*, 139–153.
3. Ortega, R.; Elipe, P.; Mora-Merchan, J.A.; Calmaestra, J.; Vega, E. The emotional impact on victims of traditional bullying and cyberbullying: A study of Spanish adolescents. *J. Psychol.* **2009**, *217*, 197–204. [CrossRef]

4. Baldry, A.C.; Blaya, C.; Farrington, D.P. *International Perspectives on Cyberbullying: Prevalence, Risk Factors and Interventions*; Palgrave-MacMillan: London, UK, 2018; pp. 1–326, ISBN 978-3-319-73262-6.

5. Gaffney, H.; Farrington, D.P.; Espelage, D.L.; Ttofi, M.M. Are cyberbullying intervention and prevention programs effective? A systematic and meta-analytical review. *Aggress. Violent Behav.* **2018**. [CrossRef]

6. Tanrikulu, I. Cyberbullying prevention and intervention programs in schools: A systematic review. *Sch. Psychol. Int.* **2018**, *39*, 74–91. [CrossRef]

7. Baldry, A.C.; Farrington, D.P.; Sorrentino, A. Cyberbullying in youth: A pattern of disruptive behaviour. *Psicol. Educ.* **2016**, *22*, 19–26. [CrossRef]

8. Waasdorp, T.E.; Bradshaw, C.P. The overlap between cyberbullying and traditional bullying. *J. Adolesc. Health* **2015**, *56*, 483–488. [CrossRef] [PubMed]

9. Sourander, A.; Klomek, A.B.; Ikonen, M.; Lindroos, J.; Luntamo, T.; Koskelainen, M.; Ristkari, T.; Helenius, H. Psychosocial risk factors associated with cyberbullying among adolescents: A population-based study. *Arch. Gen. Psychiatry* **2010**, *67*, 720–728. [CrossRef] [PubMed]

10. Ttofi, M.M.; Farrington, D.P.; Baldry, A.C. *Effectiveness of Programs to Reduce Bullying*; Swedish National Council for Crime Prevention: Stockholm, Sweden, 2008; pp. 1–92, ISBN 978-91-86027-11-7.

11. Farrington, D.P.; Ttofi, M.M. School-based programs to reduce bullying and victimization. *Campbell Callab.* **2009**, *6*, 1–149.

12. Ttofi, M.M.; Farrington, D.P. Effectiveness of school-based programs to reduce bullying: A systematic and meta-analytic review. *J. Exp. Criminol.* **2011**, *7*, 27–56. [CrossRef]

13. Ttofi, M.M.; Farrington, D.P.; Baldry, A.C. Effective programs to reduce school bullying. In *Juvenile Justice and Delinquency*; Springer, D.W., Roberts, A.R., Eds.; Jones and Bartlett Publishers: Sudbury, MA, USA, 2011; pp. 167–185, ISBN 978-0-7637-6056-4.

14. Mishna, F.; Cook, C.; Saini, M.; Wu, M.; MacFadden, R. Interventions for children, youth, and parents to prevent and reduce cyber abuse. *Campbell Syst. Rev.* **2009**, *2*, 1–54.

15. Tokunaga, R.S. Following you home from school: A critical review and synthesis of research on cyberbullying victimization. *Comput. Hum. Behav.* **2010**, *26*, 277–287. [CrossRef]

16. Slonje, R.; Smith, P.K.; Frisén, A. The nature of cyberbullying, and strategies for prevention. *Comput. Hum. Behav.* **2013**, *29*, 26–32. [CrossRef]

17. Palladino, B.E.; Nocentini, A.; Menesini, E. Evidence-based intervention against bullying and cyberbullying: Evaluation of the NoTrap! program in two independent trials. *Aggress. Behav.* **2016**, *42*, 194–206. [CrossRef] [PubMed]

18. Salmivalli, C.; Kärnä, A.; Poskiparta, E. Counteracting bullying in Finland: The KiVa program and its effects on different forms of being bullied. *Int. J. Behav. Dev.* **2011**, *35*, 405–411. [CrossRef]

19. Williford, A.; Elledge, L.C.; Boulton, A.J.; DePaolis, K.J.; Little, T.D.; Salmivalli, C. Effects of the KiVa antibullying program on cyberbullying and cybervictimization frequency among Finnish youth. *J. Clin. Child Adolesc. Psychol.* **2013**, *42*, 820–833. [CrossRef] [PubMed]

20. Gradinger, P.; Yanagida, T.; Strohmeier, D.; Spiel, C. Effectiveness and sustainability of the ViSC Social Competence Program to prevent cyberbullying and cyber-victimization: Class and individual level moderators. *Aggress. Behav.* **2016**, *42*, 181–193. [CrossRef] [PubMed]

21. Schultze-Krumbholz, A.; Wölfer, R.; Jäkel, A.; Zagorscak, P.; Scheithauer, H. Effective prevention of cyberbullying in Germany—The Medienhelden Program. In Proceedings of the 10th international Society for Research on Aggression (ISRA) World Meeting, Luxembourg, 17–21 July 2012.

22. Schultze-Krumbholz, A.; Schultze, M.; Zagorscak, P.; Wölfer, R.; Scheithauer, H. Feeling cybervictims' pain—The effect of empathy training on cyberbullying. *Aggress. Behav.* **2016**, *42*, 147–156. [CrossRef] [PubMed]

23. Wölfer, R.; Schultze-Krumbholz, A.; Zagorscak, P.; Jäkel, A.; Göbel, K.; Scheithauer, H. Prevention 2.0: Targeting cyberbullying@ school. *Prev. Sci.* **2014**, *15*, 879–887. [CrossRef] [PubMed]

24. Ortega-Ruiz, R.; Del, R.R.; Casas, J.A. Knowing, building and living together on internet and social networks: The ConRed cyberbullying prevention program. *Int. J. Confl. Violence* **2012**, *6*, 302–312.

25. Del, R.R.; Casas, J.A.; Ortega, R. The impacts of the CONRED Program on different cyberbulling roles. *Aggress. Behav.* **2016**, *42*, 123–135. [CrossRef] [PubMed]

26. Cross, D.; Shaw, T.; Hadwen, K.; Cardoso, P.; Slee, P.; Roberts, C.; Thomas, L.; Barnes, A. Longitudinal impact of the Cyber Friendly Schools program on adolescents' cyberbullying behavior. *Aggress. Behav.* **2016**, *42*, 166–180. [CrossRef] [PubMed]

27. Palladino, B.E.; Nocentini, A.; Menesini, E. Online and offline peer led models against bullying and cyberbullying. *Psicothema* **2012**, *24*, 634–639. [PubMed]

28. Menesini, E.; Nocentini, A.; Palladino, B.E. Empowering students against bullying and cyberbullying: Evaluation of an Italian peer-led model. *Int. J. Confl. Violence* **2012**, *6*, 313–320.

29. Van Cleemput, K.; DeSmet, A.; Vandebosch, H.; Bastiaensens, S.; Poels, K.; De Bourdeaudhuij, I. A systematic review of studies evaluating anti-cyberbullying programs. In Proceedings of the Etmaal Van De Communicatiewetenschap, Wageningen, The Netherlands, 3–4 February 2014.

30. Bronfenbrenner, U. Toward an experimental ecology of human development. *Am. Psychol.* **1977**, *32*, 513. [CrossRef]

31. Bronfenbrenner, U. *Ecology of Human Development: Experiments by Nature and Design*; Harvard University Press: Cambridge, MA, USA, 1979.

32. Borum, R.; Fein, R.; Vossekuil, B.; Berglund, J. Threat assessment: Defining an approach for evaluating risk of targeted violence. *Behav. Sci. Law* **1999**, *17*, 323–337. [CrossRef]

33. Fein, R.A.; Vossekuil, B. *Protective Intelligence and Threat Assessment Investigations: A Guide for State and Local Law Enforcement Officials (NIROJP/DOJ Publication No. 170612)*; Department of Justice: Washington, DC, USA, 1998.

34. Fein, R.A.; Vossekuil, B.V. Assassination in the United States: An operational study of recent assassins, attackers, and near-lethal approaches. *J. Forensic Sci.* **1999**, *44*, 321–333. [CrossRef] [PubMed]

35. Fein, R.A.; Vossekuil, B.; Holden, G.A. *Threat Assessment: An Approach to Prevent Targeted Violence*; National Institute of Justice: Washington, DC, USA, 1995; Volume 2.

36. Baldry, A.C.; Farrington, D.P.; Sorrentino, A. "Am I at risk of cyberbullying"? A narrative review and conceptual framework for research on risk of cyberbullying and cybervictimization: The risk and needs assessment approach. *Aggress. Violent Behav.* **2015**, *23*, 36–51. [CrossRef]

37. Baldry, A.C.; Sorrentino, A. Risk and needs assessment. In *The Encyclopedia of Juvenile Delinquency and Justice*; Schreck, C.J., Leiber, M., Miller, H.L., Welch, K., Eds.; Wiley-Blackwell: Hoboken, NJ, USA, 2017.

38. Baldry, A.C.; Blaya, C.; Farrington, D.P.; Sorrentino, A. The Tabby online project: The Threat Assessment of Bullying Behaviours Online approach. In *International Perspectives on Cyberbullying: Prevalence, Risk Factors and Interventions*; Baldry, A.C., Blaya, C., Farrington, D.P., Eds.; Palgrave-MacMillan: London, UK, 2018; pp. 25–36.

39. Smith, P.K.; Mahdavi, J.; Carvalho, M.; Fisher, S.; Russell, S.; Tippett, N. Cyberbullying: Its nature and impact in secondary school pupils. *J. Child Psychol. Psychiatry* **2008**, *49*, 376–385. [CrossRef] [PubMed]

40. Willard, N.E. *Cyberbullying and Cyberthreats: Responding to the Challenge of Online Social Aggression, Threats, and Distress*; Research Press: Champaign, IL, USA, 2007.

41. DeSmet, A.; Bastiaensens, S.; Van Cleemput, K.; Poels, K.; Vandebosch, H.; Deboutte, G.; De Troyer, O. Psychometric data of a questionnaire to measure cyberbullying bystander behavior and its behavioral determinants among adolescents. *Data Brief* **2018**, *18*, 1588–1595. [CrossRef] [PubMed]

42. Gliem, J.A.; Gliem, R.R. Calculating, Interpreting, and Reporting Cronbach's Alpha Reliability Coefficient for Likert-Type Scales. Available online: https://scholarworks.iupui.edu/bitstream/handle/1805/344/Gliem%20&%20Gliem.pdf?s (accessed on 16 October 2018).

43. Loewenthal, K.M. *An Introduction to Psychological Tests and Scales*, 2nd ed.; Psychology Press: London, UK, 2001; pp. 1–148, ISBN 9781317710158.

44. Raudenbush, S.W.; Bryk, A.S. *Hierarchical Linear Models: Applications and Data Analysis Methods*; Sage Publications: Thousand Oaks, CA, USA, 2002; pp. 1–485, ISBN 076191904X.

45. Bickel, R. *Multilevel Analysis for Applied Research: It's Just Regression!* Guilford Press: New York, NY, USA, 2007; pp. 1–428, ISBN 1-5938-5429-3.

46. Hedges, L.V.; Hedberg, E.C. Intraclass correlation values for planning group randomized trials in education. *Educ. Eval. Policy Anal.* **2007**, *29*, 60–87. [CrossRef]

47. Zych, I.; Baldry, A.C.; Farrington, D.P.; Llorent, V.J. Are children involved in cyberbullying low on empathy? A systematic review and meta-analysis of research on empathy versus different cyberbullying roles. *Aggress. Violent Behav.* **2018**, in press. [CrossRef]

48. Ttofi, M.; Farrington, D.P. What works in preventing bullying: Effective elements of anti-bullying programmes. *J. Aggress. Confl. Peace Res.* **2009**, *1*, 13–24. [CrossRef]

49. Juvonen, J.; Gross, E.F. Extending the school grounds?—Bullying experiences in cyberspace. *J. Sch. Health* **2008**, *78*, 496–505. [CrossRef] [PubMed]

50. Wilson, S.J.; Lipsey, M.W. The effects of school-based social information processing interventions on aggressive behaviors, Part I: Universal Programs. *Campbell Syst. Rev.* **2006**, *5*, 1–42.

51. Wilson, S.J.; Lipsey, M.W. School-based interventions for aggressive and disruptive behavior: Update of a meta-analysis. *Am. J. Prev. Med.* **2007**, *33*, S130–S143. [CrossRef] [PubMed]

52. Baldry, A.C.; Farrington, D.P. Evaluation of an intervention program for the reduction of bullying and victimization in schools. *Aggress. Behav.* **2004**, *30*, 1–15. [CrossRef]

53. Streiner, D.L.; Norman, G.R. *Health Measurement Scales: A Practical Guide to Their Development and Use*, 3rd ed.; Oxford University Press: Oxford, UK, 2003; pp. 1–276, ISBN 9780199231881.

54. Berne, S.; Frisén, A.; Schultze-Krumbholz, A.; Scheithauer, H.; Naruskov, K.; Luik, P.; Katzer, C.; Erentaite, R.; Zukauskiene, R. Cyberbullying assessment instruments: A systematic review. *Aggress. Violent Behav.* **2013**, *18*, 320–334. [CrossRef]

55. Topcu, Ç.; Erdur-Baker, Ö. Affective and cognitive empathy as mediators of gender differences in cyber and traditional bullying. *Sch. Psychol. Int.* **2012**, *33*, 550–561. [CrossRef]

56. Flay, B.R.; Biglan, A.; Boruch, R.F.; Castro, F.G.; Gottfredson, D.; Kellam, S.; Moscicki, E.K.; Schinke, S.; Valentin, J.C.; Ji, P. Standards of evidence: Criteria for efficacy, effectiveness and dissemination. *Prev. Sci.* **2005**, *6*, 151–175. [CrossRef] [PubMed]

57. Norman, G. Likert scales, levels of measurement and the "laws" of statistics. *Adv. Health Sci. Educ.* **2010**, *15*, 625–632. [CrossRef] [PubMed]

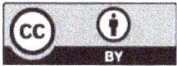

International Journal of
Environmental Research and Public Health

MDPI

Article

Pre-Service Teachers' Intervention in School Bullying Episodes with Special Education Needs Students: A Research in Italian and Greek Samples

Tatiana Begotti [1], Maurizio Tirassa [1,2] and Daniela Acquadro Maran [1,*]

[1]   Department of Psychology, Università di Torino, Via Verdi 10–10124 Torino I, Italy;
     tatiana.begotti@unito.it (T.B.); maurizio.tirassa@unito.it (M.T.)
[2]   Center of Cognitive Science, Università di Torino, Via Po 14–10123 Torino I, Italy
*   Correspondence: daniela.acquadro@unito.it

Received: 29 June 2018; Accepted: 31 August 2018; Published: 2 September 2018

Abstract: *Background*: The aim of the study was to compare the level of self-confidence in dealing with problems at school, the attitude towards bullying situations and the recommended strategies to cope with bullying in two samples of pre-service teachers (PSTs). The PSTs were in training to become teachers with special education needs students (SEN) and came from two different countries (Italy and Greece). *Methods*: A questionnaire survey was made involving 110 Italian and 84 Greek PSTs. *Results*: The results about self-confidence showed that Greek PSTs had lower outcome expectations and a higher external locus of causality than Italian PSTs. Teachers' training programs and school preventive intervention were also discussed. *Conclusions*: Because the participants in this investigation will be teachers in the near future, they require specific training on bullying in general and in students with SEN in particular.

Keywords: bullying; intervention; pre-service teachers; special education needs students

1. Introduction

Bullying is a well-known problem that involves students in primary and secondary school. The phenomenon is defined as an aggressive behaviour, repeated over time, in which the victim perceives a power imbalance [1,2]. The different forms of bullying are classified on the basis of the overt/covert dichotomy: overt bullying includes physical aggressions such as hitting, punching or kicking, or verbal aggressions such as insults or threats; covert bullying is a type of relational aggression and includes less visible actions such as gossiping, social exclusion or isolation [3,4]. Early research addressed students with Special Education Needs (SEN) and bullying victimization. Rose and Cage [5] showed students with disabilities and/or SEN to be generally more involved in the dynamics of bullying; they also turn out to be engaged in higher levels of perpetration than their peers without disabilities. Similarly, in their investigation about bullying among students with and without SEN, Fink et al. [6] argued that children with SEN are at greater risk of victimization (covert and overt) than other students. While children with SEN have a victimization rate between 30% (children with reading difficulties [7]) and 83% (children with learning difficulties [8]), children without SEN have a victimization rate of <20% [9]. Thus, SEN increases vulnerability to bullying and bullying in its turn increases distress and may inhibit the child's capability of entertaining positive social interactions in school and in other contexts [1]. McLaughlin and colleagues [10] suggested that this vulnerability was related to peer isolation, relational difficulties and poor acceptance in classrooms. In detail, the motives of the victimization are well explained by Pavri and Luftig [11]. The authors suggest that students with SEN demonstrate poor social competence: for example, delays in social development and lack of skills in initiating and sustaining positive social relationships and interpreting social cues. Moreover, they often demonstrate pervasive deficits in social functioning, exhibiting more aggressive and negative behaviours. In many ways, students with SEN have less sophisticated social skills that lead them to misinterpret social cues and to use ineffective responses [12]. Consequently, peers use covert behaviour, such as rejecting or ignoring them, instilling a sense of loneliness in students with SEN [13]. As underlined by Bryant, Smith and Bryant [14], inclusion is considered the best way to respond to the needs of students with SEN to avoid margination: inclusive education has a positive effect on social functioning [15–17]. To build an inclusive classroom and to take care of students (to respond to their emotional and psychosocial needs), teachers undoubtedly play a central role [18–20]: in the classroom, the teacher could create a context to enable students with and without SEN to learn and develop social competence, learning from each other. Moreover, because the highest victimization rate is in students with SEN, the teacher should pay particular attention to bullying [21]. Nevertheless, an analysis of the literature indicates that teachers tend to underestimate bullying episodes (particularly covert bullying) when reported by students with SEN, thus ignoring the victimization [10]. At the same time, research has shown that teachers play a key role in intervening to stop it, for example, by managing the classroom and/or suggesting ad hoc coping strategies to the victim [22,23]: fostering social development in the classroom may yield more appropriate interactions in social settings, also allowing bystanders and other third parties to intervene more often and/or more strongly in the defence of the victim.

Coping Strategies. Davis and Nixon [9] conducted an interesting study to evaluate students' perceptions about the effectiveness of the strategies used to reduce both overt and covert bullying at school. Their findings confirmed that students with SEN reported higher levels of victimization due to their disability. Regarding strategies to cope with the phenomenon, about one-third of students suggested that accessing support from peers and adults was the most helpful strategy. In particular, students appreciated adults telling them that they did the right thing to report what was happening, suggesting conflict resolution and/or the use of assertive communication. These adults listened and encouraged students, telling them that bullying was not their fault and suggesting that things would get better. However, the interventions of more than one-third of adults at school were described by victims as inefficient and did not affect their victimization. Some students reported that the intervention of one-third of adults at school made things get worse. The adults may have blamed the student for the victimization, told them to stop reporting it to adults, or instructed them to tell the bully how the victim feels (e.g., crying, venting), solve the problem him/herself (e.g., planning for revenge) and not tattle (e.g., ignoring). Scolding the victim for tattling was reported by the students as having the most negative impact in stopping the bully. Nevertheless, the authors stated that students with SEN reported that adults told them not to tattle almost twice as often as students without SEN. As emphasized by Cortes and Kochenderfer-Ladd [24], however, not only are avoidance behaviours generally ineffective but they may even have a reverse buffering effect that worsens the situation. If the teacher fails to express concern or to share appropriate advice about bullying, the students may feel uncomfortable approaching him/her not only as far as bullying is involved but also for guidance and support for other problems. On the other hand, Sokol et al. [25] examined the teachers' perspectives in responding to overt and covert bullying. Their study aimed to investigate the strategy perceived to be most effective. Their findings showed that participants were most likely to suggest to victims to report the episode to school staff. At the same time, teachers indicated that suggestions were related both to circumstances and the victim's characteristics: in some cases, the teacher recommended a contradictory approach, suggesting that they ignore the bully and express their feelings (venting). In other cases, teachers' recommendations were vague or insufficient to help the victims to stop the bullying. Thus, teachers may give conflicting and confusing messages to victims that could be perceived as useless. Therefore, because students will ask for help from adults, teachers must be ready to intervene in bullying episodes, suggesting more effective coping strategies. In particular, when students involved in bullying episodes have SEN [21], a strategy that worsens the situation could isolate them even more. The teacher's ability to intervene effectively in bullying cases was associated with the confidence that she/he has the capability to address problems at school [25–27]. As suggested by Roland and Galloway [28], students are less likely to become involved in bullying episodes when they perceive that teachers pay attention to them, particularly when a teacher is able to care for students, promote a positive environment in the classroom [29,30] and manage matters of learning and behaviour in a positive way. In the literature, the feeling of confidence was related to several explanations [25,31]. Among them, authors such Denzine, Cooney and McKenzie [32] described self-efficacy, outcome expectations and causal explanations given to each episode of bullying. According to Bandura [33], self-efficacy is the individual's perception of being able to cope with a certain task. In teachers, this perception is about his/her capability to produce outcomes (e.g., student engagement and learning) even if students are unmotivated or difficult [34]: teachers who sense a good relationship with their classroom tend to express higher level of self-efficacy. Self-efficacy is related to the chance of successfully intervening with bullying episodes. Findings from an investigation by Veenstra et al. [35] showed that classes in which teachers had a high self-efficacy also had lower occurrences of bullying. Thus, if teachers consider a bullying episode as serious, they are more likely to intervene if they have the knowledge and skills to act effectively [36,37]. A related notion is outcome expectations; that is, the belief that the behaviour will follow as a consequence of a specific outcome [38]. Teachers' expectation about students' outcomes affect the behaviour and the type and quality of interaction in the classroom [39]. If teachers have high expectations, they build a positive emotional environment [40] and increase their efforts to cope with problematic situations that occur in a classroom [41]. Social cognitivists make a distinction between outcome expectations and locus of causality [42]. The locus of causality has been described as the expectation of being able to control or reinforce the environment [43,44]. As underlined by Wang et al. [45], teachers tend to ascribe student's failure to external causes. These could be related to social and family distress or personal problems. Conversely, students' success is attributed to an internal cause, for example, the teachers' ability to challenge the student and stimulate interest in the subject. The internal locus of causality permits the teacher to intervene actively in a problematic situation that occurs in the classroom [46], such as bullying episodes. Pre-Service Teachers [PST], that is, persons who have no teaching experience but are enrolled in a training programme (like a university or post-university course) preparing them to become in-service teachers [IST], are a particularly interesting population. Authors [47] found that PSTs are more likely than ISTs to display a low external locus of causality and to ascribe positive changes in the relationships between students to their own behaviour in the classroom. PSTs may also feel more secure about their capability of supporting the victims, for example, by encouraging proactivity on the part of the bystanders [27] but not in the families' involvement. As suggested by Bagley, Woods and Woods [48], the parent's involvement is particularly important when students with SEN are bullied. PSTs may also feel that they would more likely intervene in response to overt aggression than to covert [49]; however, as described above, students with SEN are more likely to be the targets of covert bullying. This may signal that these teachers had not (or not yet) been trained and sensitized to properly address bullying, particularly when pupils with SEN are involved [47,48]. In general, too high expectations on the part of PSTs may end up in burnout when unsupported by reality [50]. Specific training on bullying, its consequences in the life of the victims, the third parties and the bullies themselves and how to recognize and effectively cope with it, could then be useful both to enable the prospective teachers to handle the actual situations in which they will likely find themselves and to help prevent consequences on their mental health and professional well-being.

Current Study. Based on this literature review, we compared two samples of pre-service teacher (PST) training to become special education teachers from two different countries (Italy and Greece) characterized by different levels of problem severity. In particular, we intended to compare (i) the level of self-confidence in dealing with problems at school (self-efficacy beliefs, outcome expectations and locus of causality) of Italian and Greek PSTs; (ii) the attitude towards bullying situations (perceived seriousness of bullying, empathy with the victims and likelihood of intervention) of Italian and Greek PSTs; and (iii) the strategies of intervention in bullying situations recommended by Italian and Greek

PSTs. (iv) We also intended to analyse the relationship between the recommended strategies to cope with bullying and the self-confidence and the attitude towards bullying in Greek and Italian PSTs. Previous research showed that PSTs perceive themselves as capable of effective intervention in bullying episodes (e.g., by encouraging viewers to be more pro-active) [27] when there was an overt episode [51]. However, Purdy and Mc Guckin [21] underlined that PSTs were not trained and sensitized to properly address the problem, particularly when the student involved in the bullying episode had SEN. In their investigation, the authors asked PSTs to describe their experience of dealing with bullying incidents (including incidents involving children with SEN) during school placement. The findings showed a lack of preparation of PSTs as a result of the lack of training on disablist bullying and "a subsequent lack of confidence in dealing with such incidents which were found to be often challenging and complex" [21] (p. 202). A European study on bullying found that in Italy, in a sample of 5042 students in secondary school, 15% declared themselves to be victims of bullying. Among 4987 students in Greece, this percentage was more than doubled (33%). The cause of bullying episodes was ascribed to a disability in 32% of cases in the Italian sample and 24% of cases in the Greek sample. Moreover, the findings showed that information about bullying (e.g., what this phenomenon is, how to cope with a bully, etc.) came mainly from school in both countries (30% in Italy, 39% in Greece). School is considered the most suitable place to talk about bullying (30% and 26%, respectively) and the most common coping strategy for victims was to ask for help from teachers (respectively 29% and 30%) [52]. Based on the above data, the aim of this study was explorative: the novelty of this work lies in the fact that, for the first time, self-confidence, attitude towards bullying and suggested strategies were compared in two PST samples of different nationalities. In particular, bullying is more common in Greece than in Italy and a greater proportion of people with disabilities are victims in Italy than in Greece.

Our expectations were the following:

1. We expected both Italian and Greek PSTs to have: (i) high levels of self-confidence in their capability of coping with problems at school, (ii) high levels of self-efficacy and expectations of outcomes and (iii) a prevalent internal locus of causality [47].
2. We (i) expected both Italian and Greek PSTs to perceive bullying, especially when overt, as a serious problem and to feel empathy toward the victims; however, (ii) we expected a higher likelihood of will to intervene in the Italian sample, due to the higher degree of victimization in Greece [52].
3. We expected in both the Italian and the Greek PSTs: (i) the strategies "Tell someone" and "Tell the bully how the victim feels" to be positively related to self-confidence, perceived seriousness of the episode, empathy with the victims and likelihood of intervention and (ii) the strategies "Solve the problem himself" and "Do not tattle" to be negatively related to the same variables [25].

To understand the perception that PSTs have both of bullying and of their own means to cope with it would allow to better tailor courses aimed at improving their relevant skills. Both the investigation and the intervention are particularly needed in countries where bullying appears to be more widespread and even more so where students with disabilities are particularly targeted.

2. Method

2.1. Ethical Statement

The study presented in this article conformed to the provisions of the Declaration of Helsinki in 1995, revised in Edinburgh 2000 [53]. All ethical guidelines were followed, as required for conducting human research, including adherence to the legal requirements of Italy. The research project was approved by the Directors of the Master. Since there was no medical treatment or other procedures that could cause psychological or social harm to participants, additional ethical approval was not required. With the approval of the Directors of the Master, participants were asked for authorization to administer the questionnaire. The cover sheet clearly explained the research aim, the voluntary nature of participation, the anonymity of the data and the elaboration of the findings. Thus, returning the questionnaires implied consent. Participants volunteered in the research without receiving any reward.

2.2. Participants

A total of 194 PSTs aged 22–52 (mean age 28 years, SD = 6.94) provided the data. The majority of respondents were female (179; 92%), confirming the trend in most countries [54,55]. Approximately 110 (57%) PSTs were Italian, aged 22–52 (mean age 27 years, SD = 6.8), with 96% females. They were recruited from the University of Torino (Italy), where they were attending the last year of the Master's course in Education. Eighty-four (43%) PSTs were Greek, aged 23–51 (mean age 29 years, SD = 6.94), with 87% females. They were recruited from the University of Torino, where they were attending a Master's course in Relational Competence in Teaching. The Greek students had courses in English, so they had to verify their knowledge of the language upon registration. Both groups (Italian and Greek students) were attending a course in preparing teachers to teach students with SEN. In most cases, Greek PSTs had work experience in teaching (68; 82.9%): for 38 PSTs, the duration of teaching experience was less than five years and for the rest of the sample, it was more than five years. Italian PSTs had teaching experience in 52 cases (47.3%): for 31 PSTs, the duration was less than five years and for 21, it was more than five years (χ^2 = 25.65; p = 0.000).

2.3. Materials

Participants were asked to anonymously fill out a self-administered questionnaire consisting of several sections. The first section described the purpose of the investigation and contained the instructions for replying, the anonymity and privacy statements and questions about the respondent's sex and age. The second part aimed to investigate the participants' self-confidence in dealing with problems at school, their attitudes towards bullying and victimisation in the case of overt and covert bullying and the strategies suggested to stop bullying. The measures used in this study were the Teacher Efficacy Scale (TES) [56], the Bullying Attitude Questionnaire [57] and the recommended strategies for coping with bullying. We used the three-factor model of TES [32], which included (i) three items measuring self-efficacy beliefs (SEB) (e.g., "If one of my students couldn't do a class assignment, I would be able to accurately assess whether the assignment was at the correct level of difficulty"); (ii) three items measuring outcome expectation (OE) (e.g., "If a student masters a new concept quickly, this might be because I knew the necessary steps in teaching that concept"); and (iii) four items measuring external locus of causality beliefs (E-LOC) (e.g., "A teacher is very limited in what he/she can achieve because of a student's home environment"). Each item was measured on a five-point scale (from 1 = strong disagreement, to 5 = strong agreement). Reliability, assessed with Cronbach's alpha, was SEB α = 0.54 (range 3–15); OE α = 0.63 (3–15); E-LOC α = 0.53 (4–20).

The Bullying Attitude Questionnaire included six scenarios hinging on either overt (such as physical or verbal) or covert (such as social exclusion) bullying episodes. Following the description of the scenarios, three items sought to evaluate the perceived seriousness of the episode (measured on a five-point scale from 1 = not serious, to 5 = very serious), the degree of empathy towards the victim (measured on a five-point scale from 1 = strong disagreement, to 5 = strong agreement) and the likelihood of intervention (measured on a five-point scale from 1 = not likely, to 5 = very likely). The six subscales were thus aimed at evaluating the three dimensions described above (perceived seriousness of the episode, empathy towards the victim and likelihood of intervention) in overt and covert bullying, each represented in three scenarios. Each subscale ranged between 3–15 points. The reliability of the subscales was measured with Cronbach's alpha: seriousness of overt bullying (α = 0.65); seriousness of covert bullying (α = 0.64); empathy in overt bullying (α = 0.82); empathy in covert bullying (α = 0.74); likelihood of intervention in overt bullying (α = 0.66); and likelihood of intervention in covert bullying (α = 0.60).

Regarding the recommended strategies for coping with bullying, participants were asked which strategies they would recommend to a child victim of bullying. Then, they were asked about their usage of ten different strategies, responding yes (score 2), sometimes (scored 1) or no (scored 0). In line with previous research [9], we divided the strategies in four categories: (1) accessing support from peers and adults (3 items, ranged 0–6; for example, "Tell parents"); (2) telling the bully how the victim feels (2 items, ranged 0–4; for example, "Crying"); (3) solving the problem him/herself (3 items, ranged 0–6; for example, "Fighting"); and (4) instructing them not to tattle (2 items, ranged 0–4; for example, "Ignoring") (Cronbach's alpha α = 0.53).

For the Italian sample, we used the Italian version of the questionnaire, which was already used in an investigation on bullying involving teachers [21]. Statistical analyses were performed with SPSS, version 22 (SPSS Inc., Chicago, IL, USA). Descriptive measures (means ± SD) were calculated for all test variables for all groups of participants. The different scores were examined using analysis of variance (ANOVA); eta squared was calculated to estimate the effect size. Correlations and regression analysis were calculated to examine the relationship between self-efficacy beliefs, outcome expectations, locus of causality, perceived seriousness of bullying, empathy with the victims, likelihood of intervention and strategies recommended to cope with bullying, in each group of participants (Italian and Greek PSTs).

2.4. Procedure

The data were collected by one of the authors of this paper and by assistants trained by the researchers. The participants were contacted through their academic courses and were informed that they were participating in a study to investigate the bullying phenomenon in their own point of view. Data collection involved completion of a structured questionnaire submitted on paper. All the participants were informed that participation was voluntary and that their responses were anonymous. The self-report questionnaire (both the Italian version and the English version) took approximately 20 min to complete. The participants were asked to insert the completed questionnaire in a slot box, so to guarantee anonymity. All the questionnaires were group administered in classrooms in a single day, with the permission of the Directors of the Master before the beginning of a lesson and were returned immediately. The response rate in both groups was 100% and all questionnaires were completely filled in. Therefore, none was excluded. The study was conducted in accordance with privacy requirements. This procedure was in accordance with the code of ethics of the Italian Association of Professional Psychologists and Italian law (the latter concerning privacy).

3. Results

The first aim of this study was to compare the level of self-confidence in dealing with problems at school (distinguishing between self-efficacy, outcome expectations and locus of causality) of Italian and Greek PSTs. The results are reported in Table 1.

Table 1. Self Confidence in dealing with problems at school. Comparison between Italian and Greek PST (one-way ANOVA).

	Italian PST (n = 110) *M (SD)*	Greek PST (n = 84) *M (SD)*	*F*	*p*	η^2
Self-efficacy beliefs (range 3–15)	9.20 (1.573)	9.17 (2.159)	0.020	n.s.	0.000
Outcome expectations (range 3–15)	10.28 (1.848)	8.90 (2.234)	14.437	0.000	0.089
External locus of causality (range 4–20)	9.99 (2.179)	11.74 (2.414)	17.542	0.000	0.107

Note. *M* = mean; *SD* = standard deviation; *F* = Fisher's ratio; *p* = *p* value; n.s. = not statistically significant; η^2 = eta square; As shown in Table 1, Greek PSTs had lower outcome expectations and a higher external locus of causality than Italian PSTs. No differences were found in self-efficacy beliefs.

The second aim of this study was to compare the attitude towards bullying situations (distinguishing between perceived seriousness of bullying, empathy with the victims and likelihood of intervention) in Italian and Greek PSTs. The results are reported in Table 2.

Table 2. Attitude toward bullying. Comparison between Italian and Greek PST (one-way ANOVA) (Range: 3–15).

	Italian PST (n = 110) M (SD)	Greek PST (n = 84) M (SD)	F	p	η^2
Seriousness (overt)	12.63 (1.842)	12.64 (1.857)	0.002	n.s.	0.000
Seriousness (covert)	12.78 (1.829)	12.82 (1.904)	0.013	n.s.	0.000
Empathy (overt)	11.71 (2.421)	10.79 (3.223)	3.409	0.048	0.151
Empathy (covert)	11.61 (2.333)	10.58 (2.992)	4.683	0.032	0.177
Intervention (overt)	12.84 (1.904)	12.67 (2.442)	0.196	n.s.	0.001
Intervention (overt)	12.82 (1.897)	12.46 (2.234)	0.925	n.s.	0.006

Note. *M* = mean; *SD* = standard deviation; *F* = Fisher's ratio; *p* = *p* value; n.s. = not statistically significant; η^2 = eta square.

As shown in Table 2, no statistically significant differences were found between Italian and Greek PSTs concerning perceived seriousness of bullying and the likelihood of intervention in cases of both overt and covert bullying. Furthermore, Greek PSTs reported a lower level of empathy than Italian PSTs in cases of both overt and covert bullying.

The third aim was to compare the strategies of intervention in bullying situations recommended to students by Italian and Greek PSTs. The results are reported in Table 3.

Table 3. Strategies of intervention. Comparison between Italian and Greek PST (one-way ANOVA).

	Italian PST (n = 110) M (SD)	Greek PST (n = 84) M (SD)	F	p	η^2
Tell someone (range 0–6)	5.66 (0.67)	5.21 (1.24)	8.14	0.005	0.053
Tell the bully how the victim feels (range 0–4)	1.91 (1.97)	1.84 (0.99)	0.14	n.s.	0.001
Solve the problem himself (range 0–6)	2.16 (0.97)	1.68 (0.88)	7.10	0.009	0.048
Do not tattle (range 0–4)	1.46 (1.33)	2.56 (1.14)	20.98	0.000	0.128

Note. *M* = mean; *SD* = standard deviation; *F* = Fisher's ratio; *p* = *p* value; n.s. = not statistically significant; η^2 = eta square.

As shown in Table 3, Greek PSTs suggested the strategies "Tell someone" and "Solve the problem himself" less than Italian PSTs, while they suggested the strategy "Do not tattle" significantly more than Italian PSTs. No difference was found in the strategy "Tell the bully how the victim feels."

The fourth aim was to analyse the relationship between recommended strategies to cope with bullying and self-confidence and the attitude towards bullying in Greek and Italian PSTs. The results are reported in Tables 4 and 5.

Table 4. Correlations among variables in Greek PST (N = 84).

	Tell Someone	Tell the Bully How the Victim Feels	Solve the Problem Himself	Do Not Tattle
Self-efficacy beliefs	0.12	−0.20	0.21	0.18
Outcome expectations	−0.06	0.24	0.19	0.16
External locus of causality	0.13	−0.16	0.35 *	0.03
Seriousness (overt)	0.18	0.19	0.18	−0.08
Seriousness (covert)	0.12	0.24	0.05	−0.16
Empathy (overt)	0.07	0.10	0.13	0.27
Empathy (covert)	0.13	0.04	0.16	0.22
Intervention (overt)	−0.06	0.04	−0.06	0.13
Intervention (covert)	0.10	−0.20	−0.24	0.03

Note: * $p < 0.05$.

As shown in Table 4, in Greek PSTs, we found a significant and positive correlation between the strategy "Solve the problem himself" and an external locus of causality. Regression analysis was performed, using "external locus of causality" as independent variable and "solve the problem himself" as dependent. Results shown a significant causal relation between variables (β = 0.35; p = 0.032; R^2 = 0.13).

Table 5. Correlations among variables in Italian PST (N = 110).

	Tell Someone	Tell the Bully How the Victim Feels	Solve the Problem Himself	Do Not Tattle
Self-efficacy beliefs	−0.13	−0.01	0.17	0.001
Outcome expectations	−0.12	0.01	0.09	0.14
External locus of causality	−0.09	0.12	0.07	0.02
Seriousness (overt)	0.07	0.05	−0.10	−0.08
Seriousness (covert)	0.16	−0.03	−0.15	0.09
Empathy (overt)	0.12	−0.04	−0.09	0.07
Empathy (covert)	0.25 **	0.04	−0.11	0.08
Intervention (overt)	0.17	0.17	−0.13	−0.08
Intervention (covert)	0.31 **	0.08	−0.10	−0.05

Note: ** $p < 0.01$.

As shown in Table 5, in Italian PSTs, we found significant and positive correlations between the strategy "Tell someone" and empathy and likelihood of intervention in cases of both overt and covert bullying. Regression analysis was performed, using "empathy (covert)"as independent variable and "tell someone" as dependent. Results did not show significant causal relation between variables (β = 0.13; p = n.s.; R^2 = 0.017). Also, the regression analysis performed with "intervention (covert)" as independent variable and "tell someone" as dependent did not show significant causal relation between variables (β = 0.10; p = n.s.; R^2 = 0.010).

4. Discussion

This study aimed to investigate the differences between Italian and Greek PSTs (students in training to become special education teachers) concerning the strategies of intervention against bullying at school. According to the literature, the ability to cope with bullying is associated with self-efficacy, outcome expectations and the causal explanation of the phenomenon. The first hypothesis of this study was partially confirmed: the results showed that there are no differences between Italian and Greek PSTs in self-efficacy: one of the main sources of self-efficacy is the direct experience of success. An explanation could be in the characteristics of the participants: because they were PSTs, they did not have direct classroom management experience (except for traineeships). However, Italians and Greeks differed in their expectations of success (higher in Italians) and the external locus of causality (higher in Greeks). This appears to imply that the Italians had a higher expectation of success in managing the class. As pointed out above, Gold & Roth [50] suggested that high expectations unsupported by reality can end up in burnout. This is likely to affect the Italian PSTs in particular. On the other hand, Greek PSTs showed a greater external locus of causality (that is a stronger tendency to attribute causal responsibility to others than to oneself): thus, they were more at risk of underestimating the importance of their role in managing the classroom, shifting responsibility to the families and/or the social context. This could also hamper the attempts to create a positive context, as free as possible from aggressive covert and overt behaviour towards students with and without SEN [18,23].

The second hypothesis of this study was partially confirmed: the findings showed that Italians and Greeks PSTs perceived bullying as a serious problem and had a high propensity for intervening, both in overt and covert episodes. This is an interesting finding because, as suggested by Zee and Koomen [36], if teachers consider a bullying episode as serious, they are more likely to consider their intervention as essential [38]. Moreover, these results are not in line with Kahn and colleagues [49] because we did not find a greater attitude to intervene in the case of overt bullying. There is, however, a difference in the case of empathy: Greek PSTs have a lower level of empathy towards the victim in both overt and covert bullying. This finding is particularly interesting: from the literature, empathy is an important predictor of intervention [3]. Finally, the lack of empathy towards the bullied pupils might influence the students' confidence in approaching the teacher about other types of problems, leading them to renounce an important guide. This is particularly true for students with SEN, who need support and information to resolve problems and difficulties [24].

Regarding strategies, the results showed a significant difference among Italian and Greek PSTs. Italian PSTs more often suggest the 'Tell someone' and 'Solve the problem him/herself' strategies, while Greek PSTs more often suggest the 'Do not tattle' strategy. An interesting finding concerns the expression of the emotion: the 'Tell the bully how the victim feels' strategy was not significantly different among Italian and Greek PSTs. Davis and Nixon [9] showed that students victims of bullying found the 'Tell someone' strategy useful, while 'do not tattle' was less effective. Thus, the suggestion of the strategy 'Do not tattle,' especially used with students with SEN, means that the victim of bullying does not feel helped, risking further isolation and a lack of understanding. In accordance with Rigby [58], the result is that victims of bullying risk experiencing frustration in the need for help.

Coming to the third hypothesis, only in few cases relations were found between self-confidence, perceived seriousness of bullying, empathy with the victim, proneness to intervention and the different strategies. In particular, the strategy 'solve the problem him/herself,' while recommended by Italian PSTs, was only related to a high external locus of causality in Greek PSTs. Regression analysis confirmed a causal relation between these two variables. This means that Greek PSTs are more likely to suggest to the victims to find a solution themselves, indicating the PST's inability to intervene effectively when they attribute an external locus of causality to the problem into the classroom. Because an external locus of causality attributes the failure to social and family distress or personal problems [45], PSTs probably suggest this coping strategy to attribute the cause (and thus the solution) to the victim.

As described above, Italian PSTs are more prone to suggesting 'Tell someone' or 'Solve the problem him/herself' than Greek PSTs. As previously mentioned, victims found that 'Tell someone' was particularly useful [9], unlike 'Solve the problem him/herself.' The strategy 'Tell someone' could be counterproductive (reverse buffering effect) [59] if the person asked for help, such as the teacher, suggests a poor strategy. This strategy was more commonly suggested by Italian PSTs with higher scores in empathy and a higher propensity to intervene in covert bullying episodes. This finding appears to be very interesting despite regression analysis did not confirm the causal relation between the variables. According to the literature, teachers tend to underestimate covert bullying [60,61] and are more likely to intervene in the cases of physical and verbal bullying and to take no action in cases of social bullying [62]. Thus, this finding is not in accordance with the literature, since Italian PSTs suggest that covert bullying victims talk about their experience. This strategy allows victims to escape the sense of isolation that characterizes bullying victims in general and the covert bullying victims in particular.

There are, of course, limitations to this study. First, since participants belonged to a sample of convenience, non-randomly selected, the results should be considered with caution and not be generalized. Moreover, the participants' possible previous experience with bullying (as a victim, bully, bystander, or other role) was not investigated: such experience, however, would likely affect one's perception [63]. Third, the questionnaire used in this research sought to investigate the PST's attitudes towards bullying in the classroom and not towards bullying in students with SEN. Future research should be addressed to investigate previous experience in bullying in PSTs and their attitude towards bullying in students with SEN. Finally, the questionnaire did not take into account the PST's confidence in dealing with cyberbullying. This, too, should be the matter of future investigations.

5. Conclusions

Despite these limitations, this investigation suggests particular strategies for Italian and Greek PST training. Because the participants in this investigation will be teachers in the near future, they require specific training on bullying in general and on bullying in students with SEN in particular. Concerning the former, training might include discussions of overt and covert bullying aimed at helping distinguish it from other forms of aggression (not repetitive, not imbalanced and/or not intentional). This could also include examples of intervention, both toward the bullies and toward the victims. Baumann and Del Rio [64] suggested to use videos, role play and other available techniques aimed at the understanding of theories and at the application of recommended strategies of intervention in simulated situations. Training could also improve the ability of promoting empathy and pro-social skills not only in bullies and victims but in the entire classroom. Furthermore, training should highlight the central role that teachers can have in stopping the phenomenon. In fact, suggesting a strategy and accepting the victim's need for help can disrupt the victim-bully relationship and influence children's attitudes on bullying and bystanding behaviour [26,65]. Specifically, students with SEN should be helped effectively and in a timely manner. These students are particularly vulnerable and need to be placed in a class that can accommodate them, not isolate them. Inclusive education itself may offer opportunities for students with SEN to interact with peers but it does not necessarily lead to positive and supportive relationships [66]. This suggestion is specific for Italian PSTs, where the bullying affects students with SEN more than in Greece. Moreover, for Italian PSTs the courses ought to take into account the issue of the high outcome expectations, so to avoid the risk, discussed above [50], that these teachers develop unrealistic expectations, unsupported by reality. Furthermore, as suggested by Bagley, Woods and Woods [48], training courses ought to stress the importance of parents' involvement in cases of bullying, especially where students with SEN are involved. This is important for all PSTs, particularly for the Greek ones, whose high external locus of causality could lead to handing over the whole responsibility of intervention to the families. This would have several negative consequences, among which the failure to build an effective alliance with them. As shown by Nicolaides, Toda and Smith [26], specific training in university courses could improve teachers' chances of a more effective intervention. These courses should focus not only on the mere concept of bullying, its nature and causes, the protagonists and the possible coping strategies with respect to the perpetrators, the victims, the classroom and others but also on the specific case when students with SEN are involved. If PSTs have expertise on the issue, they could be better able to manage and intervene effectively against bullying. This could disrupt the chain of victimization, benefiting not only the victims and the perpetrators but also the classroom as a whole and the teacher's well-being.

Author Contributions: T.B. and D.A.M. conducted the research project; T.B. analysed the data; T.B., D.A.M. and M.T. wrote the paper.

Funding: This research received no external funding.

Acknowledgments: Authors wish to thank all the participants that took part to this investigation.

Conflicts of Interest: The authors declare no conflict of interest.

References

1. Olweus, D. Victimization by peers: Antecedents and long-term outcomes. In *Social Withdrawal, Inhibition, and Shyness in Childhood*; Rubin, K.H., Asendorpf, J.B., Eds.; Psychology Press: New York, NY, USA; London, UK, 1993; pp. 315–341.
2. Olweus, D. A profile of bullying at school. *Educ. Leadersh.* **2003**, *60*, 12–17.
3. Byers, D.L.; Caltabiano, N.J.; Caltabiano, M.L. Teachers' attitudes towards overt and covert bullying, and perceived efficacy to intervene. *Aust. J. Teach. Educ.* **2011**, *36*, 105. [CrossRef]
4. Power-Elliott, M.; Harris, G.E. Guidance counsellor strategies for handling bullying. *Br. J. Guid. Couns.* **2012**, *40*, 83–98. [CrossRef]
5. Rose, C.A.; Gage, N.A. Exploring the involvement of bullying among students with disabilities over time. *Except. Child.* **2017**, *83*, 298–314. [CrossRef]
6. Fink, E.; Deighton, J.; Humphrey, N.; Wolpert, M. Assessing the bullying and victimisation experiences of children with special educational needs in mainstream schools: Development and validation of the Bullying Behaviour and Experience Scale. *Res. Dev. Disabil.* **2015**, *36*, 611–619. [CrossRef] [PubMed]
7. Sweeting, H.; West, P. Being different: Correlates of the experience of teasing and bullying at age 11. *Res. Pap. Educ.* **2001**, *16*, 225–246. [CrossRef]
8. Luciano, S.; Savage, R.S. Bullying risk in children with learning difficulties in inclusive educational settings. *Can. J. Sch. Psychol.* **2007**, *22*, 14–31. [CrossRef]
9. Davis, S.; Nixon, C. The Youth Voice Project. Preliminary Results from the Youth Voice Project: Victimization and Strategies. 2010. Available online: www.pacer.org/bullying/about/media-kit/stats.asp (accessed on 1 September 2018).
10. McLaughlin, C.; Byers, R.; Vaughn, R.P. *Responding to Bullying among Children with Special Educational Needs and/or Disabilities*; Anti-Bullying Alliance: London, UK, 2010.
11. Pavri, S.; Luftig, R. The social face of inclusive education: Are students with learning disabilities really included in the classroom? *Prev. Sch. Fail. Altern. Educ. Child. Youth* **2001**, *45*, 8–14. [CrossRef]
12. Hartley, M.T.; Bauman, S.; Nixon, C.L.; Davis, S. Responding to bullying victimization: Comparative analysis of victimized students in general and special education. *J. Disabil. Policy Stud.* **2017**, *28*, 77–89. [CrossRef]
13. Rose, C.A.; Simpson, C.G.; Preast, J.L. Exploring psychosocial predictors of bullying involvement for students with disabilities. *Rem. Spéc. Educ.* **2016**, *37*, 308–317. [CrossRef]
14. Bryant, D.P.; Smith, D.D.; Bryant, B.R. *Teaching Students with Special Needs in Inclusive Classrooms*; Pearson Education, Inc.: Boston, MA, USA, 2008.
15. Ainscow, M.; Dyson, A.; Weiner, S. From Exclusion to Inclusion: A review of international literature on ways of responding to students with special educational needs in schools. *En-clave Pedagógica Revista Internacional de Investigación e Innovación Educativa* **2013**, *13*, 13–30.
16. Banks, J.; McCoy, S.; Frawley, D. One of the gang? Peer relations among students with special educational needs in Irish mainstream primary schools. *Eur. J. Spéc. Needs Educ.* **2018**, *33*, 396–411. [CrossRef]
17. Ajuwon, P.M. Inclusive Education for Students with Disabilities in Nigeria: Benefits, Challenges and Policy Implications. *Int. J. Spéc. Educ.* **2008**, *23*, 11–16.
18. Briggs, S. *Meeting Special Educational Needs in Secondary Classrooms: Inclusion and How to Do It*; Routledge: Thames, UK, 2015.
19. Laletas, S.; Reupert, A. Exploring pre-service secondary teachers' understanding of care. *Teach. Teach.* **2015**, *22*, 485–503. [CrossRef]
20. Han, Z.; Fu, M.; Liu, C.; Guo, J. Bullying and Suicidality in Urban Chinese Youth: The Role of Teacher–Student Relationships. *Cyberpsychol. Behav. Soc. Netw.* **2018**, *21*, 287–293. [CrossRef] [PubMed]
21. Purdy, N.; Mc Guckin, C. Disablist bullying in schools: Giving a voice to student teachers. *J. Res. Spéc. Educ. Needs.* **2015**, *15*, 202–210. [CrossRef]
22. Acquadro Maran, D.; Tirassa, M.; Begotti, T. Teachers' intervention in school Bullying: A qualitative analysis on italian Teachers. *Front. Educ.* **2017**, *2*, 36. [CrossRef]
23. Tucker, E.; Maunder, R. Helping children to get along: Teachers' strategies for dealing with bullying in primary schools. *Educ. Stud.* **2015**, *41*, 466–470. [CrossRef]

24. Cortes, K.I.; Kochenderfer-Ladd, B. To tell or not to tell: What influences children's decisions to report bullying to their teachers? *Sch. Psychol. Q.* **2014**, *29*, 336. [CrossRef] [PubMed]

25. Sokol, N.; Bussey, K.; Rapee, R.M. Teachers' perspectives on effective responses to overt bullying. *Br. Educ. Res. J.* **2016**, *42*, 851–870. [CrossRef]

26. Ettekal, I.; Kochenderfer-Ladd, B.; Ladd, G.W. A synthesis of person-and relational-level factors that influence bullying and bystanding behaviors: Toward an integrative framework. *Aggress. Violent Behav.* **2015**, *23*, 75–86. [CrossRef]

27. Nicolaides, S.; Toda, Y.; Smith, P.K. Knowledge and attitudes about school bullying in trainee teachers. *Br. J. Educ. Psychol.* **2002**, *72*, 105. [CrossRef] [PubMed]

28. Roland, E.; Galloway, D. Classroom influences on bullying. *Educ. Res.* **2002**, *44*, 299–312. [CrossRef]

29. Crooks, C.V.; Jaffe, P.G.; Rodriguez, A. Increasing knowledge and self-efficacy through a pre-service course on promoting positive school climate: The crucial role of reducing moral disengagement. *Adv. Sch. Ment. Health Promot.* **2017**, *10*, 49–64. [CrossRef]

30. Vuorinen, K.; Erikivi, A.; Uusitalo-Malmivaara, L. A character strength intervention in 11 inclusive Finnish classrooms to promote social participation of students with special educational needs. *J. Res. Spéc. Educ. Needs* **2018**. [CrossRef]

31. Kandakai, T.L.; King, K.A. reservice teachers' perceived confidence in teaching school violence prevention. *Am. J. Health Behav.* **2002**, *26*, 342–353. [CrossRef] [PubMed]

32. Denzine, G.M.; Cooney, J.B.; McKenzie, R. Confirmatory factor analysis of the Teacher Efficacy Scale for prospective teachers. *Br. J. Educ. Psychol.* **2005**, *75*, 689–708. [CrossRef] [PubMed]

33. Bandura, A. *Self-efficacy: The Exercise of Control*; Freeman: New York, NY, USA, 1997.

34. Alvarez, H.K. The impact of teacher preparation on responses to student aggression in the classroom. *Teach. Teach. Educ.* **2007**, *23*, 1113–1126. [CrossRef]

35. Veenstra, R.; Lindenberg, S.; Huitsing, G.; Sainio, M.; Salmivalli, C. The role of teachers in bullying: The relation between antibullying attitudes, efficacy, and efforts to reduce bullying. *J. Educ. Psychol.* **2014**, *106*, 1135–1143. [CrossRef]

36. Dedousis-Wallace, A.; Shute, R.; Varlow, M.; Murrihy, R.; Kidman, T. Predictors of teacher intervention in indirect bullying at school and outcome of a professional development presentation for teachers. *Educ. Psychol.* **2014**, *34*, 862–875. [CrossRef]

37. Zee, M.; Koomen, H.M. Teacher Self-Efficacy and Its Effects on Classroom Processes, Student Academic Adjustment, and Teacher Well-Being A Synthesis of 40 Years of Research. *Rev. Educ. Res.* **2016**, *86*, 981–1015. [CrossRef]

38. Skinner, A.T.; Babinski, L.M.; Gifford, E.J. Teachers' expectations and self-efficacy for working with bullies and victims. *Psychol. Sch.* **2014**, *51*, 72–84. [CrossRef]

39. Rubie-Davies, C.M. Teacher expectations and student self-perceptions: Exploring relationships. *Psychol. Sch.* **2006**, *43*, 537–552. [CrossRef]

40. Weiner, B. *An Attributional Theory of Motivation and Emotion*; Springer-Verlag: New York, NY, USA, 1986.

41. Rotter, J.B. Generalized expectancies for internal versus external control of reinforcement. *Psychol. Monogr. Gen. Appl.* **1966**, *80*, 1–28. [CrossRef]

42. Woodcock, S.; Vialle, W. An examination of pre-service teachers' attributions for students with specific learning difficulties. *Learn. Individ. Differ.* **2016**, *45*, 252–259. [CrossRef]

43. Lachman, M.E. Perceived control over aging-related declines adaptive beliefs and behaviors. *Curr. Dir. Psychol. Sci.* **2006**, *15*, 282–286. [CrossRef]

44. Sarıçam, H.; Duran, A.; Çardak, M.; Hamaltov, M. The examination of pre-school teacher candidates' academic locus of control levels according to gender and grade. *Mevlana Int. J. Educ.* **2012**, *2*, 67–74.

45. Wang, H.; Hall, N.C.; Rahimi, S. Self-efficacy and causal attributions in teachers: Effects on burnout, job satisfaction, illness, and quitting intentions. *Teach. Teach. Educ.* **2015**, *47*, 120–130. [CrossRef]

46. Craig, K.; Bell, D.; Leschied, A. Pre-service Teachers' Knowledge and Attitudes Regarding School-Based Bullying. *Can. J. Educ.* **2011**, *34*, 21–33.

47. Begotti, T.; Tirassa, M.; Acquadro Maran, D. School bullying episodes: Attitudes and intervention in pre-service and in-service Italian teachers. *Res. Papers Educ.* **2017**, *32*, 170–182. [CrossRef]

48. Bagley, C.; Woods, P.A.; Woods, G. Implementation of school choice policy: Interpretation and response by parents of students with special educational needs. *Br. Educ. Res. J.* **2001**, *27*, 287–311. [CrossRef]

49. Kahn, J.H.; Jones, J.L.; Wieland, A.L. Preservice teachers' coping styles and their responses to bullying. *Psychol. Sch.* **2012**, *49*, 784–793. [CrossRef]

50. Gold, Y.; Roth, R.A. *Teachers Managing Stress and Preventing Burnout: The Professional Health Solution;* Routledge: London, UK, 1993.

51. Oldenburg, B.; van Duijn, M.; Sentse, M.; Huitsing, G.; van der Ploeg, R.; Salmivalli, C.; Veenstra, R. Teacher characteristics and peer victimization in elementary schools: A classroom-level perspective. *J. Abnorm. Child Psychol.* **2015**, *43*, 33–44. [CrossRef] [PubMed]

52. European Bullying Research. Available online: http://www.e-abc.eu/files/1/PDF/Research/School_Bullying_Italy.pdf (accessed on 1 September 2018).

53. World Medical Association. Declaration of Helsinki. Ethical principles for medical research involving human subjects. *Bull. World Health Organ.* **2001**, *79*, 373–374.

54. Leuze, K.; Strauß, S. Why do occupations dominated by women pay less? How 'female-typical' work tasks and working-time arrangements affect the gender wage gap among higher education graduates. *Work Employ. Soc.* **2016**, *30*, 802–820. [CrossRef]

55. Weldon, P.; Rowley, G.; Calnin, G.; Lawrence, A.; Houghton, J.; Thomas, J. Understanding the current teacher workforce: Supply and demand. *Prof. Voice* **2016**, *10*, 30–38.

56. Gibson, S.; Dembo, M.H. Teacher efficacy: A construct validation. *J. Educ. Psychol.* **1984**, *76*, 569. [CrossRef]

57. Craig, W.M.; Henderson, K.; Murphy, J.G. Prospective teachers' attitudes toward bullying and victimization. *Sch. Psychol. Int.* **2000**, *21*, 5–21. [CrossRef]

58. Rigby, K. *Stop the Bullying: A Handbook for Schools;* Aust Council for Ed Research: London, UK, 2003.

59. Kaufmann, G.M.; Beehr, T.A. Occupational stressors, individual strains, and social supports among police officers. *Hum. Relat.* **1989**, *42*, 185–197. [CrossRef]

60. Yoon, J.; Kerber, K. Bullying: Elementary teachers' attitudes and intervention strategies. *Res. Educ.* **2003**, *69*, 27–35. [CrossRef]

61. Yoon, J.; Sulkowski, M.L.; Bauman, S.A. Teachers' responses to bullying incidents: Effects of teacher characteristics and contexts. *J. Sch. Violence* **2016**, *15*, 91–113. [CrossRef]

62. Psalti, A. Greek In-Service and Preservice Teachers' Views about Bullying in Early Childhood Settings. *J. Sch. Violence* **2017**, *16*, 386–398. [CrossRef]

63. Kallestad, J.H.; Olweus, D. Predicting Teachers' and Schools' Implementation of the Olweus Bullying Prevention Program: A Multilevel Study. *Prev. Treat.* **2003**, *6*, 21a. [CrossRef]

64. Bauman, S.; Del Rio, A. Knowledge and beliefs about bullying in schools: Comparing pre-service teachers in the United States and the United Kingdom. *Sch. Psychol. Int.* **2005**, *26*, 428–442. [CrossRef]

65. Burger, C.; Strohmeier, D.; Spröber, N.; Bauman, S.; Rigby, K. How teachers respond to school bullying: An examination of self-reported intervention strategy use, moderator effects, and concurrent use of multiple strategies. *Teach. Teach. Educ.* **2015**, *51*, 191–202. [CrossRef]

66. Blake, J.J.; Kim, E.S.; Lund, E.M.; Zhou, Q.; Kwok, O.; Benz, M.R. Predictors of bully victimization in students with disabilities: A longitudinal examination using a national data set. *J. Disabil. Policy Stud.* **2016**, *26*, 199–208. [CrossRef]

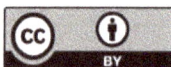

International Journal of
Environmental Research and Public Health

MDPI

Brief Report

Teacher Authority in Long-Lasting Cases of Bullying: A Qualitative Study from Norway and Ireland

Ida Risanger Sjursø [1,*], Hildegunn Fandrem [1], James O'Higgins Norman [2] and Erling Roland [1]

[1] Norwegian Centre for Learning Environment and Behavioral Research in Education, University of Stavanger, 4036 Stavanger, Norway; hildegunn.fandrem@uis.no (H.F.); erling.roland@uis.no (E.R.)
[2] The National Anti-Bullying Research and Resource Centre, Dublin City University, St. Patrick's Campus, Dublin 9, Ireland; james.ohigginsnorman@dcu.ie
*   Correspondence: ida.r.sjurso@uis.no; Tel.: +47-4158-0019

Received: 15 February 2019; Accepted: 29 March 2019; Published: 31 March 2019

Abstract: A growing body of research shows a correlation between an authoritative school climate and lower levels of bullying. One objective of this study is to conceptualize authoritative intervention in bullying cases. A second goal is to explore whether, and how, the pupils, having experienced traditional and/or cyber victimization, perceive that the class teacher is demonstrating authoritative leadership when intervening in long-lasting cases of bullying. Class teacher refers to the teacher that has a special responsibility for the class. The article presents the findings from nine semi-structured interviews with four Irish and five Norwegian pupils. The informants were between 12 to 18 years of age and had experienced either traditional victimization or both traditional and cyber victimization for 1 to 7 years. The informants were selected because their cases had been reported as resolved. The findings showed no descriptions of the class teacher that appeared to fit with the authoritative style of leadership, both high on warmth and control. The possible practical implications of these findings are discussed.

Keywords: traditional victimization; cyber victimization; bullying; teacher styles; authoritative leadership; warmth; control; class teacher

1. Introduction

Bullying can change a victim's view of the people surrounding them. It can lead to lack of trust and disappointment towards peers and a lack of involvement, but it can also evolve into disappointment in teachers. This highlights the importance of having caring and competent teachers in school who make it easier for the pupils to cope with bullying.

1.1. Authoritative Classroom Leadership

The authoritative style, which is high on control and high on warmth, appears to be the adult role that produces the best results for a child's development [1–3]. However, this important insight does not necessarily mean that such leadership is the best way to handle bullying.

When studying the concept of authoritative classroom leadership [3–6], research refers to the first of four parental styles, introduced by Baumrind [1,2]. The four styles are based on two dimensions: Degree of control/demands and degree of warmth/nurturance. Authoritative (high on warmth, high on control), authoritarian (low on warmth, high on control), indulgent (high on warmth, low on control), and neglectful (low on warmth, low on control) are the four styles [1,2]. Control could be defined as "enforcing demands for appropriate behavior" [3] (p. 123). Warmth could be defined as supporting the child's agency and individuality in addition to being sensitive and responding to the needs of the child [3].

Roland and Galloway [7] found a positive correlation between teacher authority in the classroom and low levels of bullying and that improved teacher authority in the classroom reduced bullying [8]. One study has found a relationship between victimization and classroom climate that has low levels of caring, warmth, and support [9]. Thornberg, Wänström, and Jungert [10] found that students belonging to a classroom with an authoritative climate, measured from the students' perspective, were less likely to experience victimization in school. In addition, they found that an authoritative classroom appears to be related to greater defense and less reinforcement from peers when bullying is happening.

Bullying is predominantly proactive aggression [11,12] and adult control reduces this aggression [7]. Teacher authority also tends to improve teacher–pupil relations and thereby pupil–pupil relations, which stimulates the pupils to support and protect each other [7]. This could indicate that authoritative leadership on the part of the teacher is positive when intervening with bullying, and not just for prevention. To our knowledge, there have been no studies looking directly at teacher style in relation to intervening for victims.

1.2. Perceived Authoritative Intervention

A challenge is that authoritative classroom leadership is described as how to address one unit, for example a pupil or a class [3,7]. A bullying case is a strongly differentiated social system comprising at least a bully and a victim. Furthermore, according to Marzano [13], different reactions to, or aspects of, the authoritative style is important to emphasize dependent on what behavior is shown. Thus, teacher authority may be differently perceived according to the roles one has in such a case.

Victim-perceived authoritative intervention has, therefore, to be defined according to teachers' warmth and control towards both the victim and one or more bullies, as the victim presumably sees it. It is reasonable, to assume that the victim wants the teacher to demonstrate warmth towards her or himself, in other words that the warmth dimension of authority is highly relevant for the victim. Another question is how the teacher should calibrate such empathy towards a child who is suffering from bullying. What the victims say about warmth related concerns they receive from the teacher is important.

The control dimension of authority is different from warmth when seen from the victims' perspective. When the communication with the teacher is about the ongoing bullying, the victims may feel humiliated if the teacher profiles control towards them. The control dimension is, however, interesting when related to the safety of the victim, and we suggest calling this 'perceived protective control'. By this, we mean whether the victim realizes that the teacher is willing to stop the bullying and/or capable of stopping the bullying. Again, it is interesting to disclose how the victims of long-lasting bullying discuss this.

1.3. Aims of the Study

We explored how the victims described the bullying situation, and how the cases ended. The first objective was to conceptualize authoritative intervention in bullying cases, from the assumed perspective of the victim. A second goal was to explore the experiences and understanding of pupils who have been bullied in regard to how teachers responded when the bullying was occurring.

2. Method

2.1. Sample

A convenience sample was used [14]. We used this because of the challenge of finding informants who have been victims of bullying and who were willing to be interviewed. In our case, professional connections were used, and the sample consisted of cases reported to the national centers working with bullying in Norway and Ireland. The inclusion criteria for the sample were that the cases should have been considered as bullying according to a standard definition: A negative repeated act, against someone who cannot easily defend themselves [11,12,15] resolved within the last year, the pupils had not themselves bullied others and the victim was comfortable talking about the victimization. In addition, to increase the possibility of finding informants, the age span was set from 8 to 18 years.

The informants were interviewed in Norway and Ireland in 2014. The school administration had reported the cases as resolved in Norway, and the Irish cases were resolved cases reported to the center. We interviewed 10 informants aged 8 to 18 years using semi-structured interviews: Of the 10 informants, 6 were from Norway and 4 from Ireland, including 2 boys and 8 girls. One interview provided too little information about the teacher and was therefore excluded. In all, there were 9 cases: 2 cases were victims who had experienced traditional bullying and 7 cases were victims who had experienced both traditional and cyberbullying. No cases included only cyberbullying.

2.2. Access and Ethics

The ethics committees in both Ireland and Norway received information about the study and both committees approved the study. Prior to the study, the informants and the parents received letters with information about the study. The parents with children under the age of 18 were asked to fill out a parental consent form before they were contacted by phone to set a date for the interview. All the informants below the age of 18 were given information about the study customized to their age. They were also told that they could withdraw from the study at any time. Being a member of a vulnerable group also gives these children an important voice and could, as Dalen [16] asserts, contribute to new and important information that could improve the situation for children experiencing similar events.

2.3. Data Collection

The data collection was conducted using individual qualitative semi-structured interviews, jointly constructed by the members of the research team. Originally, the interview guide was written in Norwegian and translated into English for the interviews in Ireland. Members of the research group addressing bullying were the ones conducting the interviews. In Ireland, a Norwegian, who is also fluent in English, conducted all interviews to secure the same meaning in the two countries. The interview guide had different themes that were to be explored with the participants. The main themes were: Their experience of being bullied from the beginning of the bullying to the resolution of the situation, some of the episodes they remembered well, communication about the bullying, if and how the bullying affected their life in general, the investigation and what was done by the school, what measures were attempted and what social support did they receive, how they felt emotionally and how the bullying affected their life in school and also their spare time, their relationships with the teacher, parents, and other pupils.

The interviews were held in a private setting or a private room in the school, lasted from 30 to 90 min, and were tape-recorded. The interviews started with small talk, to make the informants as relaxed as possible before they were asked to talk about their bullying experience. The same definition of bullying was presented to all the informants before starting the interview. The definition stated that bullying is a repeated aggressive act, including an imbalance of power, against someone who cannot easily defend themselves. The interviews were transcribed using standardized methods agreed upon in the research group, inspired by the description given in Kvale and Brinkmann [17].

2.4. Data Analysis

The first step in the analysis of the interviews was to read through of all the interviews to get an overview of emerging themes regarding how teachers were described. The interviews where read through a second time, and during this read through all the descriptions of the teachers were gathered under one main node 'teacher descriptions'. In further analysis, everything that was gathered under 'teacher descriptions' was read through and only the descriptions related to the class teacher were chosen for a new main node 'class teacher'. As we read through the node 'class teacher' focusing on themes relating to the class teachers support of the informants, two themes emerged; the class teacher offering emotional support, and the class teacher stopping the bullying. The second step was to use a thematic approach to identify, analyze, and report on patterns or themes that were found within the data [18]. Rather than an inductive, a theoretical approach was used, fitting the data into pre-existing coding frames [17] i.e., the two aspects of the authoritative teacher style; warmth and control. In this step of the analysis, also a semantic rather than a latent approach was used, meaning that what a participant said was more important than going beyond the semantic content of the data to identify the underlying ideas, assumptions, and conceptualizations [18]. For analysis, the qualitative data analysis software NVivo 12 (QSR International, Melbourne, Australia) was used. This program was used for storage and sorting of the data in addition to being helpful in the process of categorizing and classifying the data thematically. The first read through was done by two researchers, while the latter analysis was done by only one researcher, but with a continuous check of the interpretations by one or two other researchers in the team. If there were disagreements, a third party was involved.

3. Findings

The first section will cover descriptions of how the bullying happened and how it stopped. Further, the findings will be presented relating to the two main themes that occurred from our data: Class teacher showing control and class teacher showing warmth. As different degrees and aspects of warmth and control shown by the class teacher were described, the main node of control and warmth was divided in to lacking, low, medium, and high. A teacher that had a high or medium on both control and warmth would be categorized as authoritative. The findings, however, showed that none of the nine informants perceived their class teacher as having had a high or medium score on both warmth and control. The findings regarding the main nodes of control and warmth will, therefore, be presented separately. Later in the process, we changed control to 'protective control'.

3.1. How Did the Bullying Happen and How Did It Stop

The informants were all asked how the bullying happened. None of them described having experienced physical bullying. The most common descriptions were negative comments and exclusion, both in real life and online. For the victims that had experienced both types of victimization, the bullying was often described as starting with exclusion and negative comments in real life, which then followed to similar occurrences online for example on the social media platform, Instagram. Only one of the informants, having experienced both traditional and cyber victimization, described being victimized by someone else online than the ones they were interacting with in the school setting.

When describing how the bullying stopped, none of the informants described their class teacher being directly involved in this. Over half of the informants changed school, describing this as a new start. A couple of the informants experienced that the bullying just stopped without any special measures being done. The last informant isolated herself from the other pupils and explained that this was the reason that the bullying stopped.

3.2. Class Teachers and Perceived Protective Control

The content of all the descriptions related to the perception of the class teacher as lacking or low on protective control impacted on the victim's perceived belief that the teacher could stop the bullying. The class teachers were mainly perceived as passive or having low competence. On the question of what the teacher would do to stop the bullying, over half of the participants described their class teachers as lacking protective control: "They did not react to it" (Norwegian girl, 17), "The teachers were just completely ignoring that it happened, I didn't get anything sorted" (Irish girl, 17). In addition to experiencing that the teachers did not react to their victimization with constructive measures, also a lack of communication about what the teacher thought and would do was described: "The teachers kept it to themselves" (Irish girl, 18), "The teacher actually did not say anything to me" (Irish girl, 13). A few of the class teachers were described as low on protective control. What classified the teacher being described as low on protective control were that they tried to intervene, but the informant described that the teacher had challenges due to possible lack of experience: "She tried everything she could, but it's difficult when you don't have the experience" (Norwegian girl, 14). "The teacher talked to us and it was very time consuming, I felt it only got worse, because then we could hear what the other one felt and we ended up getting mad at each other" (Norwegian girl, 13), "The teacher tried but he gave up because there was nothing to do" (Norwegian girl, 12). None of the class teachers were described as medium or high regarding protective control.

3.3. Class Teachers and Perceived Warmth

The perceptions of the degree of warmth shown by class teachers was revealed from the extent to which the informants reported they could talk to their teachers about bullying, as well as their general relationship with the class teacher. Warmth was also described as either lacking, low, medium, or high.

High on warmth is described as a good relationship where the informants experience that the teacher is there for them and that they can tell them everything and get the feeling of being heard. In our analysis, only one class teacher was found to be described in a way that could be interpreted as high on warmth: "She tried to help me, and she knew how I was feeling in a way. It was just like she was there for me, just like a friend kind of" (Norwegian girl, 14). Medium means they have an ok relationship and the informant and can tell the teacher about the experienced victimization. The informant trusts the teacher and tells him or her about the bullying. The teacher is described as an overall nice person to everyone, but not as having an especially good relationship with the informant. A couple of the informants described their class teacher as medium on warmth: "She was nice to everyone" (Norwegian girl, 13), "I don't trust that many teachers really, but I trust my class tutor" (Norwegian girl, 12). A couple of informants also described their class teacher as low on warmth. With low, the informants described not talking much to their class teacher about having experienced the victimization and they described only telling their class teacher, but not having conversations about it: "I went to my tutor, my class tutor and I told her I was being bullied" (Irish girl, 18). Half of the informants described their class teacher in a way that could be related to a lack of warmth. To lack warmth refers to an absence of, or not a good, relationship described between the informant and their class teacher. They did not feel they could tell their class teacher what was going on. On the question if he could tell the teacher, one informant said "no" (Irish boy, 18). The informants also described it being difficult to trust their class teacher, "she pretends to be nice but she is not really" (Irish girl, 13). Another informant did not feel that she was taken seriously: "She meant I did not have a problem, so she did not listen to what I said. She only talked to me about my grades not to how I was doing" (Norwegian girl, 17). One informant described experiencing a situation where teacher supported the bullying taking place, "she encouraged the bullying. The teacher would never listen" (Irish girl, 17).

4. Discussion of Findings

One goal of the present study was to conceptualize teacher authority in responding to bullying, as perceived by the victim. We did this by relating the two main dimensions of authority—warmth and control [1,2] to the bullying core system, the victim and the bully or bullies, as perceived by the victim. From a theoretical perspective, we argued that a preferable teacher approach perceived by the victim would be warmth towards her or himself and control towards the bullies regarding their behavior. The other main goal, which was related to the first one, was to identify whether and how the class teachers demonstrate authoritative leadership in their work with long-lasting cases of bullying, from the perspective of the pupils having experienced victimization.

Our conceptualization of teacher authority related to a bullying case, as perceived by the victim, helped in analyzing the cases. The findings showed that none of these nine informants who experienced long-lasting cases of victimization gave a description of their class teacher that could be characterized as an authoritative teacher style regarding intervention to stop bullying. In other words, the nonappearance of teacher authority coincides with long-lasting bullying.

Our findings do not say that an authoritative style as conceptualized in this study would have hindered long-lasting bullying. This result is of interest and we will now focus on some of the possible reasons for the class teacher being perceived as low on control and/or low on warmth, or even lacking both aspects.

4.1. Lacking or Low on Control

The findings show that none of the participants perceived their class teachers as being medium or high on control. In fact, all participants perceived their class teachers as either lacking or low on control. There could be many reasons why a class teacher is perceived as low on control in a case of bullying. One reason could be the lack of competence in identifying bullying. Research has shown that teachers who experience bullying behavior as normative seem to be less likely to intervene and put an end to the bullying [19,20]. The teacher might not have understood that the child has been bullied and, therefore, did not find it necessary to act. Previous research has shown that teachers do not always know how to interpret what is happening, or do not know what bullying looks like [21]. Thus, a lack of competence could be related to uncertainty regarding what type of measures should be implemented. Research also has shown that when teachers believe that they lack the skills to be able to effectively intervene in a bullying situation, it decreases the possibility that they will intervene, and they are more likely to ignore the bullying [22]. One informant excuses her class teacher for not efficiently intervening in bullying as due to lack of competence: "She tried everything that she could, but it's difficult when you don't have the experience" (Norwegian girl, 14). When lacking competence, the teacher might decide to not do anything for fear of doing something that they think might be wrong. However, we argue that by not doing anything, the teachers are negative role models because they ignore bullying behavior and, in some cases, could actually be contributing to bullying children themselves [23]. One informant described her class teacher as one of the bullies: "She encouraged the bullying. The teacher would never listen so I gave up telling them" (Irish girl, 17).

4.2. Lacking or Low on Warmth

The findings show that only one participant perceived their class teachers as high on warmth, and only a couple described their class teacher as medium in this regard. Over half of the informants described their class teacher as low or lacking warmth. There could be several reasons why many of the class teachers seem to show little or no warmth towards the informants who experienced victimization. For instance, variations in teachers' responses might reflect teachers' lack of empathy [24]. Teachers who show empathy for others seem to be more likely to identify, report, and intervene when discovering bullying [22]. Some class teachers were described as not acknowledging the bullying and reacting with low empathy towards the child talking about their experience of victimization: "She meant I did not have a problem. So she did not listen to what I said" (Norwegian girl, 17). In relation to the empathy shown by the teacher, the type of bullying also seems to impact the quality of the teacher's intervention. Teachers have less empathy and intervene less when witnessing relational, verbal, or cyber victimization compared to physical victimization [24,25]. Other studies showed that relational victimization is considered to be less serious than physical and verbal bullying [22]. However, the reasons for this difference are not necessarily a sign of a lack of empathy, but could be because physical bullying is easier to observe than relational and verbal victimization. None of the informants in this study described experiencing physical bullying, which might be easier to uncover. This lack of physical bullying might be one of the reasons why the cases lasted for such a long time.

5. Limitations of the Study

This study provides important qualitative information from informants who have experienced long-term victimization; however, there are some limitations. Finding children who had experienced victimization and agreed to be interviewed is not an easy task, and, therefore, a convenience sample was used.

The study only provides a retrospective perspective of the child, and the memories can be imprecise. This may particularly have been the case for the oldest memories. It is also possible that a victim of bullying consciously hides information or presents it in certain ways, for unknown reasons. The perspective of others, for example those of the parents, teachers, and bystanders could have added valuable information.

There is also controversy regarding whether children should be used for rating teachers' behavior [26,27]. However, in the field of bullying, it is important to present the perspective of the children who have experienced the victimization in addition to their experiences of the teacher, especially in regard to how the victims are handled when they report their bullying experience. It should also be argued that the power imbalance between the child and teacher could make it even harder for the informants describing their teachers' behavior as negative.

6. Conclusion and Future Research

Our sample is small, but the findings are in many ways consistent. Most of the victims in these long-lasting cases described absence of warmth from the class teacher, which strongly indicates that such comfort from a significant adult is important in a time of great emotional distress. Furthermore, all the victims criticize the class teacher for not offering what we conceptualize as protective control. This demonstrates that these pupils expect their class teacher to protect them from the bullying.

From our study, we cannot say what approach is the best in performing protective control. One obvious goal is to stop the bullying, and effectivity in this regard is, therefore, important. Another significant issue is the impact different forms of intervention may have on the bullies' emotions and roles in class and the school community. One should consider different forms of intervention both in regard to short-term effects and long-term benefits [28]. Moreover, schools must consider whether the class teachers need some assistance in communicating with those who bully, as this is not always straight forward [29]. Protective control could possibly also be given by the class teacher via special trained personnel.

Examples of good practice from Norway and Ireland concerning bullying prevention are, for example, anti-bullying programs, such as Olweus and Respect from Norway, and the Donegal program from Ireland. In these programs, the role of the teacher in bullying prevention and intervention is emphasized [30].

A bullying case consists of the following: The perspectives of the pupils who bully, the victims, the parents of both the bully and the victim, and the teachers. These perspectives may be greatly different, as bullying cases probably are tense. Further research should address these different perspectives in general, and in particular the role of the teacher and the school, when intervention is concerned.

From this, it would be useful to try different approaches of intervention towards the whole bullying case system and evaluate short-term and longer-term effects on the different parties, using both qualitative and quantitative methods.

Author Contributions: Conceptualization, I.R.S. and E.R.; Formal analysis, I.R.S., E.R. and H.F.; Investigation, I.R.S. and E.R.; Methodology, I.R.S., H.F. and J.O.N.; Project administration, E.R.; Supervision, H.F. and E.R.; Writing—original draft, I.R.S.; Writing—review and editing, H.F., J.O.N. and E.R.

Funding: This research received no external funding.

Conflicts of Interest: The authors declare no conflict of interest.

References

1. Baumrind, D. *Parenting Styles and Adolescents Development*; Petersen, A.C., Books-Gunn, J., Lerner, R.M., Eds.; Garland: New York, NY, USA, 1991; pp. 746–758.

2.   Baumrind, D. *Authoritative Parenting Revisited: History and Current Status*; Larzelere, R.E., Morris, A.S., Harrist, A.W., Eds.; American Psychological Association: Washington, DC, USA, 2013; pp. 11–35.

3.   Walker, J. Authoritative classroom management: How control and nurturance work together. *Theory Into Pract.* **2009**, *48*, 122–129. [CrossRef]

4.   Cornell, D.; Huang, F. Authoritative school climate and high school student risk behavior: A cross-sectional multi-level analysis of student self-reports. *J. Youth Adolesc.* **2016**, *45*, 2246–2259. [CrossRef] [PubMed]

5.   Ertesvåg, S. Measuring authoritative teaching. *Teach. Teach. Educ.* **2011**, *27*, 51–61. [CrossRef]

6.   Wentzel, K.R. Are effective teachers like good parents? Teaching styles and students adjustment in early adolescence. *Child Dev.* **2002**, *73*, 287–301. [CrossRef] [PubMed]

7.   Roland, E.; Galloway, D. Classroom influences on bullying. *Educ. Res.* **2002**, *44*, 299–312. [CrossRef]

8.   Galloway, D.; Roland, E. *Is the Direct Approach to Reducing Bullying Always the Best? Bullying in Schools: How Successful Can Interventions be*; Smith, P.K., Pepler, D., Rigby, K., Eds.; Cambridge University Press: New York, NY, USA, 2004; pp. 37–53.

9.   Thornberg, R.; Wänström, L.; Pozzoli, T. Peer victimization and its relation to class relational climate and class moral disengagement among school children. *Educ. Psychol.* **2017**, *37*, 524–536. [CrossRef]

10. Thornberg, R.; Wänström, L.; Jungert, T. Authoritative classroom climate and its relations to bullying victimization and bystander behaviors. *Sch. Psychol. Int.* **2018**. [CrossRef]

11. Roland, E.; Idsøe, T. Aggression and bullying. *Aggress. Behav.* **2001**, *27*, 446–462. [CrossRef]

12. Fandrem, H.; Strohmeier, D.; Roland, E. Bullying and Victimization Among Native and Immigrant Adolescents in Norway: The Role of Proactive and Reactive Aggressiveness. *J. Early Adolesc.* **2009**, *29*, 898–923. [CrossRef]

13. Marzano, R.J. *Classroom Management that Works*; Pearson Education: Cranbury, NJ, USA, 2003.

14. Bryman, A. *Social Research Methods*; Oxford University Press: Oxford, UK, 2016.

15. Olweus, D.; Roland, E. *Mobbing—Bakgrunn og Tiltak (Bullying, Background and Measures)*; Kirke og undervisningsdepartementet: Oslo, Norway, 1983.

16. Dalen, M. *Intervju Som Forskningsmetode—En Kvalitativ Tilnærming*; Universitetsforlaget: Oslo, Norway, 2004.

17. Kvale, S.; Brinkmann, S. *Det Kvalitative Forskningsintervju*; Gyldendal Norsk Forlag: Oslo, Norway, 2010.

18. Braun, V.; Clarke, V. Using thematic analysis in psychology. *Qual. Res. Psychol.* **2006**, *3*, 77–101. [CrossRef]

19. Hektner, J.M.; Swenson, C.A. Links from teacher beliefs to peer victimization and bystander intervention: Tests of mediating processes. *J. Early Adolesc.* **2012**, *32*, 516–536. [CrossRef]

20. O'Higgins Norman, J. Equality in the provision of social, personal and health education in the Republic of Ireland: The case of homophobic bullying? Pastoral Care in Education. *Int. J. Pers. Soc. Emot. Dev.* **2008**, *26*, 69–81. [CrossRef]

21. O'Moore, M.; Cross, D.; Valimaki, M.; Almeida, A.; Berne, S.; Deboutte, G.; Fandrem, H.; Olenik-Shemesh, D.; Heiman, T.; Kurki, M.; et al. Guidelines to Prevent Cyberbullying. In *Cyberbullying through the New Media. Findings from an International Network*; Steffgen, P.K., Smith, G., Eds.; Psychology Press Taylor and Francis Group: London, UK, 2013.

22. Shuster, M.A.; Bogart, L.M. Did the Ugly Duckling Have PTSD? Bullying, its effects and the role of pediatricians. *Pediatrics* **2013**, *131*, 1–6. [CrossRef] [PubMed]

23. Troop-Gordon, W.; Ladd, G.W. Teachers' victimization -related beliefs and strategies: Associations with student's aggressive behavior and peer victimization. *J. Abnorm. Psychol.* **2015**, *43*, 45–60. [CrossRef] [PubMed]

24. Blain-Arcaro, c.; Smith, J.D.; Cunningham, C.E.; Vaillancourt, T.; Reimas, H. Contextual attributes of indirect bullying situations that influence teachers' decisions to intervene. *J. Sch. Violence* **2012**, *11*, 226–245. [CrossRef]

25. Costley, J.H.; Sueng-Lock, H.; Ji-Eun, L. Preservice teachers' responses to bullying vignettes: The effect of bullying type and gender. *Int. J. Second. Educ.* **2013**, *1*, 45–52. [CrossRef]

26. Kunter, M.; Baumert, J. Who is the expert? Construct and criteria validity of students and teacher ratings of instruction. *Learn. Environ. Res.* **2006**, *9*, 231–251. [CrossRef]

27. Den Brok, P.; Brekelmans, M.; Wubbels, T. Multilevel issues in research using students' perceptions of learning environments: The case of the questionnaire on teacher interaction. *Learn. Environ. Res.* **2006**, *9*, 199–213. [CrossRef]

28. Finne, J.; Roland, E.; Svartdal, F. Relational rehabilitation. Reducing harmful effects of bullying. *Nord. Stud. Educ.* **2018**, *38*, 352–367. [CrossRef]

29. Rigby, K.; Bauman, S. What Teachers Think Should be Done about Cases of Bullying. *Prof. Educ.* **2007**, *6*, 4–8.
30. Farrington, D.; Tofti, M. *School Based Programs to Reduce Bullying and Victimization*; Cambridge University: Cambridge, UK, 2009.

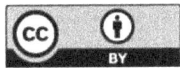

International Journal of
Environmental Research and Public Health

MDPI

Brief Report

Students' Willingness to Intervene in Bullying: Direct and Indirect Associations with Classroom Cohesion and Self-Efficacy

Sebastian Wachs [1,*] , Ludwig Bilz [2], Saskia M. Fischer [2], Wilfried Schubarth [1] and Michelle F. Wright [3,4]

[1] Department of Educational Studies, University of Potsdam, 14476 Potsdam, Germany; wilschub@uni-potsdam.de
[2] Brandenburg University of Technology Cottbus-Senftenberg, Institute of Health Sciences, 01968 Senftenberg, Germany; ludwig.bilz@b-tu.de (L.B.); saskia.fischer@b-tu.de (S.M.F.)
[3] Department of Psychology, Pennsylvania State University, PA 16802, USA; mfw5215@psu.edu
[4] Faculty of Social Studies, Masaryk University, 60200 Brno, Czech Republic
* Correspondence: wachs@uni-potsdam.de; Tel.: +49-331-977-2702

Received: 2 October 2018; Accepted: 15 November 2018; Published: 17 November 2018

Abstract: Although school climate and self-efficacy have received some attention in the literature, as correlates of students' willingness to intervene in bullying, to date, very little is known about the potential mediating role of self-efficacy in the relationship between classroom climate and students' willingness to intervene in bullying. To this end, the present study analyzes whether the relationship between classroom cohesion (as one facet of classroom climate) and students' willingness to intervene in bullying situations is mediated by self-efficacy in social conflicts. This study is based on a representative stratified random sample of two thousand and seventy-one students (51.3% male), between the ages of twelve and seventeen, from twenty-four schools in Germany. Results showed that between 43% and 48% of students reported that they would not intervene in bullying. A mediation test using the structural equation modeling framework revealed that classroom cohesion and self-efficacy in social conflicts were directly associated with students' willingness to intervene in bullying situations. Furthermore, classroom cohesion was indirectly associated with higher levels of students' willingness to intervene in bullying situations, due to self-efficacy in social conflicts. We thus conclude that: (1) It is crucial to increase students' willingness to intervene in bullying; (2) efforts to increase students' willingness to intervene in bullying should promote students' confidence in dealing with social conflicts and interpersonal relationships; and (3) self-efficacy plays an important role in understanding the relationship between classroom cohesion and students' willingness to intervene in bullying. Recommendations are provided to help increase adolescents' willingness to intervene in bullying and for future research.

Keywords: bullying; intervention; willingness to intervene; verbal bullying; relational bullying; aggression; school; classroom climate; classroom cohesion; self-efficacy

1. Introduction

Bullying in schools is a prevalent problem and can have serious physical, mental, social, and behavioral short- and long-term consequences for those involved [1–3]. Bullying is defined as any repeatedly aggressive behavior against persons or groups that cannot readily defend themselves [4]. Bullying may involve physical assault, such as hitting or kicking, verbal harassment, such as hurtful name-calling, verbal threats, and verbal abuse, as well as selectively undermining social relationships through manipulation or exclusion from social groups [5]. There are a range of different roles that adolescents can take in bullying situations, that differ from the commonly described roles of bully, victim, and bully-victim. "Assistants", for instance, join the bullies, "reinforcers" provide positive feedback to bullies (e.g., cheering), but do not actively assist the bullies, "outsiders" withdraw from bullying situations, "defenders" side with the victims and support them, and "bystanders" see the bullying occur but do not choose a side, thereby, passively enabling bullying to continue [6]. The most common way that people experience bullying is observing it as a bystander [7]. The tendency for bystanders to remain passive might be explained by, for instance, their lack of a sense of responsibility for helping the victim, fearing being judged unfavorably by peers for helping the victim, not realizing that the situation is perceived as uncomfortable, being afraid that they could also be bullied if they get involved, and lacking the skills to intervene in bullying behaviors [8]. Bystanders have received a lot of attention by scholars, because research has shown that bullying prevention and intervention programs that emphasize and encourage bystanders to defend victims result in a decrease in bullying overall and an increase the success of bullying interventions [9,10]. In addition, some research suggests that if bystanders become actively involved in bullying, on the side of the victim, then they are often successful in ending the bullying in that particular situation and they can also have positive impact on the victims' adjustment and social status [11,12]. There are additional reasons to empower bystanders to give up their passive role in bullying. There is some evidence, for instance, that witnessing bullying can affect the bystanders' mental health, school satisfaction, and increase their levels of stress and negative feelings (e.g., anxiety) [13–15]. Possible explanations for these findings might include, the cognitive dissonance they experience when faced with the discrepancy between their lack of action and their desire to intervene; a sense co-victimization; and feelings of powerlessness [13]. As there is some evidence that other students seldom intervene to defend the victims of bullying [16–18], it is important to understand which factors increase students' willingness to intervene. Such findings might help to deepen our knowledge about successful bullying prevention and intervention in schools and help us protect bystanders from experiencing negative psychological and school-related outcomes, when faced with bullying.

According to Bandura [19], self-efficacy is defined as one's "beliefs in one's capabilities to organize and execute the courses of action required to produce given attainments." (p. 3). The conviction that it is possible to cope through one's action with what is required of one socially, even under difficult conditions, is an essential motivational foundation in individuals and an important predictor of socially-competent behavior in childhood and adolescence [20]. In addition, students with high self-efficacy are more likely to challenge themselves with difficult tasks and recover faster from setbacks [19]. Students with low self-efficacy, on the other hand, often shy away from challenging tasks, because they view these tasks as threats rather than challenges that they can overcome [19]. It is possible that a domain-specific form of self-efficacy might be important in students' willingness to stand up to bullying, because if they lack confidence in their capacity to successfully intervene, they would be less likely to act [21]. The positive association between students' perceived self-efficacy, in terms of actually or potentially intervening in bullying, has been highlighted in a number of studies, using qualitative and quantitative methods, self-reports and peer nominations, and cross-sectional and longitudinal study designs [21–27].

There are a number of factors, along with self-efficacy, that play a crucial role in whether students do decide to defend bullying victims or not. From a socio-ecological perspective [28], the microsystem, which consists of structures or locations where individuals have direct interactions (i.e., family, peer group, school, and school class), has immediate influence on the active or passive behavior of bystanders [17,29,30]. In Germany, students in the fifth and sixth grade usually stay in the same classroom with the same students, during the school day. Therefore, it seems reasonable to consider the subjective perceived peer relationship, within a class, as a possible correlate of students' willingness to intervene in bullying. Indeed, previous research showed that a positive school/classroom climate which also includes aspects, such as classroom cohesion, is positively correlated with students' readiness to intervene in bullying [31–33].

Classroom cohesion understood as one facet of classroom climate, however, might not only be associated with students' willingness to intervene in bullying but also with students' self-efficacy toward intervening in bullying. In Bandura's view [19], self-efficacy affects one's behaviors and the social environments with which people are interacting, and is influenced by one's actions and significant others, such as parents, siblings, teachers, and peers. Particularly, during adolescence, peer acceptance and relationships are important to the adolescents' development of self-efficacy because peers contribute considerably to adolescents' socialization and views of themselves [34,35]. Peers provide adolescents with possibilities to learn from each other and function as role models. Thus, it can be assumed that in classrooms that are characterized by strong cohesion and mutual sympathy among classmates, students meet the right conditions to develop self-efficacy. Indeed, initial research found a positive link between the classroom student–student relationship quality and students' self-efficacy towards bullying [33].

To summarize, previous research attempted to elucidate the personal and contextual factors that explain students' willingness to intervene in bullying situations. These studies have found that the defender's self-efficacy [21–27] and school climate [31–33] might play a crucial role. There is also some evidence to suggest that school climate (i.e., cohesion) is related to students' defender self-efficacy beliefs [33]. Therefore, the present study aims to investigate whether the relationship between school climate and willingness to intervene in bullying might be mediated by self-efficacy. We expect that school climate will increase self-efficacy, which in turn increases students' readiness to intervene in bullying. More specifically, we hypothesized:

Hypothesis 1 (H1). *Classroom cohesion will be directly associated with greater self-efficacy, and students' willingness to intervene in bullying situations.*

Hypothesis 2 (H2). *Classroom cohesion will be indirectly associated with students' willingness to intervene in bullying situations via greater self-efficacy.*

2. Materials and Methods

2.1. Participants and Sampling Procedure

This study uses data from a stratified random sample (strata: three types of school) in the Eastern German federal state of Saxony. A randomized probability-proportional-to-size sampling scheme was used, where the size is equivalent to the number of students per school. There were forty-one schools initially contacted for inclusion in this study, but twenty-four agreed to participate (roughly a 60% response rate at school level). A maximum of six classes per school were asked to participate in the study, resulting in three classes in the sixth grade and three classes in the eighth grade. Only those students within these classes were invited to participate in the study.

The final sample included 2071 participants (51.2% males; $n = 1060$), in the sixth grade ($n = 1080$) and eighth grade ($n = 991$), from 114 classes across 24 schools. Of the schools, seven were secondary grammar schools, thirteen were non-academic-track secondary schools, and four schools were for children with special needs (students with emotional and behavioral disorders, and students with learning disabilities). Overall, 581 students were not included in the study because they did not have written parental consent ($n = 419$), had a doctor's note excuse on the days of data collection ($n = 109$), had an unexcused absence from school ($n = 2$), were absent because of school projects ($n = 26$), were attending internship ($n = 4$), refused to participate ($n = 8$), were on vacation ($n = 4$), and were new to the class and uninformed about the study ($n = 2$).

Age of participants ranged from 12 to 17 years ($M = 13.63$, $SD = 1.17$). The age breakdown of participants is as follows: 20.6% ($n = 427$) were 12 years old, 27.1% ($n = 562$) were 13 years old, 23.8% ($n = 493$) were 14 years old, 24.6% ($n = 509$) were 15 years old, 3.3% ($n = 69$) were 16 years old, 0.3% ($n = 6$) were 17 years old, and 0.2% ($n = 5$) did not specify their age. Most of the students (50.4%;

n = 1044) attended non-academic-track secondary schools, followed by 43.7% (*n* = 904) for secondary grammar schools, and 5.9% (*n* = 123) who attended schools for children with special educational needs. Most participants were born in Germany, with 1.9% (*n* = 40) who were not born in Germany. Demographic characteristics of participants, organized by grade, sex, and type of school are displayed in Table 1.

Table 1. Frequencies of demographic variables by grade, sex, and type of school.

Grade	Sex	Type of School							
		Grammar Schools		Non-Academic-Track Secondary School		Schools for Children with Special Needs		Total	
		n	%	*n*	%	*n*	%	*n*	%
6th grade	Boys	230	25.4	312	30.1	33	26.8	575	27.8
	Girls	250	27.7	215	20.6	37	30.1	502	24.3
8th grade	Boys	194	21.5	258	24.8	33	26.8	485	23.5
	Girls	230	25.4	255	24.5	20	16.2	505	24.4
Total		904	43.7	1040	50.3	123	5.9	2067 *	100

Note. * Four participants did not specify their sex.

2.2. Measures

2.2.1. Students' Willingness to Intervene in Bullying Situations

The questionnaire started with a definition of traditional bullying that outlined the central characteristics of bullying (intention to hurt, imbalance of power, and repetition), as postulated by Olweus [1], in order to increase the validity of responses. The vignettes used to assess students' willingness to intervene in bullying was adopted from Yoon and Kerber [36]. The first vignette assessed students' willingness to intervene in verbal bullying situations:

"You hear a sixth-grade student calling out to another: "Nerd, bootlicker, asshole". The student tries to ignore the remarks but is obviously sad. You have already observed the same thing a few days ago".

The second vignette asked for students' willingness to intervene in relational bullying situations:

"During the break, you hear a sixth-grade student say to another: "No, absolutely not. I've already told you that you can't join us." The student has no friends in class and is alone throughout the break and looks sad. It's not the first time that the student was excluded from playing".

After each vignette, participants were asked to rate how much they agree with the following statement: "When I observe something like that, I interfere and try to stop the behavior". The participants could choose from five responses—(1) "completely disagree", (2) "disagree", (3) "neither agree nor disagree", (4) "agree", and (5) "completely agree".

2.2.2. Self-Efficacy in Social Conflicts

The scale is intended to capture self-efficacy expectations when dealing with social demands and conflicts. The scale consists of three items like, "I manage to cope well even with difficult classmates" [37]. A high value expresses the conviction of a person to act competently in conflictive situations. Participants could choose between four responses—(1) "completely disagree", (2) "disagree", (3) "agree", and (4) "completely agree". Cronbach's alpha was 0.68.

2.2.3. Classroom Cohesion

To assess the extent of cohesion and mutual sympathy among students in a class, as one facet of classroom climate, a scale consisting of three items was used, including items such as "When someone says something against our class, everyone sticks together" [38]. Participants could then choose between five responses—(1) "completely disagree", (2) "disagree", (3) "neither agree nor disagree", (4) "agree" and, (5) "completely agree". Cronbach's alpha was 0.71.

2.2.4. Socio-Demographic Variables

Socio-demographics were assessed by asking for information on students' grade (6th or 8th), age, sex (1 = male or 2 = female), and type of school (non-academic-track secondary school (Oberschule), school for students with special needs (Förderschule), and grammar school (Gymnasium)). Previous research has shown significant differences regarding sex and age in students' willingness to intervene in bullying, with girls compared with boys and younger students compared with older students more likely to defend [17,18,21,25,39]. Hence, sex, and age were included as control variables.

2.3. Procedures

The data protection officer and educational authority of the federal state of Saxony in Germany approved the study. After approval, email invitations were sent to the forty-one schools. Data were collected from June 2014 to October 2014, using paper-pencil questionnaires that were administered by trained research assistants. Signed written parental consent was obtained from children who were minors. During data collection, participants were informed that their participation was voluntary and anonymous, and that they could stop participating in the study at any time, without any penalty. The total time to administer the questionnaire was 30–45 min and it was administered during normal school hours.

2.4. Data Analyses

To begin with, the mean scores were computed by averaging items on the questionnaires. Then correlation analyses and descriptive statistics were used to investigate the main study variables. In a next step, mediation analysis was conducted in structural equation modeling framework with classroom cohesion, self-efficacy, and students' willingness to intervene in bullying, as latent variables. The latent variable "willingness to intervene in bullying" was composed of the willingness to intervene in a verbal bullying incident and the willingness to intervene in a relational bullying incident. The factor loadings of these two observed variables were freely estimated, so the factor variance of the latent factor was fixed to one. Mediation analysis was used to test direct effects of classroom cohesion on self-efficacy, in social conflicts, and students' willingness to intervene in bullying, as well as indirect effects of classroom cohesion on students' willingness to intervene in bullying, via self-efficacy in social conflicts. The mediation analysis was completed in Mplus 8.0 software (Muthén & Muthén, Los Angeles, CA, USA) [40]. Since the dependent variables, willingness to intervene in verbal bullying, and willingness to intervene in relational bullying, departed from normality, in their distribution, maximum likelihood estimation with robust standard errors (MLR) was used for the analyses. The significance of indirect effects was assessed by using a bias-corrected bootstrapping procedure, with 5000 samples. Full information maximum likelihood (FIML) estimation was used to address missing data issues. To account for the multilevel structure of the data (i.e., students nested within school classes) standard errors were corrected by using the complex sampling option in Mplus (complex-option).

3. Results

3.1. Descriptive Statistics

Regarding students' willingness to intervene in verbal bullying, 20.9% (n = 428) of adolescents answered that they 'completely disagree', 22.4% (n = 458) 'disagree', 34.9% (n = 716) 'neither agree nor disagree', 16.4% (n = 337) 'agree', and 5.4% (n = 110) 'completely agree' to intervene. Similarly for students' willingness to intervene in relational bullying, 22.6% (n = 463) of adolescents answered that they 'completely disagree', 25.3% (n = 518) 'disagree', 33.4% (n = 684) 'neither agree nor disagree', 13.4% (n = 274) 'agree', and 5.2% (n = 107) 'completely agree' to intervene. Correlations between the study variables, means, and standard deviations are shown in Table 2. All correlations were in the expected direction. Higher levels of classroom cohesion were positively correlated with higher levels of self-efficacy in social conflicts, and willingness to intervene in bullying. Self-efficacy was positively correlated with willingness to intervene in bullying. There were also some significant correlations between the control and the main study variables. Girls, in comparison with boys, reported higher levels of willingness to intervene in bullying. With increasing grade, adolescents reported lower levels of willingness to intervene in verbal and relational bullying.

Table 2. Bivariate correlations between classroom cohesion, self-efficacy, intervention willingness, and control variables, means, and standard deviations.

Variables	1	2	3	4	5
1. Intervention willingness	–				
2. Self-efficacy in social conflicts	0.29 **	–			
3. Classroom cohesion	0.14 **	0.26 **	–		
4. Grade ⁸ᵗʰ ᵍʳᵃᵈᵉ	−0.10 **	0.04 *	0.01	–	
5. Sex ᶠᵉᵐᵃˡᵉ	0.07 **	0.03	0.01	0.04 *	–
Mean	2.66	2.81	3.21	–	–
SD	0.96	0.57	0.88	–	–

* $p < 0.05$. ** $p < 0.01$.

3.2. Direct and Indirect Associations between Classroom Cohesion, Self-Efficacy, and Students' Willingness to Intervene in Bullying

We investigated the direct effects of classroom cohesion on self-efficacy in social conflicts and students' willingness to intervene in bullying, as well as indirect effects of classroom cohesion on students' willingness to intervene in bullying, via self-efficacy in social conflicts. The model had an excellent fit: $\chi^2 = 56.58$ $df = 27$ $\chi^2/df = 2.09$, $p < 0.001$, comparative fit index (CFI)= 0.99, Tucker–Lewis index (TLI) = 0.98, root mean square error of approximation (RMSEA) = 0.02 (90% CI = 0.01, 0.03), standardized root mean square residual (SRMR) = 0.02. As shown in Figure 1, classroom cohesion had a direct effect on self-efficacy in social conflicts ($\beta = 0.50$, $p < 0.001$), as well as on students' willingness to intervene in bullying ($\beta = 0.10$, $p < 0.001$). There was also a direct effect of self-efficacy in social conflicts on students' willingness to intervene in bullying ($\beta = 0.35$, $p < 0.001$). The indirect effect of classroom cohesion on students' willingness to intervene in bullying, via self-efficacy in social conflicts, was also significant ($\beta = 0.18$, $p < 0.001$). The analyses also revealed significant effects of the control variables on classroom cohesion and students' willingness to intervene in bullying. Girls scored significantly higher than boys on the measures of students' willingness to intervene in bullying ($\beta = 0.15$, $p < 0.001$), as well as on classroom cohesion ($\beta = 0.07$, $p < 0.001$). Additionally, an increasing grade was negatively associated with students' willingness to intervene in bullying ($\beta = -0.19$, $p < 0.001$). Other paths in the model did not reach statistical significance. The proposed model explained 21% of variance in students' willingness to intervene in bullying ($R^2 = 0.21$) and 25.5% of variance in self-efficacy in social conflicts ($R^2 = 0.25$). Finally, we analyzed the mediation model, separately, by grade (6th vs. 8th) and sex (female vs. male), and did not find any relevant grade or sex differences in the direct and indirect effect sizes. These results can be requested from the first author.

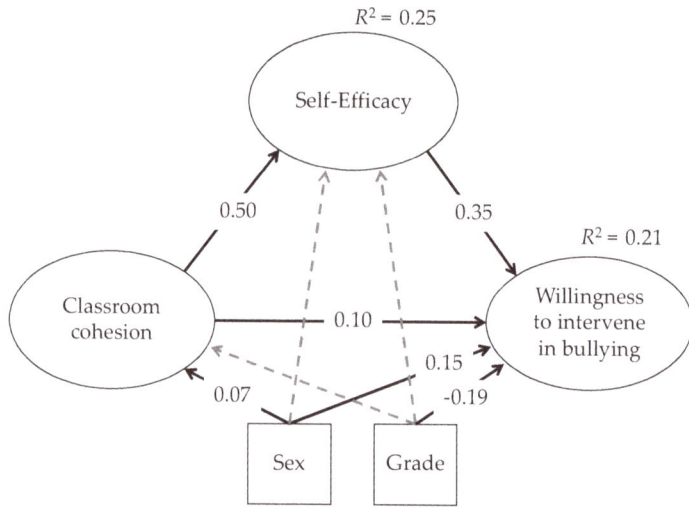

Figure 1. Direct and indirect effects of the latent variables classroom cohesion, self-efficacy, control variables, and willingness to intervene in bullying. Notes: Dash arrows—non-significant path coefficients.

4. Discussion

The present study aimed to investigate the direct and indirect associations between classroom cohesion, self-efficacy in social conflicts, and students' willingness to intervene in bullying, among German students. Several interesting findings emerged.

A first important finding of the present study was that personal and contextual factors need to be considered, in order to better understand students' readiness to intervene in bullying situations. We found support for our prediction that self-efficacy in social conflicts and classroom cohesion would be directly associated with students' willingness to intervene in bullying situations (H1). The analyses also showed that the effect of self-efficacy in social conflicts ($\beta = 0.35$) on students' intervention willingness was nearly the same as the effect of classroom cohesion (total effect: direct effect, $\beta = 0.10$ + indirect effect, $\beta = 0.18$) on students' intervention willingness. This finding further underlines that both predictors are nearly equally important to explain students' willingness to intervene in bullying. Overall, our findings are consistent with previous research revealing the relationships between students' willingness to intervene in bullying and self-efficacy [21–27], and school climate [31–33]. Self-efficacy regarding social conflicts might be vital for understanding students' willingness to intervene in bullying. Support for this proposal is found in previous research suggesting that students with high self-efficacy in social conflicts are less inhibited when intervening in bullying, are more likely to tackle difficult tasks, and recuperate much quicker from setbacks [19–21]. Positive peer relationships might influence students' readiness to intervene because classroom cohesion characterized by positiveness, mutual respect, and warmth, might be a solid fundament for positive peer group norms. In these classes, rejection and exclusion of single students might be less tolerated and respectful interaction promoted. Taken together, these findings suggest that efforts to address students' willingness to intervene in bullying should involve measures to encourage interpersonal relationships and support within the school classes, and students' efficacy to deal with social conflicts.

We add valuable knowledge to the literature on bystander behavior in bullying, regarding the indirect association between classroom cohesion and students' willingness to intervene in bullying via self-efficacy, in social conflicts. Hence, we found support for our hypothesis that classroom cohesion would be indirectly associated with students' willingness to intervene in bullying, via greater self-efficacy in social conflicts (H2). This finding was consistent for different age groups (6th vs.

8th graders) and for boys and girls, as shown by differential analyses of grade and sex. A possible explanation for the indirect effect might be that students learn from their peers how to intervene from each other and that some peers function as role models to students, within a class. Indeed, vicarious experience has been shown to be an important source of self-efficacy [19]. Thus, observing peers successfully intervening in bullying may also contribute to enhancing self-efficacy, in social conflicts such as bullying. Intervention and prevention programs to increase students' intervention willingness should aim to foster positive relationships within the school class. This might positively influence students feeling to be efficacious towards social conflicts, which in turn increases the willingness for intervention in bullying. It is worth mentioning that the indirect effect of classroom cohesion on students willingness to intervene in bullying ($\beta = 0.18$) was larger than the direct effect of classroom cohesion on students willingness to intervene ($\beta = 0.10$). This means that a substantial amount of the effect between classroom cohesion and students' willingness to intervene can be explained by self-efficacy. Our findings also highlight the important role of classroom cohesion for self-efficacy, in social conflicts, in intervening in bullying among adolescents, which has also been shown by previous research on the development of general self-efficacy [34,35] and initial research on students' defending behavior [33].

Another noteworthy result was that nearly half of the students reported that they would not intervene in verbal (43%) and relational bullying (48%) situations. The finding that students often did not believe they would intervene, is in accordance with previous research from other countries [16–18]. Reasons to remain passive might be the absence of feeling responsible for helping the victim, fearing unfavorable judgment by peers when helping the victim, not realizing that the situation is perceived as uncomfortable, being afraid that they could also be bullied if they get involved, and the lack of skills to intervene in bullying behaviors [8]. Regarding sex and grade differences, we found that girls were more likely to intervene in bullying situations, when compared to boys, and with increasing grades, students were less likely to intervene in bullying situations. These differences are also similar to what has been reported by past research [17,18,21,25,39]. However, previous research found girls to have higher levels of moral sensitivity and lower moral disengagement than boys [21]. In addition, girls are more likely than boys to interpret bullying situations as emergencies and report bullying to an adult and ask for social support, which can increase their readiness to stand up for the victims [11,12]. On the one hand, the grade differences found are somewhat counterintuitive because with increasing age social and cognitive skills are further developed [23]. On the other hand, the results are in line with past research that showed that bullying increases among students between 11 to 13 years old [8]. Possible explanations for the grade differences might be that younger adolescents might underestimate the potentially negative social consequences of interventions, whereas older students are more reluctant as they believe that interventions could make them the next target and might seem like they are violating peer norms [43]. In addition, with increasing age, students believe that victims should be able to solve their problems by themselves and, therefore, they do not want to solidarize with the socially-stigmatized victims, often against a powerful, perceived bully, within the peer network [44]. Finally, the students in our sample were 12 to 15 years old. This might have limited the possibilities to draw any conclusion for age differences regarding intervention willingness.

Taken together, it appears to be important to raise awareness among students that they can be successful to end bullying and that their actions could have a positive impact on the victims' adjustment. Particularly, boys and older students need to be addressed in intervention prevention measures to increase their willingness to intervene in bullying. However, the findings of the present study highlight that awareness is most likely not a sufficient condition. Students need also the right social environment, characterized by positive peer-peer relationships and the confidence that they are capable to deal with bullying, efficaciously.

5. Limitations and Outlook on Future Research

First, in the present study we measured behavioral intentions, rather than actual intervention behavior. This means, we assessed how students believe they would intervene in a given situation, but not necessarily how they have actually intervened. To overcome this shortcoming, future studies should measure actual intervention behavior by asking students to recall a specific bullying situation and how they behaved in that situation. Second, the present study relies exclusively on self-reports to assess bystander behavior. Therefore, social desirability might be a concern because students might tend to hide their true behavior about not helping the victim. Follow-up research should try to replicate the findings of the present study by using peer-nominations or a combination of peer- and self-reports. Third, because of the cross-sectional design of this study, it is not possible to determine the temporal ordering among classroom cohesion, self-efficacy, and students' willingness to intervene in bullying. Follow-up studies should include a longitudinal study design with at least three measurement points to further substantiate the mediating relationships tested in the present study. Fourth, we assessed only one facet of classroom climate, namely cohesion, and we used a general measurement of self-efficacy in social conflicts and not a specific self-efficacy scale concerning bullying, both of which might have deflated the estimates. Future studies should try to replicate our findings by using a multifaceted-scale, for measuring classroom climate, and a domain-specific self-efficacy scale which measures students' readiness to intervene in bullying. In addition, both scales showed relatively low reliabilities, as measured by Cronbach's alpha. Finally, in addition to verbal and relational bullying scenarios, used in the present study, future research should include physical and cyber bullying and compare students' potential or actual intervention behavior, among a wider range of student bullying behavior. Finally, future studies could also investigate whether self-efficacy and classroom cohesion play the same role in sexual, racial, or homophobic harassment situations.

6. Conclusions

To understand which factors increase students' willingness to intervene in bullying might deepen current knowledge concerning the success of bullying prevention and intervention in schools, and protect bystanders from experiencing adverse health and school-related outcomes. The present study revealed that self-efficacy in social conflicts and classroom cohesion were directly associated with students' willingness to intervene in bullying situations. Furthermore, this study was one of the first to examine the indirect associations among classroom cohesion, self-efficacy in social conflicts, and students' willingness to intervene in bullying. Findings indicate that the more positive the students' perceived peer-to-peer relationships within the classroom, the more efficacious students felt towards social conflicts, and the more likely they were to intervene in bullying situations. This finding was consistent for different age groups and girls and boys. Another finding was that a high percentage of students reported that they would never or rarely intervene in bullying, with boys and older students being less likely to intervene. Thus, we conclude that (1) it appears crucial to increase students' motivation to intervene in bullying; (2) efforts to address students' willingness to intervene in bullying should promote students' confidence in dealing with social conflicts and interpersonal relationships within school classes; and (3) self-efficacy plays an important role in understanding the relationship between classroom cohesion and students' willingness to intervene in bullying.

Author Contributions: W.S. and L.B. designed this study. S.W. drafted the manuscript and performed the statistical analyses. L.B., S.M.F., W.S., and M.F.W. provided constructive feedback on drafts of the manuscript. S.W. processed all feedback from the coauthors and reviewers. All authors read and approved of the manuscript.

Funding: This research was funded by the German Science Foundation (DFG, reference number BI 1046/6-1). We acknowledge the support of the Deutsche Forschungsgemeinschaft and Open Access Publishing Fund of University of Potsdam.

Conflicts of Interest: The authors declare no conflict of interest.

References

1. Kowalski, R.M.; Giumetti, G.W.; Schroeder, A.N.; Lattanner, M.R. Bullying in the digital age: A critical review and meta-analysis of cyberbullying research among youth. *Psychol. Bull.* **2014**, *140*, 1073–1137. [CrossRef] [PubMed]

2. Bauman, S.; Toomey, R.B.; Walker, J.L. Associations among bullying, cyberbullying, and suicide in high school students. *J. Adolesc.* **2013**, *36*, 341–350. [CrossRef] [PubMed]

3. Eslea, M.; Menesini, E.; Morita, Y.; O'Moore, M.; Mora-Merchán, J.A.; Pereira, B.; Smith, P.K. Friendship and loneliness among bullies and victims: Data from seven countries. *Aggress. Behav.* **2004**, *30*, 71–83. [CrossRef]

4. Olweus, D. Cyberbullying: An overrated phenomenon? *Eur. J. Dev. Psychol.* **2012**, *9*, 520–538. [CrossRef]

5. Solberg, M.E.; Olweus, D. Prevalence estimation of school bullying with the Olweus Bully/Victim Questionnaire. *Aggress. Behav.* **2003**, *29*, 239–268. [CrossRef]

6. Salmivalli, C. Participant role approach to school bullying: Implications for interventions. *J. Adolesc.* **1999**, *22*, 453–459. [CrossRef] [PubMed]

7. Salmivalli, C. Bullying and the peer group: A review. *Aggress. Viol. Behav.* **2010**, *15*, 112–120. [CrossRef]

8. Wachs, S.; Schubarth, W.; Scheithauer, H.; Hess, M. *Mobbing an Schulen: Erkennen-Handeln-Vorbeugen*; Kohlhammer Verlag: Stuttgart, Germany, 2016; ISBN 3-17-030042-3.

9. Salmivalli, C. Participant roles in bullying: How can peer bystanders be utilized in interventions? *Theory Pract.* **2014**, *53*, 286–292. [CrossRef]

10. Wachs, S.; Bilz, L.; Niproschke, S.; Schubarth, W. Bullying Intervention in Schools: A Multilevel Analysis of Teachers' Success in Handling Bullying from the Students' Perspective. *J. Early Adolesc.* **2018**. [CrossRef]

11. Sainio, M.; Veenstra, R.; Huitsing, G.; Salmivalli, C. Victims and their defenders: A dyadic approach. *Int. J. Behav. Dev.* **2011**, *35*, 144–151. [CrossRef]

12. Lynn Hawkins, D.; Pepler, D.J.; Craig, W.M. Naturalistic observations of peer interventions in bullying. *Soc. Dev.* **2001**, *10*, 512–527. [CrossRef]

13. Rivers, I.; Poteat, V.P.; Noret, N.; Ashurst, N. Observing bullying at school: The mental health implications of witness status. *Sch. Psychol. Q.* **2009**, *24*, 211–223. [CrossRef]

14. Wachs, S. Moral disengagement and emotional and social difficulties in bullying and cyberbullying: Differences by participant role. *Emot. Behav. Diffic.* **2012**, *17*, 347–360. [CrossRef]

15. Evans, C.B.; Smokowski, P.R.; Rose, R.A.; Mercado, M.C.; Marshall, K.J. Cumulative Bullying Experiences, Adolescent Behavioral and Mental Health, and Academic Achievement: An Integrative Model of Perpetration, Victimization, and Bystander Behavior. *J. Child Fam. Stud.* **2018**, 1–14. [CrossRef] [PubMed]

16. Craig, W.M.; Pepler, D.J. Observations of bullying and victimization in the school yard. *Can. J. Sch. Psychol.* **1998**, *13*, 41–59. [CrossRef]

17. Espelage, D.; Green, H.; Polanin, J. Willingness to intervene in bullying episodes among middle school students: Individual and peer-group influences. *J. Early Adolesc.* **2012**, *32*, 776–801. [CrossRef]

18. Rigby, K.; Johnson, B. Expressed readiness of Australian schoolchildren to act as bystanders in support of children who are being bullied. *Educ. Psychol.* **2006**, *26*, 425–440. [CrossRef]

19. Bandura, A. *Self-Efficacy: The Exercise of Control*; Freedom and Company: New York, NY, USA, 1997; ISBN 0716728508.

20. Connolly, J. Social self-efficacy in adolescence: Relations with self-concept, social adjustment, and mental health. *Can. J. Behav. Sci.* **1989**, *21*, 258. [CrossRef]

21. Thornberg, R.; Jungert, T. Bystander behavior in bullying situations: Basic moral sensitivity, moral disengagement and defender self-efficacy. *J. Adolesc.* **2013**, *36*, 475–483. [CrossRef] [PubMed]

22. Thornberg, R.; Tenenbaum, L.; Varjas, K.; Meyers, J.; Jungert, T.; Vanegas, G. Bystander motivation in bullying incidents: To intervene or not to intervene? *West. J. Emerg. Med.* **2012**, *13*, 247. [CrossRef] [PubMed]

23. Pöyhönen, V.; Juvonen, J.; Salmivalli, C. What does it take to stand up for the victim of bullying? The interplay between personal and social factors. *Merrill-Palmer Q.* **2010**, *56*, 143–163. [CrossRef]

24. Pöyhönen, V.; Juvonen, J.; Salmivalli, C. Standing up for the victim, siding with the bully or standing by? Bystander responses in bullying situations. *Soc. Dev.* **2012**, *21*, 722–741. [CrossRef]

25. van der Ploeg, R.; Kretschmer, T.; Salmivalli, C.; Veenstra, R. Defending victims: What does it take to intervene in bullying and how is it rewarded by peers? *J. Sch. Psychol.* **2017**, *65*, 1–10. [CrossRef] [PubMed]

26. Gini, G.; Albiero, P.; Benelli, B.; Altoe, G. Determinants of adolescents' active defending and passive bystanding behavior in bullying. *J. Adolesc.* **2008**, *31*, 93–105. [CrossRef] [PubMed]

27. Pozzoli, T.; Gini, G. Active defending and passive bystanding behavior in bullying: The role of personal characteristics and perceived peer pressure. *J. Abnorm. Child Psychol.* **2010**, *38*, 815–827. [CrossRef] [PubMed]

28. Bronfenbrenner, U. *The Ecology of Human Development*; Harvard University Press: Cambridge, MA, USA; London, UK, 1979; ISBN 0-674-22457-4.

29. Espelage, D.L. Ecological theory: Preventing youth bullying, aggression, and victimization. *Theory Pract.* **2014**, *53*, 257–264. [CrossRef]

30. Polanin, J.R.; Espelage, D.L.; Pigott, T.D. A Meta-Analysis of School-Based Bullying Prevention Programs' Effects on Bystander Intervention Behavior. *Sch. Psychol. Rev.* **2012**, *41*, 47–65.

31. Wernick, L.J.; Kulick, A.; Inglehart, M. Influences of peers, teachers, and climate on students' willingness to intervene when witnessing anti-transgender harassment. *J. Adolesc.* **2014**, *37*, 927–935. [CrossRef] [PubMed]

32. Goldammer, L.; Swahn, M.H.; Strasser, S.M.; Ashby, J.S.; Meyers, J. An examination of bullying in Georgia schools: Demographic and school climate factors associated with willingness to intervene in bullying situations. *West. J. Emerg. Med.* **2013**, *14*, 324. [CrossRef] [PubMed]

33. Thornberg, R.; Wänström, L.; Hong, J.S.; Espelage, D.L. Classroom relationship qualities and social-cognitive correlates of defending and passive bystanding in school bullying in Sweden: A multilevel analysis. *J. School Psychol.* **2017**, *63*, 49–62. [CrossRef] [PubMed]

34. Schunk, D.H.; Meece, J.L. Self-efficacy development in adolescence. In *Self-Efficacy Beliefs of Adolescents*; Pajares, F., Urdan, T., Eds.; IAP: Greenwich, CT, USA, 2006; Volume 5, pp. 71–96. ISBN 1-59311-366-8.

35. Schunk, D.H.; Miller, S.D. Self-efficacy and adolescents' motivation. In *Academic Motivation of Adolescents*; Pajares, F., Urdan, T., Eds.; IAP: Greenwich, CT, USA, 2002; Volume 2, pp. 29–52. ISBN 1-931576-62-9.

36. Yoon, J.S.; Kerber, K. Bullying: Elementary teachers' attitudes and intervention strategies. *Res. Educ.* **2003**, *69*, 27–35. [CrossRef]

37. Jerusalem, M.; Klein-Heßling, J. Soziale Selbstwirksamkeitserwartung. In *Skalendokumentation der Lehrer- und Schülerskalen des Projektes, Sicher und Gesund in der Schule (SIGIS)*; Humboldt-Universität zu Berlin: Berlin, Germany, 2002.

38. Fend, H.; Prester, H.G. *Dokumentation der Skalen des Projektes Entwicklung im Jugendalter*; Universität Konstanz: Konstanz, Germany, 1986.

39. Trach, J.; Hymel, S.; Waterhouse, T.; Neale, K. Bystander responses to school bullying: A cross-sectional investigation of grade and sex differences. *Can. J. Sch. Psychol.* **2010**, *25*, 114–130. [CrossRef]

40. Muthen, L.K.; Muthen, B.O. *Mplus [Computer Software]*; Muthén & Muthén: Los Angeles, CA, USA, 1998.

41. Naylor, P.; Cowie, H.; del Rey, R. Coping strategies of secondary school children in response to being bullied. *Child Psychol. Psychiatry Rev.* **2001**, *6*, 114–120. [CrossRef]

42. Jenkins, L.N.; Nickerson, A.B. Bullying participant roles and gender as predictors of bystander intervention. *Aggress. Behav.* **2017**, *43*, 281–290. [CrossRef] [PubMed]

43. Nucci, L. Classroom management for moral and social development. In *Handbook of Classroom Management: Research, Practice, and Contemporary Issues*; Evertson, C., Weinstein, C., Eds.; Lawrence Erlbaum Associates Publishers: Mahwah, NJ, USA, 2011; pp. 711–731. ISBN 978-0805847536.

44. Juvonen, J.; Galván, A. Peer influence in involuntary social groups: Lessons from research on bullying. In *Duke Series in Child Development and Public Policy. Understanding peer Influence in Children and Adolescents*; Prinstein, M.J., Dodge, K.A., Eds.; Guilford Press: New York, NY, USA, 2008; pp. 225–244.

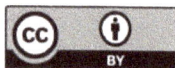

MDPI

St. Alban-Anlage 66

4052 Basel

Switzerland

Tel. +41 61 683 77 34

Fax +41 61 302 89 18

www.mdpi.com

International Journal of Environmental Research and Public Health Editorial Office

E-mail: ijerph@mdpi.com

www.mdpi.com/journal/ijerph

www.ingramcontent.com/pod-product-compliance
Lightning Source LLC
Chambersburg PA
CBHW051846210326
41597CB00033B/5793